D1757817

BM

Health P... ...on

...ter care

, working (

.u are accer

turned to t'

·d until the

ı items ca

ıother

POST

.ne

ns

BRITISH MEDICAL ASSOCIATION

WITHDRAWN
FROM LIBRARY

1000520

Health Protection
Principles and Practice

Edited by

Sam Ghebrehewet
Consultant in Communicable Disease Control and Deputy Director
for Health Protection, Public Health England, Liverpool, UK

Alex G. Stewart
Consultant in Health Protection, Public Health England, Liverpool, UK

David Baxter
Consultant in Communicable Disease Control and Director of Medical
Education, Stockport NHS Foundation Trust, UK

Paul Shears
Consultant Microbiologist, Wirral University Teaching Hospital,
Wirral, UK

David Conrad
Consultant in Public Health (Evidence & Intelligence), Hertfordshire
County Council, UK

Merav Kliner
Consultant in Communicable Disease Control, Public Health England,
Manchester, UK

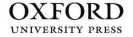

OXFORD

UNIVERSITY PRESS

Great Clarendon Street, Oxford, OX2 6DP,
United Kingdom

Oxford University Press is a department of the University of Oxford.
It furthers the University's objective of excellence in research, scholarship,
and education by publishing worldwide. Oxford is a registered trade mark of
Oxford University Press in the UK and in certain other countries

© Oxford University Press 2016

The moral rights of the authors have been asserted

First Edition published in 2016

Impression: 1

All rights reserved. No part of this publication may be reproduced, stored in
a retrieval system, or transmitted, in any form or by any means, without the
prior permission in writing of Oxford University Press, or as expressly permitted
by law, by licence or under terms agreed with the appropriate reprographics
rights organization. Enquiries concerning reproduction outside the scope of the
above should be sent to the Rights Department, Oxford University Press, at the
address above

You must not circulate this work in any other form
and you must impose this same condition on any acquirer

Published in the United States of America by Oxford University Press
198 Madison Avenue, New York, NY 10016, United States of America

British Library Cataloguing in Publication Data

Data available

Library of Congress Control Number: 2016943987

ISBN 978–0–19–874547–1

Printed and bound by
CPI Group (UK) Ltd, Croydon, CR0 4YY

Oxford University Press makes no representation, express or implied, that the
drug dosages in this book are correct. Readers must therefore always check
the product information and clinical procedures with the most up-to-date
published product information and data sheets provided by the manufacturers
and the most recent codes of conduct and safety regulations. The authors and
the publishers do not accept responsibility or legal liability for any errors in the
text or for the misuse or misapplication of material in this work. Except where
otherwise stated, drug dosages and recommendations are for the non-pregnant
adult who is not breast-feeding

Links to third party websites are provided by Oxford in good faith and
for information only. Oxford disclaims any responsibility for the materials
contained in any third party website referenced in this work.

This book is dedicated to the memory of Dr Marko Petrovic (1963–2015), late Consultant in Communicable Disease Control in Greater Manchester, a humble and inspiring colleague.

Foreword

"Health protection" is a recent description of a long established set of functions which act to protect individuals, groups and populations from the impact of infectious diseases, radiation, chemical and environmental hazards. Being a term which has come recently to common usage, it is particularly interesting that the authors have had to create their own definition of health protection.

Of course, public protection from hazard is steeped in the history of public health. Medical officers of health were appointed to local and national government from the early 19th century, advising and implementing strategies to reduce rates of infection, improve housing, ensure clean water and clean air, support basic standards of hygiene and infection control, and act on individual and social risk factors for poor health. Vaccination reduced the burden of infectious disease, John Snow described an outbreak of cholera and controlled the source, and the Clean Air Acts of the 1950s reduced the obvious impact of a major environmental hazard on the public.

Nevertheless, developments which aim to bring public health practice up to date frequently make the assumption that the control of infectious disease and environmental hazards is needed less now than in the past. We think of the "waves" of public health where great public works were superseded in turn by refinement of the scientific approach, institutional reform and restructuring, a focus on individual risk factors for disease (smoking, diet, exercise, alcohol), and most recently a shift from illness to wellness, addressing the wider determinants and root social causes of illness and a focus on the assets within communities. These are vital developments in the way we improve the health of individuals, communities and populations, but they must be accompanied by a renewed focus on the basics of how we protect our communities from infectious diseases and environmental hazards. The past decades have too many examples of this being given too little focus, resulting in episodes like the mishandled Stanley Royd salmonella outbreak and the Stafford Hospital Legionnaires' disease outbreak of the 1980s, which led to the creation of the role of the Consultant in Communicable Disease Control in England. The Health Protection Agency was established in 2003 at a time when there were many single handed health protection specialists in local health authorities and serious weaknesses in the system, needing professionals to be brought together in larger health protection teams. More recently, WHO Member States have been surprised by the ability of an infectious disease, Ebola, to cause extensive outbreaks when not controlled quickly and effectively, and have moved to strengthen systems to detect and respond to new emerging hazards globally when previously the WHO's focus was shifting from infectious disease control to act on the major problems of chronic diseases worldwide.

Most countries address health protection by relying on national specialist institutes of infectious diseases or environmental hazards which are separate from, but offer advice to, those who deliver the control of these hazards in local communities. In the UK we are fortunate to have an integrated set of functions delivered through local health protection teams which act on both infectious diseases and environmental hazards and work alongside local government and the health service, each with their own specific roles in hazard control. These local multidisciplinary teams are supported by national specialists in aspects of infectious disease and environmental hazard control including surveillance, epidemiology, diagnostics, genomics, emergency response and disease modelling, as well as specialists in individual infectious diseases and environmental hazards. Given the growing importance of antimicrobial resistance, concerns about bio-terrorism and the need to maintain a competent and efficient set of services which act together to protect the health of our communities, this is a critical system for the future. It needs to constantly modernise, take on new technologies, and adapt to the changing environment in which it operates.

This book is the first to describe these functions in a single dedicated text book of health protection, taking an inclusive, all-hazards approach. As such it is a very welcome and indeed a vital development. It is a step in the wider recognition of health protection as a distinct discipline which brings together many different specialists and disciplines with common purpose - to protect individuals, groups and the population from infectious disease and environmental hazards. I pay tribute to the editors for their prescience in making this book a reality, and thank all the contributors for their essential contributions.

Professor Paul Cosford CB
Director of Health Protection & Medical Director
Public Health England
June 2016.

Preface

This book is intended to be an accessible and practical core text on the three domains of health protection: Communicable Disease Control, Emergency Preparedness Resilience and Response (EPRR), and protection of the public from environmental hazards (Environmental Public Health).

We have written the book for students, health protection practitioners, and general public health professionals. The book will also be helpful for health protection specialists. No prior medical or clinical knowledge is assumed in any chapter, and supporting information for more technical issues is available throughout the book.

As well as introducing the essential principles of health protection work, the book guides the reader in dealing with real incidents through a combination of representative case studies and quick reference action checklists (called SIMCARDs in the book from the acronym—see below).

We have attempted to develop an "all-hazards approach" in dealing with health protection situations. Most health protection books confine themselves to one of the three domains, whereas this book presents a practical and generic approach to the wide range of possible hazards, with some account of the principles of health protection on which day-to-day practice rests.

Health protection covers a broad range of topics and while some may wish to read the full contents of the book in order, others may seek to improve their knowledge of particular topics, or use the book quickly to find relevant information when faced with a real-life situation. For this reason, each chapter has been designed as much as possible to be self-contained. The first section, however, which succinctly sets out the essential basics of health protection, should be the starting point for any reader who does not already possess a broad familiarity with the field. The remaining sections and chapters of the book can effectively be read in any order.

Each case study chapter immerses the reader in a common health protection scenario which develops in stages, in much the same way as health protection cases and incidents develop in real life. As the story unfolds, the reader will learn about the nature and significance of the specific threat to population health, the practical steps and issues involved in an effective public health response and the health protection principles underpinning that response.

Each case study chapter follows the same basic format, including:

♦ *Background facts* about the topic

♦ *What's the story?* setting out the initial realistic scenario which the chapter will work through

♦ Sections covering *What action should be taken?* and additional *Information* helping the reader to think through the public health response required

♦ *Update* sections describing new developments in the scenario

♦ *What if …?* briefly describing common variations on the scenario featured in the chapter

♦ *Lessons learned*—summarizing key learning points from the chapter

♦ *Unanswered questions* and *Further thinking* sections covering gaps in current knowledge on the topic and issues for further consideration or reflection

♦ *Additional reading*, pointing the reader to other sources of information

The case study chapters (scenarios) are followed by chapters that provide a deeper understanding of the key tools and mechanisms used in day-to-day health protection work, and insights into new and emerging health protection issues.

Three appendices of practical checklists, called SIMCARDs, give a quick-reference tool covering more than 180 common or important topics which can arise in health protection practice (including those featured in the case study chapters). They offer concise and practically focused information for practitioners needing a simple guide which can be used by all, including non-specialists, in time-pressured situations.

The variety of chapters covered throughout the book on Communicable Diseases, Emergency Preparedness Resilience and Response, and Environmental Public Health, offer a unique perspective borne out of practical experience, which is not easily accessible elsewhere.

The acronym SIMCARD stands for:

S = Signs and symptoms/situation

I = Incubation Period & Infectivity (= lead time in environmental issues)

M = Mode of transmission/exposure

C = Confirmation/Criteria, both clinical and laboratory

A = Action (including immediate and essential public health actions)

R = Report/Communication on a need-to-know basis

D = Disease clusters and outbreaks/outcome patterns

SIMCARD is a simple, memorable approach which captures all relevant information which is needed to enable a public health practitioner methodically to assess the issue, provide advice and act. The SIMCARD approach also allows clinicians to provide immediate public health advice to fellow professionals and patients, and provide the relevant information to their local health protection or public health team for prevention and control actions.

Public health trainees preparing for the Membership of the Faculty of Public Health examinations, non-specialist health protection staff, and, hopefully, other healthcare professionals, such as general practitioners, Infection Prevention and Control teams, and hospital clinicians, will find these chapters particularly useful.

It is also envisaged that SIMCARDs will serve as an essential first port of call for other professionals, including undergraduate and postgraduate medical students, and others who are interested in identifying accurate information to guide or inform public health action.

Acknowledgements

We would like to thank all of the volunteers who freely gave time and energy to read the chapters and supported the editors and authors on technical issues, breadth of the subject matter, readability, and writing style. The reviewers consisted of:

Yasmin Ahmed-Little, David Alexander, Stephen Ashmore, John Astbury, Carole Billington, Linda Booth, Kate Brierley, Mark Brown, Suzanne Calvert, Nic Coetzee, Emer Coffey, Jen Connelly, Richard Convey, Richard Cooke, John Cunniffe, Paul Davison, Andrew Dodgson, Richard Elson, Nesta Featherstone, Diane Fiefield, Kirsty Foster, Ivan Gee, Mike Gent, Sarah Harrison, Guy Hayhurst, Jon Hobday, Jason Horsely, Tom Keegan, Peter Kenny, David Kirrage, Matt Innerd, Ben Leaman, Andy Lui, Peter MacPherson, Helen McAuslane, Rosemary McCann, David McConalogue, Sarah McNulty, Frances Maguire, Glynn Marriott, Gill Marsh, Laura Mitchem, Rachel Musgrave, Ken Mutton, Allie Nash, Ebere Okereke, Helen Oulton, Matthieu Pegorie, Nick Phin, Kristina Poole, Ian Rufus, Tracy Ruthven, Ashley Sharp, Theresa Shryane, David Sinclair, James Smith, Rachel Smith, Katrina Stevens, Charlotte Stevenson, Hayley Teshome Tesfaye, Liz Tyler, Graham Urquhart, Neville Verlander, William Welfare, Ewan Wilkinson, Peter Williams, Toni Williams, and Tiffany Yeung.

We would also like to thank those who were equally generous in sharing their knowledge and experience in developing and checking the SIMCARDs, including: Elspeth Anwar, Suzanne Calvert, Melissa Campbell, Anna Donaldson, Kirsty Foster, Jon Hobday, Rita Huyton, Rebecca Ingham, Peter Macpherson, Shilpa Nayak, Wendy Philips, Anjila Shah, Hayley Teshome Tesfaye, Barry Walsh, and Yvonne Young.

In addition, we are deeply grateful to Peter MacPherson and Ewan Wilkinson for freely sharing their time, knowledge, and expertise without any reservations.

As ever, responsibility for any errors rests with us; any merit this book may have is shared by all those who supported us.

The Editors

Contents

Appendices

Abbreviations

A&E	Accident & Emergency department		CQC	Care Quality Commission
ACDP	Advisory Committee on Dangerous Pathogens		CRCE	Centre for Radiation, Chemical and Environmental Hazards
ACM	Asbestos Containing Material		CRP	C-Reactive Protein (CRP)
AFB	Acid Fast Bacilli		CRS	Congenital Rubella Syndrome
AGPs	Aerosol Generating Procedures		CSF	Cerebrospinal Fluid
AMR	Antimicrobial Resistance		DATER	Detection, Assessment, Treatment, Escalation and Recovery
AMRHAI	Antimicrobial Resistance and Healthcare Associated Infections (laboratory)		DECC	Department of Environment and Climate Change
AMSTAR	Assessment of Multiple SysTemAtic Reviews		DECIDE	Developing and Evaluating Communication strategies to support Informed Decisions and practice based on Evidence
APHA	Animal and Plant Health Agency			
AQC	Air Quality Cell			
AQMA	Air Quality Management Area		Defra	Department for Environment Food & Rural Affairs
ATT	Anti Tuberculosis Treatment		DIF	Direct Immunofluorescence
BAL	Bronchioalveolar Lavage (washings)		DIPC	Director of Infection Prevention and Control
BCG	Bacille Calmette-Guèrin vaccine			
BCM	Business Continuity Management		DNA	Deoxyribonucleic Acid
BSE	Bovine Spongiform Encephalopathy		DOT	Directly Observed Therapy
CAP	Community Acquired Pneumonia		DPH	Director of Public Health
CASC	Clinical Audit Support Centre		DRR	Disaster Risk Reduction
CASP	Critical Appraisal Skills Programme		DWI	Drinking Water Inspectorate
CCA	Civil Contingencies Act		EA	Environment Agency
CCDC	Consultant in Communicable Disease Control		EBS	Event-based Surveillance
			EBV	Epstein-Barr Virus
CDC	Centers for Disease Control and Prevention		ECDC	European Centre for Disease Prevention and Control
CHEMET	Chemical Meteorology		EFSA	European Food Safety Authority
CMO	Chief Medical Officer		EHO	Environmental Health Officer
CO	Carbon Monoxide		EIA	Enzyme Immunoassay
COMAH	Control of Major Accident Hazards (Regulations)		ELDSNet	European Legionnaires' Disease Surveillance Network
COMEAP	Committee on the Medical Effects of Air Pollutants		ELISA	Enzyme-linked Immunosorbent Assay
			EM	Electron Microscopy
COPD	Chronic Obstructive Pulmonary (airways) Disease		EPHT	Environmental Public Health Tracking (integration of environmental surveillance within a public health service)
CoSSH	Control of Substances Hazardous to Health Regulations			
			EPP	Exposure-Prone Procedures
CPE	Carbapenemase Producing Enterobacteriaciae		EPRR	Emergency Preparedness, Resilience and Response
CPH	Consultant in Health Protection			

ESBL	Extended-Spectrum Beta-Lactamase
EU	European Union
FFC	Flood Forecasting Centre
FGS	Flood Guidance Statement
FPH	Faculty of Public Health
FRS	Fire and Rescue Service
FSA	Food Standards Agency
GIS	Geographic Information System
GP	General Practitioner
Gr +ve	Gram positive bacteria
Gr –ve	Gram negative bacteria
GRADE	Grading of Recommendations Assessment Development and Evaluation
HAIRS	Human and Animal Infections and Risk Surveillance
HAV	Hepatitis A Virus
HBeAg	Hepatitis B e Antigen
HBIG	Hepatitis B Immunogolobulin
HBsAg	Hepatitis B surface Antigen
HBV	Hepatitis B Virus
HCAI	Healthcare Associated Infections
HCV	Hepatitis C Virus
HCW	Healthcare Worker
HDU	High Dependency Unit
HES	Hospital Episode Statistics
HEV	Hepatitis E Virus
HIA	Health Impact Assessments
HiB	Haemophilus influenzae Type B
HIV	Human Immunodeficiency Virus
HNIG	Human Normal Immunoglobulin
HPA	Health Protection Agency
HPV	Human Papilloma Virus
HQIP	Health Quality Improvement Partnership
HSE	Health and Safety Executive
HSV	Herpes Simplex Virus
HUS	Haemolytic Uraemic Syndrome
ICC	Infection Control Committee
ICD	Infection Control Doctor
ICT	Incident Control Team
ICU	Intensive Care Unit
ID	Intradermal
IDD	Iodine Deficiency Disorders
IDU	Injecting Drug User
IFA	Indirect Immunoflourescent Antibody test

IgG	Immunoglobulin class G
IgM	Immunoglobulin class M
IGRA	Interferon-gamma Release Assay
IHR	International Health Regulations
ILI	Influenza-like illness
IM	Intramascular
IMT	Incident Management Team
IPCN	Infection Prevention & Control Nurse
IPCT	Infection Prevention and Control Team
IPV	Inactivated Polio Vaccine
JESIP	Joint Emergency Services Interoperability Principles
LA	Local Authority
LGV	Lymphogranuloma Venereum
LHRP	Local Health Resilience Partnership
LRF	Local Resilience Forum
LTBI	Latent TB Infection
MAFP	Multi-Agency Flood Plan
MDR TB	Multi-Drug Resistant TB
MERS	Middle East Respiratory Syndrome
MERS-CoV	Middle East Respiratory Syndrome Coronavirus
MHRA	Medicines and Healthcare products Regulatory Agency
MMR	Measles, Mumps and Rubella vaccine
MRSA	Methicillin-resistant Staphylococcus aureus
MTB	Mycobacterium tuberculosis complex
NAAT	Nuclei Acid Amplification Test
NHSE	National Health Service England
NICE	National Institute of Health and Care Excellence
OCT	Outbreak Control Team
OECD	Organisation for Economic Co-operation and Development
OOH	Out-Of-hours
OPV	Oral Poliovirus Vaccine
PCR	Polymerase Chain Reaction
PEP	Post-Exposure Prophylaxis
PFGE	Pulse Field Gel Electrophoresis
PHE	Public Health England
PHN	Postherpetic Neuralgia
PM	Particulate Matter
PPE	Personal Protective Equipment
PrP	Prion Proteins
PVL	Panton-Valentine Leukocidin (toxin)
QOF	Quality and Outcomes Framework

RCEP	Royal Commission on Environmental Pollution
RCG	Recovery Coordinating Group
RCGP	Royal College of General Practitioners
RCT	Randomized Controlled Trial
REACH	Registration, Evaluation, Authorisation and restriction of Chemicals (Regulations)
RNA	Ribonucleic Acid
RSV	Respiratory Syncytial Virus
SARS	Severe Acute Respiratory Syndrome
SCG	Strategic Coordinating Group
SICPs	Standard Infection Control Precautions
SIR	Standardized Incident Ratio
SitReps	Situational Reports (SitReps)
SMR	Standardized Mortality Ratio
SPC	Statistical Process Control
SSPE	Subacute Sclerosing Panencephalitis
STAC	Scientific and Technical Advice Cell
STIs	Sexually Transmitted Infections
SyS	Syndromic Surveillance
TB	Tuberculosis
TBE	Tick-Borne Encephalitis
TBPs	Transmission-Based Precautions
TCG	Tactical Coordinating Group
TSE	Transmissable Spongioform Encephalopathy
TST	Tuberculin Skin Test
TT	Tetanus Toxoid
UK	United Kingdom of great Britain and Northern Ireland
UNFCCC	United Nations Framework Convention on Climate Change
UNISDR	United Nations International Strategy on Disaster Reduction
vCJD	variant Creutzfeldt–Jakob disease
VHF	Viral Haemorrhagic Fever
VNTR	Variable Number Tandem Repeat
VRE	Vancomycin Resistant Enterococci
VTEC	Verocytotoxin-producing Escherichia coli
VZIG	Varicella-zoster Immunoglobulin
VZV	Varicella-Zoster Virus
WGS	Whole Genome Sequencing
WHO	World Health Organization
WISH	Waste Industry Safety and Health forum
WNV	West Nile Virus

About the editors

Dr Sam Ghebrehewet MD, MPH, FFPH

Dr Ghebrehewet has been working as a Consultant in Communicable Disease Control and health protection team lead in Cheshire and Merseyside (UK) for over 15 years. He graduated from medical school in Ethiopia, where he worked as a GP and Regional Director of Public Health Programmes. Dr Ghebrehewet has extensive experience in health protection, with specialist interests in immunisation, Emergency Preparedness, Resilience and Response (EPRR), environmental public health practice, and wider health protection strategy and policy development. He has published widely, and is the lead for Health Protection Module in the Masters of Public Health at the University of Liverpool and lead health protection trainer in Cheshire & Merseyside, North West, UK.

Dr Alex G Stewart MBChB, DTM&H, FHEA, MPH, MFPHMI

Following a successful career of around 20 years in the northern mountains of Pakistan as a rural GP, Dr Stewart returned to the UK where he trained in Public Health in Cheshire and Merseyside. He was a Consultant in Health Protection for eleven years, with special interest in the acute and long-term effects of the environment on health. He has investigated and responded to many complex public health issues, and has developed an understanding of how to support local and national agencies and the public in the face of limited information, incomplete understanding and often great uncertainty. He has published extensively and continues to teach undergraduate and postgraduate students in health protection and public health.

Dr David Baxter MBChB, DTM&H, DPH, MSc, PhD, FFPH

Dr Baxter has been a Consultant in Communicable Disease Control for 20 years, working in the Stockport and Greater Manchester area. Over the last 25 years he has run successfully the UK National Immunisation Conference for Health Care Workers, attracting more than 100 delegates every year from all over the country, and delivered by key national and international experts. Dr Baxter has published extensively, and his research focuses on health protection and the epidemiology and control of infectious diseases, with a particular emphasis on vaccine preventable infections and sexually transmitted diseases. He continues to provide a specialist immunisation clinics at a District General Hospital receiving referrals from GPs and hospital clinicians from a wide catchment area. Dr Baxter has supervised several PhD theses, and continues to teach and deliver courses to both undergraduate medical students and post graduates on health protection.

Dr Paul Shears MBBS, MD, FRCPath

Dr Shears is a former consultant medical microbiologist and Director of Infection Prevention and Control at Arrowe Park Wirral University Hospital, North West, UK. He has a special interest in the epidemiology and control of health care associated infections. Dr Shears was previously senior lecturer in medical microbiology at Liverpool University/Liverpool School of Hygiene & Tropical Medicine, with postgraduate teaching responsibilities and public health microbiology projects in Sudan and Bangladesh. Dr Shears was a member of WHO working groups on antimicrobial resistance, and public health laboratory development. He is the author of over 60 peer reviewed publications, has contributed chapters in several books, and is an Assistant Editor of the Journal of Hospital Infection. In the 1980s he was a medical officer in refugee programmes in Somalia, Ethiopia, Rwanda and Lebanon.

Mr David Conrad MA, MSc, MPH, FFPH

Mr Conrad is a Consultant in Public Health at Hertfordshire County Council. He has published papers on a broad range of public health topics and, in collaboration with colleagues from the Centre for Men's Health at Leeds Beckett University, has previously edited three books: Men's Health: How To Do It (Radcliffe), Promoting Men's Mental Health (Radcliffe) and Sports-Based Health Interventions: Case Studies from Around the World (Springer).

Dr Merav Kliner BA(hons), MBChB, MPH, MFPH

Dr Kliner graduated from University of Leeds with a degree in Medicine, and a BA in Healthcare Ethics. She has an interest in infectious diseases, and in particular TB and HIV, which developed during clinical training, guideline development work with WHO, and academic work within Good Shepherd Hospital in Swaziland, with the University of Leeds. She currently works as a Consultant in Communicable Disease Control in Greater Manchester.

List of Contributors

Dr Musarrat Afza
Consultant in Communicable Disease
Control, West Midlands Public Health
England Centre, UK

Dr Amina Aitsi-Selmi
Consultant in International Public Health
Public Health England, UK

Dr David Baxter
Consultant in Communicable Disease
Control and Director of Medical Education
Stockport NHS Foundation Trust Stockport,
UK

Dr Angie Bone
Consultant in Public Health Medicine
Extreme Events and Health Protection
Public Health England, UK

Dr Joanna Cartwright
Consultant in Communicable Disease
Control, Cheshire & Merseyside Public
Health England Centre, UK

Dr Paul Cleary
Consultant Epidemiologist, Field
Epidemiology Services
Public Health England, UK

Mr David Conrad
Consultant in Public Health
(Evidence & Intelligence)
Hertfordshire County Council, UK

Mr Alec Dobney
Head of Unit (Birmingham/Manchester)
Environmental Hazards and Emergencies
Department, UK

Mr Alex J. Elliot
National Scientist Lead (Syndromic
Surveillance), Real-time Syndromic
Surveillance Department
Public Health England, UK

Prof Andrew Fox
Director of the Public Health England Food
Water and Environmental Laboratory Preston,
UK

Dr Sam Ghebrehewet
Consultant in Communicable Disease
Control and Deputy Director for Health
Protection, Cheshire and Merseyside
Public Health England Centre, UK

Mrs Henrietta Harrison
Unit Head, Environmental Hazards
and Emergencies Department
Public Health England, UK

Dr David Harvey
Consultant Microbiologist
Wirral University Teaching Hospital, UK

Mr Greg Hodgson
Head of Unit (Nottingham), Environmental
Hazards and Emergencies Department, UK

Mrs Rita Huyton
Senior Health Protection Nurse
Cheshire & Merseyside Public Health
England Centre, UK

Dr Richard Jarvis
Consultant in Health Protection
Cheshire & Merseyside Public Health
England Centre, UK

Dr Merav Kliner
Consultant in Communicable Disease
Control, Greater Manchester
Public Health England Centre, UK

Dr Ken Lamden
Consultant in Communicable Disease
Control, Cumbria & Lancashire
Public Health England Centre, UK

Mrs Andrea Ledgerton
Associate Director of Nursing Infection
Prevention and Control, Wirral University
Teaching Hospital, UK

Dr Giovanni Leonardi
Head of Epidemiology Department
Centre for Radiation, Chemical
and Environmental Hazards
Public Health England, UK

Dr Peter MacPherson
Lecturer (Clinical) in Public Health University
of Liverpool & Specialist Registrar in Public
Health, Cheshire & Merseyside Public Health
England Centre, UK

Ms Gill Marsh
Senior Health Protection Nurse Practitioner
Cheshire & Merseyside Public Health
England Centre, UK

Dr Laura Mitchem
Principal Environmental Public Health
Scientist, Centre for Radiation
Chemical and Environmental Hazards
Public Health England, UK

Prof Virginia Murray
Consultant in Global Disaster Reduction
Public Health England, and Vice-chair of
UNISDR Scientific and Technical Advisory
Group, UK

Ms Falguni Naik
Surveillance Coordinator (Scientist)
Respiratory Diseases Department
Centre for Infectious Disease Surveillance
and Control, Public Health England, UK

Dr Marko Petrovic
Consultant in Communicable Disease
Control, Greater Manchester Public
Health England Centre, UK

Prof Nick Phin
Interim Head, Respiratory Diseases
Department, Centre for Infectious Disease
Surveillance and Control, Public Health
England, UK

Prof John Reid
Visiting Lecturer, Centre for Public Health
Liverpool John Moores University, UK

Mr Sam Rowell
Health Protection Practitioner, Cumbria &
Lancashire Public Health England Centre, UK

Mr Ian Rufus
Regional Emergency Preparedness Manager
Public Health England North Region, UK

Dr Amal Rushdy
Consultant in Public Health Medicine Quality,
Governance and Service Improvement, Public
Health England, UK

Dr Anjila Shah
Consultant in Communicable
Disease Control, Cheshire & Merseyside
Public Health England Centre, UK

Dr Paul Shears
Consultant Microbiologist
former Director of Infection Prevention
Control, Wirral University Teaching Hospital,
UK

Dr Elaine Stanford
Legionella Scientist, Respiratory Diseases
Department, Centre for Infectious Disease
Surveillance and Control, Public Health
England, UK

Dr Alex G Stewart
Consultant in Health Protection
Cheshire & Merseyside Public Health
England Centre, UK

Dr Roberto Vivancos
Consultant Epidemiologist
Field Epidemiology Services
Public Health England, UK

Prof Ewan Wilkinson
Professor, The Institure of Medicine
University of Chester, UK

Mr Alan Wilton
Head of Emergency Planning
Lancashire County Council, UK

Section 1

The basics

Chapter 1

What is health protection?

Sam Ghebrehewet, Alex G. Stewart, and Ian Rufus

OVERVIEW
....

After reading this chapter the reader will be familiar with:

• the definition of health protection,
• the domains of health protection,
• the scope of health protection, and
• its history in the English context.

1.1 Introduction to health protection

As early as the beginning of the twentieth century, a comprehensive definition of public health was formulated by C.-E.A Winslow (1920), following a response to two Yale undergraduate medical students seeking career advice. They wanted to know something about the field of public health, what it included, the nature of the work involved, the necessary qualifications and financial rewards, and what were the more intangible emoluments to be expected by those who may enter this career. It is impossible to summarize the full response without compromising the vision, which meticulously and eloquently articulated the potential, the opportunities, and the future of public health. The full response included the following wide-ranging definition of public health:

> Public health is the science and the art of preventing disease, prolonging life, and promoting physical health and efficiency through organised community efforts for the sanitation of the environment, the control of community infections, the education of the individual in principles of personal hygiene, the organisation of medical and nursing service for the early diagnosis and preventive treatment of disease, and the development of the social machinery which will ensure to every individual in the community a standard of living adequate for the maintenance of health.

In 1988, a succinct summary of the above definition of public health was put forward by the former Chief Medical Officer of the United Kingdom (Acheson 1988): 'the science and art of preventing disease, prolonging life and promoting health through organized efforts of society.'

The UK Faculty of Public Health further categorized public health into three domains: health protection, health improvement and health-care public health (Faculty of Public Health 2010).

Although health protection is a distinct domain, in practice it is not, and should not be, delivered in isolation from the other domains of public health; this is illustrated by our working definition of health protection:

> The protection of individuals, groups and populations through expert advice and effective collaboration to identify, prevent and mitigate the impacts of infectious disease, and environmental, chemical and radiological threats.

In England, health protection is delivered by Public Health England (PHE). PHE is the expert public health agency with statutory duty to protect health, address inequalities, and promote the health and wellbeing of the nation (Public Health England 2013). In the rest of the UK, Health Protection Scotland (Health Protection Scotland 2005), Public Health Wales (Public Health Wales 2010), and the Public Health Agency for Northern Ireland (Public Health Agency 2011) provide similar health protection functions. There are similar organizations in other countries: e.g. Centers for Disease Control and Prevention (CDC) in the United States, National Institute for Public Health and the Environment (RIVM) in The Netherlands, Robert Koch Institute (RKI) in Germany, Public Health Agency of Canada (PHAC) in Canada, Swedish National Institute of Public Health and Swedish Institute for Communicable Disease Control in Sweden, Institute for Public Health Surveillance (InVS) and National Institute for Prevention and Health Education (INPES) in France. The public health and health protection responsibilities of these agencies are outlined in a recent report that was commissioned by Public Health England (RAND Europe 2014).

Just as the accident and emergency department (A&E) is the front line of health care that deals with acute and sudden health problems, so health protection is the front line of public health, dealing with acute public health emergencies, involving communicable or non-communicable disease. However, unlike A&E, health protection also deals with chronic public health situations (e.g. contaminated land, air, or water), which may have acute or chronic manifestations. Furthermore, health protection concerns itself with gathering evidence and providing intelligence and support to prepare for emergencies as well as anticipating future issues, incidents, emergencies, and other threats to health.

The UK has a defined, local specialist health protection service as part of a national specialist health protection system. The delivery of health protection at both local and national levels is multi-agency, working with other public bodies such as the National Health Service, local authorities, the Food Standards Agency, etc.

1.2 Domains of health protection

Health protection consists of three main domains: communicable disease control; emergency preparedness, resilience and response (EPRR); and environmental public health.

1.2.1 Communicable disease control

Communicable disease control involves prevention, investigation, control, and management of infections through local, regional, and national specialist health protection teams.

1.2.2 EPRR

EPRR involves preparation, prevention, investigation, control, and management of events that threaten serious damage to human welfare. This includes communicable disease as well as environmental public health situations. The practice of EPRR also includes business continuity planning and recovery to normality.

1.2.3 Environmental public health

Environmental public health does not have an agreed definition. A working definition that was used as part of a review of environmental public health functions by the North West Health Protection Team (Ghebrehewet and Stewart, 2014) is:

> The identification, characterisation and provision of a safe and sustainable response, both immediate and prospective, to any kind of threat to health from issues in the natural and man-made environment.

Environmental public health issues are often complex, change with time and involvement and have a unique solution ('wicked problems', Head and Alford 2013; Redford et al. 2013). Environmental public health differs from communicable disease control:

♦ The investigation process is not as well developed and tested.

♦ Issues can take months or years to resolve.

♦ Evidence is not so well developed and what is well known (e.g. the effects of particles on respiratory and cardiovascular disease) may be difficult to demonstrate at local level due to the number of people and changes in environmental concentrations required to demonstrate an effect.

♦ There is a frequent lack of specific, diagnostic symptoms, syndromes, and diagnostic tools, particularly in low-level exposures.

♦ The multiplicity of factors and interactions result in the need for a multi-agency response, often led by a non-health agency in most environmental situations.

1.3 The scope of a specialist health protection service

Health protection responsibility can be seen as starting with protecting the individual, through their families and communities, to the wider population. There is a spectrum in health protection from single cases of communicable disease to incidents, clusters, and outbreaks. Planning for outbreaks is part of EPRR through the development of robust plans, but the spectrum continues through planning for major incidents (including chemical spills), into the realm of what may be called environmental public health, which looks into the impact of the environment on health. Examples of the scope of a specialist health protection are considered in the following sections.

1.3.1 Communicable disease

This may range from an individual case of *E. coli* infection to a large measles outbreak in a community with multiple smaller outbreaks in schools, impacting on the local hospital patients, staff, nearby communities and beyond.

1.3.2 EPRR

The scope may vary from an incident where three residents living in a house above a restaurant are exposed to carbon monoxide, to a massive chemical incident with a smoke plume containing noxious substances blowing over a large residential community containing nursing homes, health centres, and schools. Furthermore, the scope and range of EPRR services extend beyond planning and preparedness for local, regional, and national situations (e.g., incidents, outbreaks, and epidemics), to preparing and responding to pandemics.

1.3.3 Environmental public health

The scope of environmental public health ranges from an enquiry about an alleged impact of power lines on the health of the residents of a few houses to a complex, ongoing issue involving contaminated land from which the pollutants are leaking into the air and water, with health effects which may be physical, psychological, or perceived but require investigation, reassurance, and long-term follow-up.

1.3.4 **Common features of the three main domains**

The provision of health protection services, in whichever domain and whether large or small in scope, are supported and underpinned by:

- good surveillance,
- strong multi-agency partnerships,
- clear and robust epidemiology,
- supportive science (microbiology, toxicology, environmental sciences, clinical sciences, and radiation science),
- timely audit,
- focused research,
- clear communication strategy, and
- learning and development.

Learning and development is important at all levels, from the individual through the team, agency, multi-agency to national and even international levels, while the sciences are supported locally by regional and national experts.

Health protection effectiveness is judged by a lack of incidents, clusters/outbreaks, new and emerging diseases, events, situations/disasters. Although it could be argued that some of the significant incidents that have occurred in recent years could have been predicted and/or prevented, in practice not all are preventable or predictable. For example:

- the catastrophic fire in Buncefield, UK, 2005 (Buncefield Major Incident Investigation Board Report 2008),
- pandemic influenza, 2009 (Hine 2010),
- a leak of highly toxic gas (methyl isocyanate) from a pesticide plant in 1984, Bhopal, India (Broughton 2005),
- uncontrolled radioactive iodine and caesium releases in 1986, following an explosion and fires at the Chernobyl nuclear plant in Ukraine (IAEA 2006; Cardis and Hatch 2011), and
- devastating outbreaks of Ebola (Shears and O'Dempsey 2015).

Nevertheless, the discipline of health protection includes planning and preparing for similar situations, assessing their immediate and long-term impacts, reflecting and learning from previous situations, and mounting a robust response in order to mitigate their impact and protect the health of the population.

1.4 **Brief history of health protection in England**

The development of the domains and scope of health protection can be illustrated by its history in England.

In 1984, an outbreak of Salmonella in Stanley Royd Hospital, a large psychogeriatric hospital in Wakefield, Yorkshire, claimed the lives of 19 patients (Department of Health and Social Security 1986). Six months later, an outbreak of Legionnaires' disease at Stafford District General Hospital caused 28 deaths (O'Mahonya et al. 1990). Few health authorities in England had written plans for dealing with outbreaks of food poisoning or communicable disease. Public enquiries followed, resulting in 1988 in the Chief Medical Officer, Donald Acheson, establishing the post of Consultant in Communicable Disease Control (CCDC), a local public health doctor with responsibility for investigating outbreaks of communicable diseases in the community (Kapila and Buttery 1986; Keeble 2006).

These CsCDC worked independently in health authorities, with a small team of nurses and administrative staff, until the establishment of the Health Protection Agency (HPA) in 2003 in England through the Chief Medical Officer, Liam Donaldson's report *Getting Ahead of the Curve* (Department of Health 2002). The existing functions of the Public Health Laboratory Service and three other national bodies (the National Radiological Protection Board, the Centre for Applied Microbiology and Research, and the National Focus for Chemical Incidents) were integrated to protect the health of the public against infectious diseases as well as chemical and radiological hazards. The report further announced that, at local level, health protection services would be delivered by the new agency, working with the NHS and local authorities. Similar organizations were created in the devolved administrations in the UK.

With the establishment of the CCDC post, planning for outbreaks of communicable disease became standardized across the health service and the public health community. In 2004, local arrangements for civil protection (Civil Contingencies Act 2004) widened the response from outbreak planning to EPRR: planning for an emergency, ensuring essential services continue, and answering the crisis (HM Government, CCA 2004 Regulations (2005); HM Government, CCA 2004 and its associated Regulations (2006) and Non-Statutory).

The HPA and its similar organizations in devolved administrations created opportunities for CsCDC and other health protection staff to work together across larger boundaries providing the same support to local and health authorities as before, but in a strengthened, systematic, and resilient manner. Similar to general practitioners, who work in teams, know their local community, and coordinate specialist care, CsCDC also work in teams, and know the local epidemiology of infectious diseases and environmental health threats in their community, while integrating public health and specialist health protection knowledge, skills, and competencies. Health protection teams are often faced by the growing nature of health protection challenges. Nevertheless, local health protection teams have developed a reputation in their communities for reliability, sound advice, strong leadership, and commendable partnership working.

In April 2013, as a result of the Health and Social Care Act 2012, the HPA was combined with other public health services into Public Health England. PHE is an Executive Agency of the Department of Health, tasked with protecting and improving the nation's health and well-being, and reducing health inequalities. This is the first time in England that responsibilities for public health in all its many forms have been brought together within a national organization, creating an opportunity for the delivery of integrated public health at local, regional and national levels.

1.5 **Conclusions**

We have used a comprehensive definition of health protection, that outlines the scope and domains of the subject, while offering a practical approach that describes the subject in a recognizable manner.

Within health protection there are three domains that are interrelated, especially at the local level. They function in parallel, allowing professionals, partner agencies, and stakeholders one port of entry to a consistent and integrated local service with access to expert advice and support.

The scope of health protection is wide, covering communicable disease control, environmental public health and EPRR. These domains are integrated horizontally and vertically, both in planning and delivery, from local to national levels. In all three domains, it is vital to practice and integrate the art (e.g. relationship with partners, influencing behaviour, using resources wisely) and science (e.g. surveillance, epidemiology, modelling, environmental and social sciences) of public health to achieve the best possible protection of the health of the public.

References

Acheson, D. 1988. *Public Health in England: The Report of the Committee of Inquiry into the Future Development of the Public Health Function.* London: HMSO.

Broughton E. 2005. The Bhopal disaster and its aftermath: a review. *Environmental Health,* 4:6. doi:10.1186/1476-069X-4-6

Buncefield Major Incident Investigation Board. 2008. *The Buncefield Incident 11 December 2005: The Final Report of the Major Incident Investigation Board.* Sudbury: HSE Books: Vol. 1. http://www.hse.gov.uk/comah/buncefield/miib-final-volume1.pdf (accessed 16 March 2016).

Cardis E, M Hatch. 2011. The Chernobyl accident—an epidemiological perspective. *Clinical Oncology,* 23(4): 251–60.

Department of Health. 2002. *Getting Ahead of the Curve: A Strategy for Combating Infectious Diseases.* London: Department of Health.

Department of Health and Social Security. 1986. *Report of the Committee of Inquiry into an Outbreak of Food Poisoning at Stanley Royd Hospital.* London: HMSO.

Faculty of Public Health. 2010. *What is public health?* http://www.fph.org.uk/what_is_public_health (accessed 5 March 2016).

Ghebrehewet S, AG Stewart. 2014. *North West Environmental Public Health Practice Review: Discussion Paper.* Liverpool: Cheshire and Merseyside Public Health England Centre Report.

Head BW, J Alford. 2013. Wicked problems: implications for public policy and management. *Administration & Society,* 28 March. doi:10.1177/0095399713481601

Health and Social Care Act. 2012. London: The Stationery Office.

Health Protection Scotland. 2005. http://www.hps.scot.nhs.uk/about/index.aspx (accessed 5 March 2016).

Hine DD. 2010. *The 2009 Influenza Pandemic: An independent review of the UK Response to the 2009 Influenza Pandemic.* London: Cabinet Office.

HM Government. 2005. *The Civil Contingencies Act 2004 (Contingency Planning) Regulations 2005.* London: The Stationery Office.

HM Government. 2006. *Emergency Preparedness. Guidance on Part 1 of the Civil Contingencies Act 2004, Its Associated Regulations and Non-Statutory Arrangements.* https://www.gov.uk/government/publications/emergency-preparedness (accessed 5 March 2016).

IAEA. 2006. *Chernobyl's Legacy: Health, Environmental and Socio-Economic Impacts and Recommendations to the Governments of Belarus, the Russian Federation and Ukraine.* Vienna: International Atomic Energy Agency. https://www.iaea.org/sites/default/files/chernobyl.pdf (accessed 5 March 2016).

Kapila M, R Buttery. 1986. Lessons from the outbreak of food poisoning at Stanley Royd Hospital: what are health authorities doing now? *BMJ (Clin Res Ed),* **293:** 321–32.

Keeble B. 2006. Sleep walking to another Stanley Royd? *BMJ,* **333:** 557.

O'Mahonya CM, ER Stanwell-Smith, HE Tillett, et al. 1990. The Stafford outbreak of Legionnaires' disease. *Epidemiology and Infection,* **104**(3): 361–80.

Public Health Agency. 2011. http://www.publichealth.hscni.net/ (accessed 5 March 2016).

Public Health England. 2013. *Our priorities for 2013/14.* https://www.gov.uk/government/uploads/system/uploads/attachment_data/file/192676/Our_priorities_final.pdf (accessed 5 March 2016).

Public Health Wales. 2010. http://www.wales.nhs.uk/sitesplus/888/home (accessed 5 March 2016).

RAND Europe. 2014. *The future of public health: A horizon scan.* http://www.rand.org/pubs/research_reports/RR433.html (accessed 5 March 2016).

Redford KH, W Adams, GM Mace. (2013). Synthetic biology and conservation of nature: wicked problems and wicked solutions. *PLoS Biology,* **11**(4): e1001530.

Shears P, TJD O'Dempsey. 2015. Ebola virus disease in Africa: epidemiology and nosocomial transmission. *Journal of Hospital Infection,* **90**(1): 1–9.

Winslow CEA 1920. The untilled fields of public health". *Science,* **51** (1306): 23–33. http://www.jstor.org/stable/1645011 (accessed 16 March 2016).

Chapter 2

Who is involved in health protection?

Sam Ghebrehewet and Alex G. Stewart

OVERVIEW

After reading this chapter the reader will be familiar with:

• the key players in health protection,
• their roles and functions, and
• the criteria for the local footprint of specialist health protection teams.

2.1 Introduction to the participants in health protection

Protecting the nation's health relies on involvement and meaningful engagement of the general public, professionals, media, politicians, and many other parties. It is important to engage the wider community and workforce in health protection, and consider the wider health of the local population. However, at the same time, a line needs to be drawn for practical purposes of legislation, responsibility, accountability, and efficient service management, and in some situations, particular individuals may be required to undertake specific functions. For example, caring for an ill patient is not just restricted to doctors and nurses but includes family members, neighbours, voluntary agencies, and the like. However, there are some functions, such as giving intravenous fluids, which require particular individuals (nurses) to undertake.

Similarly, contributions to health protection functions and activities are not limited to those who practise health protection professionally, but include, for example, those who provide clean water and sewage removal (including the labourers and plumbers), from the water utility companies, through regulators such as the Environment Agency or the Drinking Water Inspectorate, local authority planners, to those who prepare and plan for emergencies.

Although the examples given in this chapter of how different roles play a part in health protection are taken from the UK, the basic principles apply in other countries, even though job titles and organizational names and structures will of course vary.

2.2 Roles and functions

An individual may undertake different roles or functions, all contributing to the protection of health. Every person's contribution is important and combines to form a comprehensive health protection response: from a hospital cleaner to the Director of Infection Prevention and Control in a health care setting; from administrative staff to a Consultant in Health Protection or Communicable Disease Control; from a refuse collector to the local authority chief executive; from a laboratory technician to a Consultant Medical Microbiologist.

Nevertheless, it is easy to overlook the contribution that the variety of staff, professional and non-professional individuals and groups make to the protection of the population's health. If their contribution is not fully acknowledged then opportunities to develop staff groups and enhance their contribution to the wider public health protection will not be realized. In addition, wider staff groups often bring a different perspective and can help to approach a problem in a different way. This contribution can be revolutionary: for example, the contribution of hospital cleaners to the reduction of health-care-associated infection is key and could be improved if recognized by senior staff. Giving hospital cleaners status (even changing their title to Hygiene Specialists) and recognizing their important contribution by involving them in meetings and strategy can revolutionize their contribution, as they see the impact they make in partnership with other professional groups. The view of the other professionals will also change, both to cleaning and to the prevention and management of health-care-associated infection.

2.3 Health protection professionals

Health protection professionals, who deliver recognized health protection functions, have responsibilities and accountability for protecting the health of the population through the provision of public health advice and the application of regulatory powers as appropriate. For example, in the UK, the local authority has advisory, scrutiny, and regulatory functions that are discharged through departments such as public health, planning, environmental health, children and adult social services, and legal.

Examples of national and international specialist health protection organizations include Public Health Wales, Health Protection Scotland, Public Health England, Public Health Agency for Northern Ireland (UK), Centers for Disease Control and Prevention (USA), Public Health Agency Canada (PHAC), Netherlands National Institute for Public Health and the Environment (Rijksinstituut voor Volksgezondheid en Milieu; RIVM), and European Centre for Disease Prevention and Control (ECDC), to mention but a few.

Health protection professionals can be categorized into two groups: those whose main role is health protection (regular functions) and those whose main role is outside health protection but who, at different times and in various ways, become involved with health protection issues as an occasional part of their role (supporting function). Most, if not all, of these organizations encourage participation from trainees in various specialities relevant to Health Protection (Table 2.1).

2.4 Health protection at a local geographical footprint

The argument is often made for working at the lowest possible level (local). But local has many shapes and sizes. For example, there is a 31-fold difference between populations in local authorities in England (<50,000 to >1,000,000; ONS 2013) and a 200-fold difference in geographical area (LGBC 2015). Therefore, it is important to determine the local population and geographical footprint in order to optimize the delivery of high-quality, safe, effective, and efficient health protection functions.

The following criteria could help define the footprint:

◆ **Population size:** defines the appropriate scale of local surveillance in order to produce valid, meaningful and applicable intelligence.

◆ **Geography:** the size of the area and the resulting distance from the local team to key partners and population.

◆ **Local relationships:** relationships between the specialist team and local professionals need to be developed and maintained in order to ensure health protection services are robust, resilient, and capable of protecting the local population. Multi-agency working relationships are critical for preparedness, planning, and response.

◆ **Organizational alignment with key partners:** responsibility and accountability cannot be discharged independently by any team. In addition, when boundaries of different health and government agencies are not coterminous there are challenges in coordinating preparedness and response to public health emergencies.

Table 2.1 Examples of organizations and staff providing health protection functions for communicable disease control, emergency preparedness, resilience and response, and environmental public health from a UK perspective

Local	*Local Authority*	*Health Care*	*Specialist Health Protection*	*Other groups*
	Regular functions: Environmental Health Officers; Emergency Planners; Planning Officers; Director of Public Health and team; Port Health Officers; police, ambulance, fire & rescue **Supporting role:** Adult and Children Social Services (e.g. safeguarding; care home issues) Legal Services (e.g. advice on LA responsibilities to mitigate and respond to risk to protect public health)	**Regular functions:** Health Care (and public health) Commissioners; Health Care Providers (particularly microbiologists, infectious disease staff, Accident & Emergency staff, infection control nurses, practice nurses, health visitors, district nurses, screening and immunization coordinators, school nurses; cleaners); Health & Safety staff **Supporting role:** Paediatric team; maternity and child health staff; clinical toxicologist; dentists; radiation physicist; cleaner in non-health care settings; occupational health, etc.	**Regular function:** Health Protection Agencies clerical staff, Health Protection Practitioners; surveillance and epidemiology analysts; project managers; Emergency Planners; Consultants in Communicable Disease Control; information technologists; Veterinary Public Health; some academia e.g., those who work for health protection research units (HPRUs) in England	**Supporting role:** Academics; chemical and environmental scientists; toxicologists; radiation specialists; Department of Communities and Local Government; industry; charitable organizations; military; Environment agencies; utility companies
Regional	*Regional Government organizations*	*Health Care*	*Specialist Health Protection*	*Regional Non-Government Organizations*
	Regular functions: Regional staff in Public Health authority and Environment Agency; Department for Communities and Local Government staff; Food Standard Agency (FSA); utility companies (water company staff); Animal and Plant Health Agency (incorporating Animal Health and Veterinary Laboratory Agency)	**Regular functions:** Regional public health and health protection authorities and agencies; regional strategic networks (e.g., TB, zoonoses). **Supporting role:** Regional strategic networks (e.g. cancer); specialist commissioning (e.g. HIV).	**Regular function:** Microbiological reference laboratories; Field Epidemiology Services (including administrative, scientist, data entry, epidemiologist staff); regional EPRR staff	**Regular functions:** Clean Air (London), utility companies, academics, chemical and environmental scientists, toxicologists, radiation specialists

(continued)

Table 2.1 Continued

	National Government organizations	Health Care	Specialist Health Protection	Other Groups
National	**Regular functions:** Central Government, Departments of Health and staff of Chief Medical Officers; National public health body staff; Minister for Public Health and team, Department of Food, Environment and Rural Affairs staff, Health & Safety Executive: Drinking Water Inspectorate (DWA); Department of Transport. Department of Energy and Climate Change	**Regular functions:** National healthcare commissioning and policy development staff; national audit, quality improvement and performance management staff **Supporting role:** National Poisons Information Service	**Regular functions:** National Health Protection/Public Health Directorate such as PHE; specialist health protection departments (e.g. Emergency Response Division, Centre for Radiation Chemicals and Environment, Centre for Infectious Disease Surveillance and Control); Food Standard Agency (FSA)	**Regular functions:** Charities—e.g. Meningitis Now, National Society for Clean Air and Environmental Protection **Supporting role:** Pressure group members
International	**International Government Organizations** **Regular functions:** World Health Organization (WHO); Roll Back Malaria; United Nations Programme on HIV/AIDS; UNICEF **Supporting role:** World Bank	**Regular functions:** International Committee of the Red Cross; Médecins Sans Frontières	**Specialist Health Protection** European Centre for Disease Prevention and Control (ECDC); WHO; United Nations International Strategy on Disaster Reduction (UNISDR); European Environment Agency; European Food Standards Agency; Blacksmith Institute, Global Alliance on Health and Pollution	**Other Groups** **Regular functions:** Stop TB Partnership; Bill & Melinda Gates Foundation; Global Health Program; OXFAM; Voluntary Service Overseas (VSO)

From experience over many years of planning for and managing a variety of health protection situations with multi-agency colleagues, a population footprint of between two and three million is workable, if not ideal, for a health protection team. The team should be consultant-led, specialist health protection nurse-delivered. Small population footprints can result in duplication and variation in health protection responses and can lead to difficulties with robustness of data. Large population footprints can bring difficulties in maintaining relationships, providing close scrutiny of data, and timely intelligence. Economies of scale are often presented as the reason for teams covering larger areas, i.e. without a clearly defined upper or lower limit. The limitations of economies of scale are often less clearly recognized or evaluated, such as the ability to (1) deliver a good, high-quality, and efficient service; (2) maintain a safe service; and (3) establish and develop resilient working relationships (personal and professional networks).

While the above criteria may help to establish the footprint of health protection services, in order to determine the appropriate size and skill mix of the specialist health protection staff, factors such as deprivation, local disease epidemiology, environmental health, and economic/historical situations need to be taken into account. For example, areas with a high prevalence of TB may need more TB control nurses, an area with a historical legacy of environmental issues or the chemical industry may need more environmental public health input, while an area with a major airport may need extra port health support.

The importance of specialist health protection teams delivering key health protection functions in all three domains (communicable disease control, emergency preparedness, resilience and response, environmental public health; see Chapter 1) at the right footprint cannot be underestimated. This could have significant implications for establishing meaningful and resilient relationship with key professionals, partners, and stakeholders, something that is critical to improving and maintaining quality, safety, confidence, and assurance in any given geographical area. In addition, the right footprint should create an environment conducive to maintaining meaningful and supportive relationships with neighbouring teams, including sharing good practice and learning, while at the same time having good vertical relationships to maintain administrative and technical support both regionally and nationally.

Health protection service delivery, of course, depends on available resources, with the result that small teams covering large geographical areas are likely to be more reactive than larger teams with relatively smaller areas per team member. These larger teams can be more strategic, but need greater resources.

2.5 Conclusions

Health protection encompasses a wide range of professionals, with a complex skill mix, in a wide variety of fields, across all domains of public health, and in every corner of the globe. The health protection functions delivered by specialized professionals are complemented by members of the community from the lowest operator to the highest strategist.

References

Local Government Boundary Commission. 2015. *Local Authorities in England*. https://www.lgbce.org.uk/records-and-resources/local-authorities-in-england (accessed 8 March 2016).

Office for National Statistics. 2013. *UK Population Estimates 2013*. http://www.ons.gov.uk/ons/rel/pop-estimate/population-estimates-for-uk--england-and-wales--scotland-and-northern-ireland/2013/sty-population-estimates.html (accessed 8 March 2016).

Chapter 3

Key principles and practice of health protection

Sam Ghebrehewet, Alex G. Stewart, and Ian Rufus

OVERVIEW

After reading this chapter the reader will be familiar with:

- the key principles and practice of health protection,
- the essential health protection functions, and
- the integrated public health risk assessment.

3.1 Introduction to the principles and practice of health protection

Health protection protects the health of the local population from threats to individuals and communities from communicable disease, emergencies, and environmental issues. As a result of the unpredictability in time, space, and scope of health protection issues, the provision of a 24/7 local service across the spectrum of communicable disease control, emergency preparedness, resilience, and response (EPRR), and environmental public health is essential.

These three domains of health protection (communicable disease control, EPRR, environmental public health) follow similar principles in their organization, development, and delivery. All three domains are delivered by one team at the local level, within a national structure, with different skills and competencies, in collaboration with local, regional, and national agencies.

This "all-hazards" approach can be clearly seen in the three domains of health protection as they follow the same principles, whether dealing with individual issues and cases or large incidents and outbreaks:

1. planning and preparedness,
2. prevention and early detection,
3. investigation and control, and
4. wider public health management and leadership (including communication to professionals and the public).

3.2 Health protection principles

3.2.1 Planning and preparedness

Planning and preparedness are the bread and butter of daily health protection practice, where most time and resources are, or should be, committed.

3.2.1.1 Communicable disease control

In communicable disease control, this entails working with partners in developing plans and strategies to prevent or mitigate the impact of health threats from new cases or outbreaks.

Development of a local business case in the context of national business plans means clear objectives and targets which can be reviewed, monitored, and developed, for example, to improve immunization uptake and reduce the incidence of vaccine-preventable diseases such as measles or meningitis.

Underpinning all communicable disease control is the agent-host-environment concept, which provides a framework for understanding any communicable disease and the resulting control measures. For example:

+ agents: the measles virus is relatively stable, whereas the influenza virus continually mutates,

+ hosts (people) become more susceptible when their immunity is compromised (e.g. illness, drugs, nutrition, age), and

+ environments can encourage microbiological agents to survive or flourish (e.g. cholera vibrio survives in seawater between outbreaks).

3.2.1.2 Emergency Prepardness Resilience and Response (EPRR)

EPRR works with a wider group of multi-agency partners, focusing on preparedness for challenging situations. Local and national risk registers are maintained, supporting the development and testing of plans, such as for pandemic influenza or major chemical pollution incidents.

The underpinning frameworks in EPRR are the agent-host-environment concept (above) and the source-pathway-receptor concept (below).

3.2.1.3 Environmental public health

Environmental public health is less well developed, but takes a similar multi-agency approach to the development of strategy and plans, business case development, and risk register maintenance. For example, planning to improve air quality includes multi-agency work on transport, industry, power generation, and waste management. Unlike communicable diseases, the lead organization in planning and prevention within EPRR and environmental public health is likely to be a non-health agency.

Underpinning environmental issues in EPRR and environmental public health is the source-pathway-receptor framework. In any environmental situation, there needs to be a defined source of the chemical spill or the hazard that is threatening health (traffic, flood, fire); receptors (people) may vary in their susceptibility (elderly and children are usually at greater risk than healthy adults, but distance to source may also affect vulnerability); sources and receptors need linking by pathways (inhalation, ingestion, skin/eye contact). If any one of the three elements is missing then there is no risk to human health.

3.2.2 **Prevention and early detection**

Prevention and early detection sit comfortably between planning and preparedness on the one hand and investigation and control on the other; they may be undertaken by professionals other than specialist health protection professionals.

3.2.2.1 Communicable disease control

Communicable disease control examples include preventative programmes of infection control in health care settings, as well as childhood vaccination and immunization programmes, the provision of clean water, and the safe disposal of household waste. Early detection examples include antenatal screening programmes for syphilis, hepatitis B, and human immunodeficiency virus (HIV), hospital screening of new patients for methicillin resistant staphylococcus aureus (MRSA) and other drug-resistant organisms or for new cases in outbreaks.

3.2.2.2 Emergency Prepardness Resilience and Response (EPRR)

Annual maintenance of boilers and other fuel-driven combustion sources to reduce carbon monoxide exposure and poisoning is an example of risk mitigation as part of the EPRR prevention strategy, as is the action of the Health and Safety Executive in large industrial sites to identify and manage risks of catastrophes. The use of carbon dioxide and fire alarms, whether domestic or industrial, constitutes early detection mechanisms.

3.2.2.3 Environmental public health

Prevention is seen in statutory risk assessments (e.g. asbestos in industrial sites, legionella in hospitals and other sites), while early detection examples include radon surveys available to householders and air quality monitoring by local authorities. Action against air pollution also fits here.

3.2.3 Investigation and control

3.2.3.1 Communicable disease

Investigation and control is well developed and practised in communicable disease. The response of health protection teams to enquiries and notifications of infectious diseases depends on the collection, collation, analysis and interpretation of information, placed within the local context and epidemiology. This allows the investigation and control of new and emerging infections and situations such as a measles outbreak where there have been no previous cases or a case of *E. coli* indicative of a breakdown of infection control measures on a farm. Note that the diseases that are statutorily notifiable vary from country to country.

3.2.3.2 EPRR

In EPRR, investigation and control follows a similar route. Intelligence arising from observations, mostly from local emergency services, about a threat to the health of the local population (e.g. from a fire in a warehouse that contains chemicals) needs the collection, collation, analysis, and interpretation of relevant information within local contexts and epidemiology. The intelligence should follow well-recognized protocols to identify the location, nature of incident (e.g. fire, flood) hazard (present or potential), accessibility for emergency services, numbers of casualties, and the emergency services response (Joint Emergency Services Interoperability Principles: JESIP, http://www.jesip.org.uk/). Control measures include timely public health advice to those at risk: e.g. shelter, evacuation, and/or prophylaxis as appropriate (such as iodine prophylaxis following nuclear accidents).

3.2.3.3 Environmental public health

In environmental public health, investigation and control is complex and may take months to years. As with planning and prevention, the lead organization is likely to be a non-health agency. For example, the investigation and control of possible chemical contamination of an allotment from historical industry is the responsibility of the local authority. Specialist health protection advice can help develop an appropriate sampling regime and control measures, with relevant and targeted public health communications to the public and local health services.

3.2.4 Public health management and leadership

Public health management and leadership bring the other three principles—planning and preparedness, prevention and early detection, investigation and control—together. Reflection is important, particularly on outbreaks and incidents, but also on single issues, as well as surveillance reports. Reflection encourages the integration of identified lessons, the science and the supporting systems into better personal understanding, service and systems and can be incorporated into continuing professional development, corporate vision, evaluation and monitoring tools, stakeholder relationships, and improved case management and surveillance systems.

There are several leadership roles, all of which are crucial in ensuring adequate preparation for, and response to, public health emergencies. All require particular competence and capability. One way of thinking about these is as strategic, tactical, and operational leadership, in line with emergency response principles, but useful in communicable disease control and environmental public health. At local level, strategic leadership is provided by the local Director of Public Health and the director of the local specialist health protection service. Local tactical leadership is provided by consultants in health protection from the specialist health protection team and the local authority Chief Environmental Health Officer. Operational leadership is provided by health protection practitioners and environmental health officers. These examples relate to local authority and public health. However, a similar approach can be applied to infection prevention and control in health care, whereby the Director of Infection Prevention and Control in a local health agency provides strategic leadership and infection prevention and control nurses provide tactical leadership and nurse practitioners provide operational leadership. Of course, these leadership roles are not mutually exclusive. For example, a consultant in health protection could provide strategic leadership in the management of an outbreak, and operational leadership in a significant major incident when providing telephone support to emergency responders and health care workers.

Beyond this, there is also a need for 'health protection partnership leadership' in EPRR, communicable disease control and environmental public health. Evidence indicates that service failure problems often occur at the borders between one organization or team and another (Healthcare Commission 2008). Similarly, in communicable disease prevention and control, partnership occurs between the local authority, NHS and specialist health protection services to develop joint plans, surveillance, and service response. In our experience, the local partnership leadership role in environmental public health needs further development, since the interaction between agencies is highly dependent on the situation. For example, in contaminated land or air pollution issues, the local authority background work often lacks systematic public health/health protection input as the leadership role has not developed in parallel to EPRR and communicable disease control.

At regional and national levels, health protection leadership is provided by senior public health/health protection professionals in the UK, or a similar post in other countries. In addition to providing support to the local teams, these roles include establishing and providing health protection direction to government and non-government agencies, supported by administrative (corporate services) and technical teams that provide regional services of surveillance (including syndromic surveillance, and environmental tracking), epidemiology, toxicological and environmental sciences (including poison information), specialist radiation, EPRR, references laboratories (microbiology, toxicology), international liaison, workforce development (including human resources), information and communication technology. Members of the local team may provide some of the regional/national level support networks, groups, and committees as appropriate.

3.3 **Health Protection Practice**

3.3.1 **Cross-cutting activities**

Specialist health protection practice in all three domains requires competencies and skills that range from providing direct public health advice to individual enquiries through to managing significant, challenging incidents/outbreaks that require influencing, advocacy, systems leadership, and advanced communication skills. Specialist health protection practice can be illustrated through essential health protection functions (adapted from Department of Health 2013).

1. Responding to cases, enquiries and providing advice.
2. Responding to, and managing, incidents and outbreaks.
3. Undertaking surveillance and epidemiological studies.
4. Managing stakeholders' relationships.
5. Contributing to, and influencing, national strategies.
6. Contributing to research and development.
7. Underpinning activities (include corporate functions, quality and governance activities, learning and development, business planning and performance management).

These functions directly represent communicable diseases practice, as well as those in EPRR and environmental public health, although, in some cases (e.g. environmental surveillance (tracking) and environmental epidemiology), this needs further development.

3.3.2 **EPRR**

The core principle activities of Integrated Emergency Management (anticipation, assessment, prevention, preparation, response, recovery) (Figure 3.1) apply to the preparation and response to outbreaks of infectious disease (e.g. measles) as much as to chemical spills, environmental hazards, and terrorist events. Indeed, they forge the link that unites communicable disease control to environmental public health, moulding health protection into one, unified whole. EPRR practitioners' skills and practice in leading debrief sessions and reflective activities covering the whole situation are particularly valuable in identifying lessons from an incident/outbreak/situation.

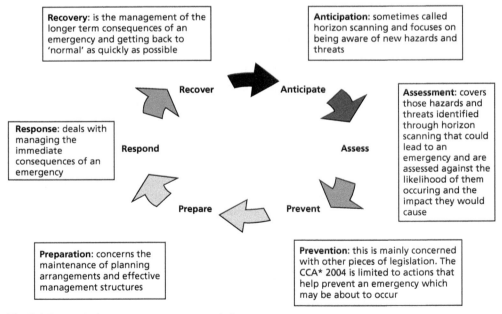

Recovery: is the management of the longer term consequences of an emergency and getting back to 'normal' as quickly as possible

Anticipation: sometimes called horizon scanning and focuses on being aware of new hazards and threats

Assessment: covers those hazards and threats identified through horizon scanning that could lead to an emergency and are assessed against the likelihood of them occuring and the impact they would cause

Response: deals with managing the immediate consequences of an emergency

Preparation: concerns the maintenance of planning arrangements and effective management structures

Prevention: this is mainly concerned with other pieces of legislation. The CCA* 2004 is limited to actions that help prevent an emergency which may be about to occur

Recover   Anticipate   Respond   Assess   Prepare   Prevent

Fig. 3.1 Integrated emergency management steps

Source: data from NHS, NHS Commissioning Board Emergency Preparedness Framework 2013 (Leeds, NHS, 2013), http://www.england.nhs.uk/wp-content/uploads/2013/03/eprr-framework.pdf.
*Civil Contingencies Act.

EPRR is both outward facing to the community and inward facing to the business continuity needs of the organization. It operates under the Civil Contingencies Act (2004), which:

- defines emergency,
- clarifies:
  - duty to assess, plan, and advise
  - assistance to the public
  - what actions can be taken
  - disclosure of information
  - urgency of response

- outlines enforcement action,
- details provision of information, and
- categorizes responders.

Organizations are classified as Category 1 or Category 2 responders. Specialist health protection services are Category 1 ('first') responders and are subject to the full set of civil protection duties. Amongst other duties, they will be required to assess risks to communities and plan to deal with emergencies cooperatively (others include emergency services, some health services, local authorities), and put in place business continuity management arrangements. Category 2 organizations (e.g. utilities, other health services) support Category 1 organizations through cooperation and sharing of information. All such organizations collaborate in a Local Resilience Forum based on police force areas to enable local cooperation and coordination, where partnership leadership is crucial to safe and efficient working. Health organizations collaborate in Local Health Resilience Partnerships which act similarly for health emergencies.

3.3.3 Environmental public health

The practice of environmental public health involves:

- identifying any source-pathway-receptor linkages,
- characterizing such linkages using relevant environmental, toxicological, epidemiological sciences,
- evaluating perceptions of professionals and the public concerning the situation,
- searching for and assessing other relevant information which impinges on the situation or its understanding,
- integrating all information in a multi-agency context,
- making judgements in the context of uncertainty concerning causes, solutions and possible health outcomes of the situation, and
- communicating with all relevant partners and the public in a timely and open manner.

3.3.4 Public Health Risk Assessment

In any incident or outbreak, it is useful to consider wider issues than those that arise from examination of the basic sciences, microbiology, toxicology, environmental sciences, or epidemiology. In all three health protection domains, but especially EPRR and environmental public health, any such technical risk assessment needs to be set in the context of anything that might possibly adversely affect the outcome of the investigation and control measures. Similarly, it is important to identify and understand, but not necessarily agree with, the outlook and expectations of as wide a

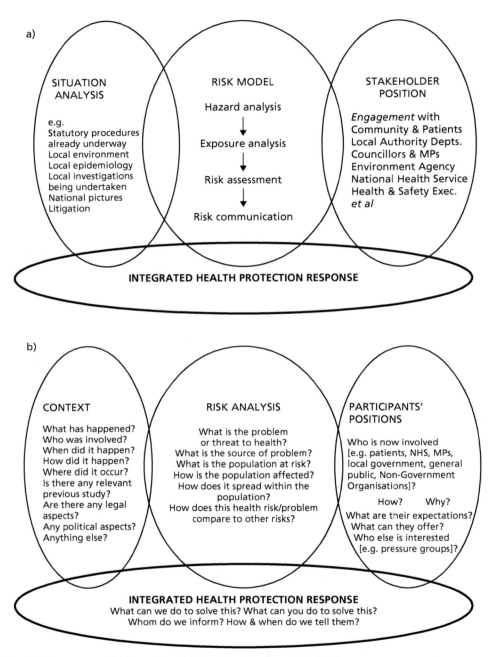

Fig. 3.2 The process of integrated public health risk assessment: (a) the summary approach: an outline of methods; (b) the practical approach: questions to be asked.

(a) Adapted with permission from Reid JR, Jarvis R, Richardson J, and Stewart AG. Responding to chronic environmental problems in Cheshire & Merseyside – Systems and Procedures, in: Health Protection Agency. Chemical Hazards and Poisons Report. May 2005, Issue 4, p. 30–5, Copyright © 2005 Chemical Hazards and Poisons Division, Health Protection Agency, UK, https://www.gov.uk/government/uploads/system/uploads/attachment_data/file/202984/rep_CHAPR4May2005.pdf; b) Reproduced with permission from Mahoney G, Stewart AG, Kennedy N, Whitely B, Turner L, and Wilkinson E. Achieving attainable outcomes from good science in an untidy world: case studies in land and air pollution. Environmental Geochemistry and Health, Volume 37, Issue 4, pp. 689–706, Copyright © 2015 Springer Science+Business Media Dordrecht.

variety of stakeholders in the situation as much as possible, again to ensure that investigation and response is as appropriate and applicable as possible (Figure 3.2). For example, without an appreciation of the culture of an immigrant community, the identification and engagement of healthy but exposed controls may not be easy (Stewart et al. 2012). An appreciation of local industrial history and community concerns can help focus questions that drive health investigations (Reeve et al. 2013). This fuller risk assessment gives more solid understanding for action which is likely to succeed than simply using the science without taking other factors into consideration (Reid et al. 2005; Mahoney et al. 2015).

3.4 **Conclusions**

The UK was at the forefront of the development of public health and communicable disease control and continues to deliver a robust service in communicable disease control. It has also been one of the first countries to integrate EPRR into the health service and emergency response (UNISDR 2013).

To date, many health protection organizations, whether international or national, concentrate their resources and attention on communicable diseases and EPRR for historical and practical reasons, including experience and well-developed science. Therefore, the practice of environmental public health, especially in the management of major, complex, chronic situations, has not developed in parallel. Nevertheless, the principles which drive communicable disease control and EPRR can be applied to environmental issues. The health effects of climate change (WHO 2015), air pollution (REVIHAAP 2013), and contamination of land and the built environment (Blacksmith Institute annual reports) continue to increase globally; the UK is not exempt from these changes and has an unknown burden on health from historical industry. Further development of effective and safe environmental public health practice could revolutionize the public health approach to chronic disease and the effect that poor environmental quality, such as air quality, has on public health.

References

Blacksmith Institute annual reports. http://www.blacksmithinstitute.org/ and http://www.worstpolluted. org/ (accessed 8 March 2016).

Department of Health. 2013. *Protecting the Health of the Local Population: The New Health Protection Duty of Local Authorities under the Local Authorities (Public Health Functions and Entry to Premises by Local Healthwatch Representatives) Regulations 2013*. https://www.gov.uk/government/uploads/system/uploads/attachment_data/file/199773/Health_Protection_in_Local_Authorities_Final.pdf (accessed 8 March 2016).

Healthcare Commission. 2008. *Annual Report 2008/09. Our Work to Improve Healthcare for Patients and the Public*. London: The Stationery Office.

NHS. 2013. *NHS Commissioning Board Emergency Preparedness Framework 2013*. http://www.england.nhs.uk/wp-content/uploads/2013/03/eprr-framework.pdf (accessed 18 December 2015).

Mahoney G, AG Stewart, N Kennedy, et al. 2015. Achieving attainable outcomes from good science in an untidy world: case studies in land and air pollution. *Environmental Geochemistry & Health*, 37: 689–706. doi:10.1007/s10653-015-9717-9.

Reeve NF, TR Fanshawe, TJ Keegan, AG Stewart, PJ Diggle. 2013. Spatial analysis of health effects of large industrial incinerators in England, 1998–2008: a study using matched case–control areas. *BMJ Open*, 3:e001847

Reid JR, R Jarvis, J Richardson, AG Stewart. 2005. Responding to chronic environmental problems in Cheshire & Merseyside—Systems and Procedures. *Chemical Hazards and Poisons Report*, 4: 33–35.

REVIHAAP. 2013. *Review of Evidence on Health Aspects of Air Pollution—REVIHAAP*. Bonn: WHO Regional Office for Europe.

Stewart AG, A Keenan, R Vivancos, C Theodore C. 2012. A point source outbreak of food poisoning in a defined community. In *Case Studies in Food Safety and Authenticity: Lessons from Real-Life Situations*, edited by J Hoorfar. Cambridge, UK: Woodhead Publishing Ltd.

UNISDR. 2013. *United Kingdom Peer Review Report 2013—Building Resilience to Disasters: Implementation of the Hyogo Framework for Action (2005–2015)*. http://www.unisdr.org/files/32996_32996hfaukpeerreview20131.pdf (accessed 8 March 2016).

WHO. 2015. *Climate Change and Human Health—Risks and Responses: Summary*. http://www.who.int/globalchange/summary/en/index12.html (accessed 8 March 2016).

Chapter 4

The basics of infection microbiology

Paul Shears and David Harvey

OVERVIEW

After reading this chapter the reader will be familiar with:

- the natural history of infections including endogenous and exogenous infection, incubation period, infectivity, and outcome,
- the classification of pathogenic micro-organisms in relation to diagnosis and disease investigation,
- the role of the laboratory in disease investigation and management, and
- the increasing problem of antimicrobial resistance, and its effect on both hospital and community infections.

4.1 Introduction to the basics of infection microbiology

Although detailed microbiology support will be provided to health protection staff by local and regional laboratories, a basic knowledge of microbiology and infection is essential for disease prevention and control.

4.1.1 The natural history of infections

Not all microorganisms cause disease, and not all humans develop clinical infections from a particular pathogen. The natural history of an infection describes the interaction between the pathogen and the host, and the resulting infection that has to be managed and controlled.

The development of an infection involves colonization of the host by the pathogen, local or systemic invasion of the pathogen, and either development of disease or resolution, depending on the presence or level of host immunity to the pathogen. Some infections, particularly in hospital, may arise from bacteria with which the patient is already colonized; this is endogenous infection. Most infections in the community will be exogenous, where the pathogen is acquired from another person, from the environment, or a source such as food or water.

The incubation period of an infection is the time between acquiring the pathogen, and developing symptoms; this may be two to three days as in the case of norovirus, or up to 21 days as in the case of mumps. The infectivity period, when the infection can be transmitted to another susceptible person, may often occur only after the development of symptoms, but may, as in chickenpox, begin a few days before the symptoms appear.

The outcome of infection depends on both the virulence of the pathogen, and degree of relevant immunity in the host. Many infections, such as respiratory virus infections, will resolve spontaneously. Most bacterial infections, though sometimes clinically severe, will respond to appropriate antimicrobial treatment. However, if treatment is delayed, apparently treatable bacterial infections may have a fatal outcome.

In some infections, variations in very specific components of immunity may lead to different outcomes with the same pathogen, which is the case in meningococcal disease.

4.2 **Micro-organism classification in relation to infections**

4.2.1 **Classification of bacteria of common importance**

Most bacteria are classified according to two simple microscopic properties: their colour, and their shape, in the Gram staining process. Bacteria may be Gram positive (Gr +ve), giving a blue/black colour on staining, or Gram negative (Gr –ve), giving a pink colour on staining, and their shape either round (cocci) or rod-like (bacilli). Mycobacterium infection, including the cause of human TB, does not fit into this Gram stain classification, as a different staining method is used.

Figure 4.1 shows the bacteria and their infections that occur in routine UK practice. The list is not exhaustive, and a comprehensive handbook such as the *Control of Communicable Diseases Manual* should be referred to where necessary (Heymann 2014).

The Gram stain classification is not just of interest to laboratory and clinical staff. It also provides a framework for public health and other staff to understand the pathogens causing the diseases they are investigating, and for understanding the laboratory results necessary for disease management and control. The majority of bacterial infections in the community and in hospital are caused by a relatively small number of bacterial types.

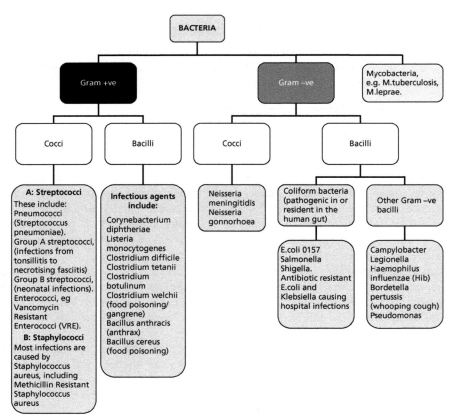

Fig. 4.1 Classification of bacteria according to Gram stain appearance

4.2.2 **Classification of viruses in relation to infection**

All viruses have a similar structure: an outer shell and a protein core in the centre of which is the genetic material. Viruses are classified based on genetic material and mode of replication into: DNA viruses (e.g. hepatitis B, herpes and adenoviruses), or RNA viruses (e.g. measles, mumps and rubella). DNA and RNA viruses can be classified further depending on the structure and symmetry of the protein, and the presence or absence of an envelope.

Some community virus infections have very specific symptoms and clinical signs, such as mumps or measles, and disease-specific laboratory investigations can be requested if a confirmed diagnosis is necessary. However, health protection staff may be faced with an outbreak in a school of fever and rash, or acute respiratory disease. In these situations, no single virus is obviously responsible, but rather than asking for 'general virology', it is invaluable for the investigation to know which possible viruses may be responsible, and to understand which tests the laboratory can undertake. Table 4.1 shows the viruses that are responsible for different syndromes, and the specimens required for diagnosis.

Table 4.1 Virus infections: syndromes and diagnoses

Syndrome	Causes	Diagnosis
Rash May be macular ('pink/red' skin rash) or macular papular (raised rash) or vesicular (small blisters).	Rubella Parvovirus B 19 Enteroviruses Adenoviruses Measles Human Herpesvirus 6 & 7 Chickenpox/Zoster Herpes simplex virus (HSV) Coxsackie A	Diagnosis is often clinical, or serological. For measles, salivary samples may detect acute antibodies (IgM)
Virus infections/exposures in pregnancy	Rubella Parvovirus B19 Cytomegalovirus Herpes simple Measles Chickenpox	Virology advice for investigation Can check antibody levels on bloods taken at start of pregnancy (booking bloods)
Respiratory disease	Influenza A or B Parainfluenza Respiratory syncytial virus Adenoviruses	<2yr: nasopharyngeal aspirate for PCR Older patient: throat swab, respiratory secretions, or serology.
Meningitis or encephalitis	*Encephalitis:* HSV-2 most common *Meningitis:* Enterovirus Mumps	Cerebrospinal fluid (CSF) sample for virus PCR
Hepatitis	Hepatitis A & E (faecal oral route) Hepatitis B & C (blood-borne)	Blood sample for antibody testing and PCR
HIV	Human immunodeficiency virus (HIV)	Blood sample for HIV antibody and antigen tests; viral load (RNA PCR) and CD4 counts to monitor treatment

(continued)

Table 4.1 Continued

Syndrome	Causes	Diagnosis
Gastrointestinal/diarrhoea	Adults: Norovirus most common. Children <18mths, and sometimes in elderly: Rotavirus most common	Stool sample for viral PCR
Other virus infections	Mumps Epstein Barr virus (glandular fever)	Serology for specific viral IgM antibody
Virus infections of global concern	Viral haemorrhagic fevers (e.g. Ebola, Lassa, dengue) Severe Acute Respiratory Syndrome coronavirus (SARS Co-V) Middle East respiratory virus (MERV) Zika virus infection	Follow national/WHO guidelines for assessment, diagnosis and management of suspected cases

4.2.3 **Other microorganisms causing human disease**

While bacteria and viruses cause most human infections seen in UK practice, other types of microorganisms are occasionally encountered. These include:

- Fungi: these are free-living organisms and cause a wide variety of diseases ranging from minor superficial skin infection (e.g. athlete's foot) to invasive infection in immunocompromised patients (aspergillus cluster during hospital renovation).
- Protozoa: these are single-celled organisms (e.g. cryptosporidium, amoeba and Giardia).
- Helminths: these are large multicellular organisms commonly known as parasitic worms (e.g. threadworm infestations, tapeworms, and hookworms).

Many tropical infections are caused by protozoa (malaria, leishmaniasis, amoebic dysentery) and helminths (schistosomiasis) and must be considered in returning travellers and asylum seekers from tropical areas. While the descriptions given here cover important current pathogens, it is also important to be aware of new and emerging infections that may occur in the future (see Chapter 26).

4.3 **The role and use of the laboratory in the investigation and control of infections relevant to public health, including new diagnostics**

4.3.1 **The microbiology laboratory**

Pathology modernization is resulting in larger centralized laboratories based on the hub and spoke model. Laboratories follow national standard methods to provide consistency. For certain tests, designated laboratories act as regional or national reference laboratories.

4.3.2 **The range of tests available**

Table 4.2 shows the range of laboratory diagnostic tests and the turnaround times for results. Bacteria and fungi can be detected directly from clinical samples using microscopy and culture. If

Table 4.2 Examples of different tests available and turnaround times

Laboratory test	Description	Interpretation	Turnaround time
Bacterial diagnosis			
Microscopy/Gram stain	Direct microscopy of stained specimens such as sputum, wound exudates, cerebrospinal fluid (CSF)	Detects shape (cocci/bacilli) & Gram appearance. Cannot give full identity	1–2 hours
Bacterial culture	Specimens are incubated on growth medium to provide bacterial colonies for further testing	Detects colony shape & Gram appearance. Can give presumptive identification	24–48hrs*
Bacterial identification	Biochemical tests done on colonies to give full identification	Identification to species level, eg. *E.coli, Staph. aureus*	A further 24–48 hours
Molecular tests for bacterial identification (nucleic acid amplification tests, NAATs)	Tests such as the polymerase chain reaction (PCR) may detect bacteria directly from specimens (e.g. CSF), or from preliminary cultures (e.g. TB)	Many rapid tests with high accuracy increasingly used in diagnostic laboratories	2–4 hours if equipment in receiving laboratory
Antimicrobial sensitivity testing	Colonies from initial culture incubated in presence of antimicrobials to determine sensitivity/resistance	Testing for complex antimicrobial resistance (e.g. ESBLs, CPEs)	24 hours after initial culture
Bacterial typing to investigate cross infection and outbreaks	Molecular methods to determine genomic differences (e.g. Variable number tandem repeat (VNTR), whole genomic sequencing (WGS))	Results can give high discrimination assisting epidemiological investigation	Usually performed at reference laboratories, so possible extended turnaround times
Virus diagnosis			
Antibody tests	Blood serum (serology) to detect virus-specific antibodies. Saliva can be used for some infections to detect antibodies	IgM indicates acute or recent viral infection. IgG is present 1–2 weeks after infection and then persists, as a marker of past infection or immunity (e.g. vaccination)	Automated methods make it possible for most diagnostic laboratories to undertake a range of serology tests. Same-day results 4–6 hours
Virus antigen detection using labelled antibody markers	Mainly used for respiratory samples from throat swabs and nasopharyngeal aspirates	Available in laboratories without molecular methods	2–4 hours
Molecular methods (NAATs)	Increasingly available tests to detect and monitor virus infections from blood sample (HIV, Hepatitis B, parvovirus) & CSF (HSV, enteroviruses, mumps)	Provide rapid and accurate results for diagnosis, monitoring treatment, and disease progression	As with serological tests, increasingly available in diagnostic laboratories. 2–4 hours if available

*These are guidelines. Some cultures will fall outside these parameters, but those will be the exceptions (e.g. *Mycobacterium tuberculosis*, i.e. AFB (Acid Fast Bacilli) standard culture takes 6–12 weeks and liquid culture can take 2–3 weeks).

an organism grows, further tests are then performed to confirm the identification and antibiotic susceptibilities. Baron et al. (2013) provide a useful review of the role of the laboratory in infection diagnosis.

Infections caused by viruses may be diagnosed by detection of the virus in suitable specimens, or by serology, where specific antibodies to the virus are detected. Molecular methods for virus (and some bacteria) detection using nucleic acid amplification tests (NAATS) such as the polymerase chain reaction (PCR) are being increasingly used.

When interpreting laboratory results, it is important to relate the results to the clinical and epidemiological situation. Bacteria may be grown, but may not necessarily be clinically significant.

As well as diagnosing infections in individual patients, the laboratory plays an important role in the investigation of disease outbreaks and clusters (Sabat et al. 2013). Within a specific bacterial species (e.g. *E.coli, N.meningitidis*) bacterial typing is used to determine if a single strain within the species is causing a cluster or outbreak. For example, in an outbreak of *E.coli* in a neonatal unit, strain typing may show that the strains from clinical samples were the same as those occurring in ventilator equipment. Most typing methods are now molecular, and some are only performed in reference laboratories.

On rare occasions, contamination of samples, or of reagents in the laboratory, may give rise to a pseudo-outbreak, where a pathogen is reported, but was not present in the suspected cases. An example would be laboratory reagents that are contaminated with environmental mycobacteria, giving false positive tuberculosis results.

4.4 The problem of antimicrobial resistance

Antibiotic resistant bacteria are an increasing problem in both hospital and community infections (World Health Organization 2014). Examples include methicillin-resistant *S.aureus* (MRSA), vancomycin-resistant enterococci (VRE), carbapenemase-producing enterobacteriaceae (CPE), and resistant strains of gonorrhoea and tuberculosis. Bacteria are constantly evolving new ways of resistance under the pressure of antibiotic use, by mutations and by the transfer of genes between bacteria. Bacteria are often multiply resistant, carrying a set of genes providing resistance to a range of antibiotics. Infections caused by multiply resistant bacteria are increasingly difficult to treat, often requiring antibiotics with significant side effects.

4.4.1 Priority hospital and community resistance problems

Extended spectrum beta lactamases (ESBLs) are enzymes produced by bacteria that inactivate penicillin and cephalosporin antibiotics, and are often linked to other resistant genes such as resistance to quinolones (e.g. ciprofloxacin). They occur in bacteria such as *E.coli* and *Klebsiella* and the bacteria are often just called ESBLs. ESBLs are widely distributed in hospital patients. In the community they are a particular problem (in urinary tract and venous ulcer infections) as they may result in no oral antibiotics being suitable.

Carbapenemases are similar to ESBLs, with added resistance to meropenem, a carbapenem antibiotic which was one of the only antibiotics to treat highly resistant ESBLs. Carbepenemases occur mostly in Enterobacteria such as *E.coli and Klebsiella*. There are many types of carbapenemase genes: important ones include NDM-1, VIM, KPC, and OXA-48. In dealing with a hospital outbreak, this detailed information may be necessary to identify links between cases (Dortet et al. 2014). Medical tourism has been an important factor in introducing carbapenemase-producing bacteria into European hospitals. CPEs are an emerging resistance problem that demonstrates the complexity that results from patients having multiple admissions to hospitals and nursing/residential homes. Estimated mortality from infections caused by CPE's is up to 50 per cent (Ben-David et al. 2012).

MRSA remains important in hospitals and increasingly in the community. Multiple antibiotic resistance in gonorrhoea and tuberculosis will continue to be important public health problems.

4.4.2 Action areas for combating antimicrobial resistance (AMR)

This requires initiatives building on the foundation of proven health strategies identified in the UK Chief Medical Office Annual Report (Department of Health 2011), and UK 5 Years AMR Strategy (Department of Health 2013). These include:

- optimizing infection prevention and control in human and animal health,
- improving antibiotic prescribing,
- education, training and public engagement,
- developing new tests and treatments,
- building on the use of surveillance,
- identifying and prioritizing resistance research,
- collaboration at all levels from local to international,
- preserving the efficacy of existing antimicrobials (e.g. antibiotic stewardship programmes, stricter infection prevention and control), and
- addressing risks from imported infections, and developing alert systems to trigger screening and appropriate containment measures to minimize the risk of spread of AMR.

4.5 Microbial pathogens and human disease

Understanding the classification of pathogens and their laboratory diagnosis is an essential component in the investigation and control of communicable diseases and infections. The public health practitioner may be concerned with an individual case, particularly if it is of high severity, but is mainly concerned with infections, or the potential of infection, in groups of people, whether in the community or hospital.

The UK Advisory Committee on Dangerous Pathogens (ACDP) groups pathogens into four categories, related to their pathogenicity to humans, and the laboratory level of safety required for safe specimen handling. Category 1 is non-pathogenic for humans. Category 2 includes the majority of organisms responsible for infection in the UK. Category 3 includes infections that are more severe, examples being typhoid fever, tuberculosis, and hepatitis B and C. Category 4 covers those virus diseases of high virulence for which there are currently no vaccines or proven treatments, the main examples being Ebola and Marburg virus.

4.6 Conclusions

Microbial diseases and their diagnosis are continually evolving, and it is essential to keep up to date with new infections, with developing antimicrobial resistance, and with future laboratory strategies. The overview provided in this chapter should provide non-specialists with sufficient background to use the more specific chapters in the investigation and management of infection-related health protection issues.

References

Baron EJ, JM Miller, MP Weinstein, et al. 2013. Executive summary: a guide to utilization of the microbiology laboratory for diagnosis of infectious diseases: 2013 recommendations by the Infectious

Diseases Society of America (IDSA) and the American Society for Microbiology (ASM). *Clinical Infectious Diseases*, **57**: 485–488.

Ben-David D, R Kordevani, N Keller, et al. 2012. Outcome of carbapenem resistant Klebsiella pneumoniae bloodstream infections. *Clinical Microbiology and Infection*, **18**(1): 54–60.

Department of Health. 2011. *Annual Report of the Chief Medical Officer. Vol. 2: Infections and the Rise of Antimicrobial Resistance.* https://www.gov.uk/government/publications/chief-medical-officer-annual-report-volume-2 (accessed 8 March 2016).

Department of Health. 2013. *UK Five Year Antimicrobial Resistance Strategy (2013 to 2018).* https://www.gov.uk/government/uploads/system/uploads/attachment_data/file/244058/20130902_UK_5_year_AMR_strategy.pdf (accessed 8 March 2016).

Dortet L, L Poirel, P Nordmann. 2014. Worldwide dissemination of the NDM-type carbapenemases in Gram-negative bacteria. *BioMed Research International*, 249856. doi: 10.1155/2014/249856

Heymann, DL. 2014. *Control of Communicable Diseases Manual.* 20th edition. Washington, DC: American Public Health Association.

Sabat AJ, A Budimir, D Nashev, et al. 2013. Overview of molecular typing methods for outbreak detection and epidemiological surveillance. *Eurosurveillance*, **18**(4): pii = 20380. http://www.eurosurveillance.org/ViewArticle.aspx?ArticleId=20380 (Accessed 8 March 2016).

World Health Organization. 2014. *Antimicrobial Resistance: Global Report on Surveillance 2014.* http://www.who.int/drugresistance/documents/surveillancereport/en/ (accessed 8 March 2016).

Further reading

Kudesia G and T Wreghitt. 2009.*Clinical and Diagnostic Virology.* Cambridge University Press.

Spicer WJ. 2008. *Clinical Microbiology and Infectious Diseases: An Illustrated Colour Text.* 2nd edition. Churchill Livingstone.

Section 2

Infectious disease control case studies and scenarios

Chapter 5

Vero cytotoxigenic *Escherichia coli* (VTEC) O157

Ken Lamden, Sam Rowell, and Andrew Fox

OVERVIEW

After reading this chapter the reader will be familiar with:

• dealing with single cases of VTEC;
• responding to outbreaks of VTEC; and
• dealing with cases of VTEC in an educational institution (nursery) and in food premises.

Terms

Index case The first case in an outbreak.
Vero cytotoxin (also known as shiga-like toxins) A toxin that damages red blood cells.
Contact A person with significant risk of direct or indirect exposure to the excreta of an infectious or asymptomatic case.
Exclusion period 48 hours after the last normal stool. This extends to include microbiological clearance for high-risk contacts.
Microbiological clearance The individual is no longer carrying the organism. In the case of *E.coli* O157, this is two negative faecal specimens 24 hours apart.
Health and safety prohibition notice A legal notice, using health and safety legislation, to prohibit any activity which poses a risk of serious injury.
(See further list of terms in the Glossary.)

5.1 Background facts of *E.coli* O157

◆ *E.coli* O157 is unlike the majority of *E.coli*, which are non-pathogenic for humans, and a relatively rare bacterial cause of infectious gastroenteritis. Its public health importance relates to its severity (in particular in children) and its propensity to cause outbreaks.

◆ Post-recovery, young children can excrete *E.coli* O157 for several months.

◆ The bacteria produces vero toxins (VTs) that target endothelial cells, hence the name vero cytotoxigenic *E.coli* O157. Less commonly, other *E.coli* serogroups also produce vero cytotoxin (O26, O111, O103).

◆ *E.coli* O157 infection ranges from mild diarrhoea to bleeding from the bowel (haemorrhagic colitis) and/or acute kidney failure (haemolytic uraemic syndrome, HUS).

◆ The average incubation period for *E.coli* O157 is three to four days but can be as long as 14 days (Health Protection Agency 2011a).

◆ In the UK, infectious bloody diarrhoea, food poisoning and haemolytic uraemic syndrome (HUS) are notifiable diseases (see Appendix 4), all of which may be caused by *E.coli* O157.

5.1.1 **Clinical signs and symptoms of _E.coli_ O157**

The early features are similar to other causes of infectious gastroenteritis but the presence of bloody diarrhoea should raise the possibility of _E.coli_ O157. The early features include: diarrhoea (with or without blood), abdominal pain, and reduced urine output. The most severe complication is HUS, involving haemolytic anaemia and renal failure.

Antibiotics are not generally used for _E.coli_ O157 as they may worsen the condition.

5.1.2 **Epidemiology of the infection**

- Between 2009 and 2012 there were approximately 900 cases of VTEC O157 in England annually of which 40% occurred in children under 15, mostly under 4 years. Sixty per cent of cases were sporadic (i.e. single unlinked cases) of which 9% were secondary infections (i.e. acquired from another case). Twenty percent of cases were part of an outbreak.
- Thirty-four percent of cases were hospitalized and HUS occurred in 6%—of which three-quarters were under 14 years.
- Twenty per cent of cases were acquired overseas.
- There is a marked seasonal variation with two-thirds of infections occurring between May and September, often associated with outbreaks.
- The incidence of VTEC O157 varies geographically. Within England and Wales the highest rates occured in the Yorkshire and Humber region and within the UK the highest rates are in Scotland.
- The infectious dose is very low—ingestion of as few as 50 organisms can cause illness.
- All isolates of _E.coli_ O157 are referred to the PHE _E.coli_ reference unit for further characterization including phagetyping. The most common phagetypes in the United Kingdom are PT 21/28, 8, and 2.

5.1.3 **Risk factors for infection**

E.coli O157 lives harmlessly in the intestine of many farm animals including cattle, goats, and sheep. Infection can be transmitted to humans through contact with animals or the farm environment, through consumption of contaminated meat or other foods, unpasteurized dairy products or contaminated drinking water, or directly from person-to-person within a household or other setting.

Incidence of VTEC O157 is four times higher in rural than urban dwellers and exposure to livestock and their faeces is twice as common in rural than urban cases.

5.2 **What's the story?**

- A hospital laboratory notifies a case of presumptive _E.coli_ O157 in an 8-year-old child with a two-day history of being unwell with bloody diarrhoea and abdominal pain.
- The child has been admitted to hospital and is having intravenous fluid replacement.
- Laboratory investigation shows that kidney function is impaired.

5.2.1 **Key scenario information**

5.2.1.1 Case definition

Immediate public health action is required when a suspected or presumptive case of _E.coli_ O157 is reported.

A **suspected** case is notified on clinical suspicion of the diagnosis. A case is classed as **presumptive** based on evidence from a hospital laboratory—for example typical colony morphology on appropriate selective medium and positive *E.coli* O157 identification by serological-latex agglutination to confirm serotype as O157 and biochemical tests to confirm identity as *E.coli*.

5.2.2 **Top tips**

The following information should be provided by the person making the notification:

◆ patient and GP details,

◆ admission details (place, time, consultant),

◆ basic clinical details including date of onset of signs and symptoms,

◆ relevant laboratory test results if available,

◆ whether the case has travelled abroad, and

◆ any relevant risk factors for infection.

This information is important for deciding on, and undertaking, the necessary public health actions. Be prepared to prompt the person notifying the case for the information you need!

5.2.3 **Tools of the trade**

All stool specimens from patients in England with diarrhoea are tested for *E.coli* O157 along with campylobacter, salmonella, shigella, and cryptosporidium.

Hospital laboratories should refer all isolates of *E.coli* O157 to the national reference laboratory for confirmation and characterization by phagetyping and genotyping.

E.coli O157 can be diagnosed from a blood sample in cases of HUS by detection of antibodies to the O157 determinant but is usually only carried out some time after the acute phase of infection when it is no longer possible to isolate the organism.

Public health and environmental health staff work jointly to undertake a public health investigation of all cases of *E.coli* O157, to collect information on potential exposures and identify people who may be at risk of infection from the same source or from secondary transmission.

In England, a national VTEC O157 surveillance questionnaire is completed for all cases.

5.2.4 **What immediate action(s) would you take?**

◆ Undertake a rapid risk assessment from the information readily available. This should include details of activities undertaken in the seven days prior to onset of infection (average incubation period) to give clues about the source of infection.

◆ Work jointly with the environmental health department to interview the patient or relatives/carers. Complete the VTEC O157 questionnaire obtaining information on risk factors including nursery, school, occupation, and links to other possible cases in the area.

◆ The most important assessment is whether there is an ongoing risk of infection to the public.

  • **Identify close contacts of the patient as soon as possible** (see section 5.2.5 for the definition of a close contact). Provide a leaflet and hygiene information to reduce the risk of secondary spread.

  • **Ensure that close contacts in risk groups are excluded from nursery or work and asked to provide two faecal specimens.** This is to prevent infection being transmitted

Box 5.1 Close contact high-risk groups

- **Group A**: People with doubtful personal hygiene (e.g.) adults or children aged 6–7 years who cannot practise good personal hygiene as assessed by public health in conjunction with parents, teachers, or carers.

- **Group B**: Children aged 5 years old or under who attend school, preschool, nursery or other similar child care or minding groups.

- **Group C**: People whose work involves preparing or serving unwrapped foods not subjected to further heating.

- **Group D**: Clinical, social care, or nursery staff with direct contact with highly susceptible patients or persons for whom a gastrointestinal infection could have serious effects.

in high-risk environments or to vulnerable people. High risk groups are described in Box 5.1.
- **Identify other possible cases,** for example in children who attend the same nursery or in people who attended the same social function or activity.

5.2.5 What is a 'contact'?

A **contact** is any person who is believed to have had significant risk of direct or indirect exposure to the excreta of an infectious person.

People who should be classed as 'contacts' include:

- those who live in the same household as the case or who have visited frequently,

- a person who has regularly eaten food prepared by the index case during the infectious period, and

- any person who has been involved in nappy changing or assistance with toileting of the index case during the infectious period.

High risk contacts, groups A to D are described in Box 5.1.

5.3 Scenario update # 1

- The environmental health officer reports that the child visited a petting farm with his family two days before becoming ill. He fed the lambs and petted goats.

- The environmental health officer has visited the farm and identified problems with infection control practice. The risk of cross-infection from animals and the farm environment to visitors is unacceptable because of uncontrolled animal contact in the lamb feeding area and the goat pens. Handwashing facilities are some distance from the animal contact areas.

- A neighbouring environmental health department reports that five days ago a case of *E.coli* O157 was notified and had visited the same farm.

5.3.1 What further action(s) would you take?

- Call an outbreak control team meeting—this will enable the key partners (health protection, environmental health, health and safety, laboratory, and communications) to decide on the investigation required and institute appropriate control measures.

◆ Inform the Animal and Plant Health Agency (APHA) who may wish to join the outbreak control team.

◆ Agree with the proprietor a series of actions required to reduce cross-infection risk and improve handwashing facilities. Failure to implement these could result in legal action.

◆ The OCT should consider urgent control measures which may include the use of an immediate health and safety prohibition notice—prohibiting the farm from allowing contact between animals and visitors. These notices can only be served by the local authority or the Health and Safety Executive.

◆ Issue an alert to inform hospitals, general practitioners (GPs), and environmental health departments of an increased risk of cases in the next few days from people who have visited the farm.

◆ A holding press statement should be prepared for use as required.

5.4 **Scenario update # 2**

◆ Five more cases of presumptive *E.coli* O157 who have visited the farm are notified over the next three days. One of them, a 2-year-old girl, attends a nursery where a number of children and staff have been unwell with diarrhoea.

◆ A waiter at the farm café becomes unwell and is diagnosed with *E.coli* O157.

◆ The index case has developed kidney failure and is transferred to the specialist renal dialysis unit but dies three days later.

5.4.1 **Key scenario information**

◆ Practical guidance on managing the risk of infection from animals at visitor attractions has been produced by the industry (FACE 2012).

◆ Local authorities have enforcement options under the Health and Safety at Work Act 1974 (and regulations made thereunder) or Part 2A of the Public Health (Control of Disease) Act 1984.

◆ Guidance is available for general practitioners on the management of bloody diarrhoea in children (Health Protection Agency 2011b).

5.4.2 **What further information do you need?**

◆ What activities did the five cases undertake at the farm? Have they been exposed to any other risk factors in the seven days before onset—it should not be assumed that the farm is the source for all the cases.

◆ What is the situation in the nursery? Is the outbreak there consistent with possible transmission of *E.coli* O157, or is it more likely to be due to another organism, for example norovirus?

◆ How significant is the waiter's infection? Could there be a foodborne explanation for the outbreak? It should not be assumed that animal contact was the source for the outbreak.

◆ What further investigation is needed to identify the source of infection and likely transmission route(s)?

◆ When can the child return to nursery and the waiter return to work?

5.4.3 **Tools of the trade**

5.4.3.1 Outbreak investigation

Formulate a case definition—for example:

Possible case—a person who attended the farm and has diarrhoea.

Probable case—a person with presumptive *E.coli* O157 who attended the farm; or who attended the farm and has bloody diarrhoea; or has bloody diarrhoea and an epidemiological link to a confirmed case.

Confirmed case—a person with *E.coli* O157 of the outbreak strain confirmed by the reference laboratory, who attended the farm.

5.4.3.2 Epidemiological investigation

Describe the cases in terms of:

- place (where do they live, have they visited other places within the country or overseas in the incubation period),
- person (basic information about the individual (age, sex, etc.), signs and symptoms, history of activity at the farm and any other potential exposure(s) during the incubation period), and
- time (date of onset, date of farm visit, and timeline of illness).

5.4.3.3 Microbiological investigation

Ensure all the relevant specimens (faeces or serum in HUS cases) are obtained and referred for characterization to the reference laboratory to establish or rule out a link between cases.

5.4.3.4 Environmental investigation

This includes the physical layout of the farm, the location and number of handwashing facilities, potential cross-contamination activities (e.g. feeding or other contact with animals or an environment contaminated by animal faeces), the route around the farm and how visitors are managed, the cleanliness of play areas (a particular risk for young children), the effectiveness of signage, supervision, and verbal advice given to parents and carers/teachers with toddlers and young children. As part of the investigation, environmental samples may be taken (e.g. swabs from toilet areas, fencing, play equipment, and food preparation areas).

5.4.3.5 Veterinary investigation

In England support may be available from the Animal and Plant Health Agency. Faecal specimens from within the animal pens and public areas will provide important evidence of an animal source if they are positive for the outbreak strain of *E.coli* O157. The veterinary investigation may also identify any animal health and welfare issues.

5.4.3.6 Microbiological clearance of cases and contacts

Secondary spread of *E.coli* O157 from cases to their contacts is common, so handwashing and personal hygiene advice must be provided. Cases require an **exclusion period** from work or school of 48 hours after the first normal stool. In addition, cases in **high-risk groups** should be excluded until they have provided two negative faecal specimens taken at intervals of not less than 24 hours.

Contacts with symptoms should submit a faecal specimen and all contacts in **high-risk groups**, with or without symptoms, should be excluded until they have provided two negative faecal specimens taken at intervals of not less than 24 hours.

5.5 **Scenario update # 3**

- Of the five new presumptive cases, two stroked the lambs and two fed the goats; the other case did not visit the farm but was the brother of the index case. None of the cases had consumed food at the farm café.

- The outbreak of diarrhoea illness in the nursery has subsided. Faecal specimens from four children and one nursery nurse were positive for norovirus.

- The waiter revealed that he also worked on the farm removing straw from the animal pens and feeding the goats and lambs. The waiter was excluded from work until he had provided two negative faecal specimens 24 hours apart.

- Faecal specimens from the 2-year-old child remained positive for *E.coli* O157 for two weeks. The child was excluded until there were two negative faecal specimens 24 hours apart.

- The reference laboratory reports that following detailed strain characterization (increasingly this is by whole genome sequencing (WGS)), all the human isolates are the same strain of *E.coli* O157—known as the outbreak strain.

- Two environmental samples from the shoe rack at the children's play area were positive for the outbreak strain.

- The outbreak strain was isolated from 6/10 animal faecal samples from the lamb pens and 4/8 faecal samples from the goat pens.

5.5.1 **What further action(s) would you take?**

- The combined epidemiological, environmental, microbiological, and veterinary investigation indicates the outbreak was caused by cross-infection from the lambs and goats to human cases—there is no plausible alternative explanation. The proprietor is happy to work with the environmental health department to institute a plan of work to reduce cross-infection risk to the public.

- The outbreak control team should advise when animal contact can recommence at the farm. The risk assessment must focus on the animal contact areas. The greater the degree of animal contact the more difficult it can be to control the risk. Improvement notices served under health and safety legislation can be used to gain compliance with the standards set out in the industry code of practice. At that stage animal contact could be permitted again.

5.5.2 **Key scenario information**

E.coli O157 has been detected in one or more species of animal in 61% of visitor farms investigated following a human case (Pritchard et al, 2009).

It is important to regard all ruminants as potentially infected since there are no clinical signs of infection in animals. Shedding of *E.coli* O157 by animals is intermittent. Some cattle act as 'super shedders' and pose a higher risk of infection as they can shed significantly more organisms over longer periods of time.

Despite the high prevalence of VTEC O157, the risk of acquiring the infection on open farms and other animal premises is very small in relation to the large numbers of visitors (estimated 10 million) each year. Visits to petting farms provide education and enjoyment to vast numbers of children every year.

Between 1994 and 2008, 23 outbreaks of *E.coli* O157 were associated with petting farms (Gov. UK 2010). Petting farms have also been associated with outbreaks of cryptosporidiosis. It is impossible to prevent cross-infection to farm visitors but risk can be minimized by adherence to industry best practice.

5.5.3 **Top tips**

Remember that there is a need to act quickly and prioritize the most important public health actions. Preventing contact between animals and humans needs to be considered immediately pending the findings of a more detailed investigation.

5.6 **Scenario update # 4**

- There have been no further cases for two weeks and the outbreak is declared over.
- Several schools have cancelled their visits to the farm and others have contacted public health for advice. Worried parents have also contacted public health.

5.6.1 **How would you respond to the schools and parents?**

- Communicate with the schools directly. Speak to the head teacher or school health and safety officer. Speak to the parents directly as well.
- Stress that the farm is now compliant with health and safety standards and that there is no reason to restrict access for members of the public.
- Highlight the educational and enjoyment value of the farm visit for children.
- Explain that no visit to a farm can be risk free but given the large numbers of people visiting farms every year serious infection is rare. Compliance with instructions at the farm and supervised handwashing will help to reduce the risk to a minimum.
- Provide information via email, leaflet, or web link.

5.6.2 **Top tips**

Before speaking to schools or parents liaise with the environmental health department and other partners to ensure a consistent message.

5.7 **What if ... ?**

5.7.1 **There was a second case of *E.coli* O157 in the nursery?**

- This is a worrying development. An outbreak investigation is required to identify the transmission route and any lapses in infection control, and to advise on control measures.
- Consideration should be given to excluding all children and staff from the nursery and requiring microbiological clearance before returning. The nursery would require a thorough (deep) clean.
- Characterization of the isolate by the reference laboratory is required to determine if it is a sporadic case or a secondary case linked to the farm outbreak.

5.7.2 **Three of the cases had eaten food at the café?**

- This opens the possibility that the outbreak is foodborne.
- The outbreak investigation should be widened to include menus, food hygiene practice, food supply chain, sampling of food handlers, and targeted food sampling.

◆ The small number of cases makes it difficult to do an analytical epidemiological study (case-control study) so it might not be possible to determine epidemiologically whether food or animal contact or both were the source of the outbreak.

◆ Control measures should focus on food hygiene practice in addition to the control measures implemented on the farm.

5.7.3 The proprietor did not undertake remedial work as required by the environmental health department?

◆ The local authority may consider taking legal action. This can be a difficult situation to resolve as legal action is likely to be drawn out and costly and despite strong evidence the prosecution can fail.

◆ Ultimately it is for the proprietor to demonstrate that they have conducted a suitable and sufficient risk assessment and that risk has been controlled or reduced to a satisfactory level. The environmental health department can intervene if either the risk assessment or the controls are inadequate.

◆ Legal powers are available under the Health and Safety at Work Act 1974 (and regulations made thereunder) or Part 2A of the Public Health (Control of Disease) Act 1984. However despite these legal controls some uncooperative operators may still chose to ignore the legal requirements and their statutory obligations.

5.8 Lessons learned

◆ A single case of *E.coli* O157 linked to a farm visit is a 'red flag' for a possible outbreak.

◆ Coordinated and prompt action is essential; this may include a visit to the premises for risk assessment.

◆ Do not automatically exclude other sources of infection when investigating cases linked to animal contact at a visitor farm.

5.9 Further thinking

◆ How can we reduce or prevent future farm-related outbreaks of *E.coli* O157?

◆ How can we best utilize genotyping technology for surveillance to identify outbreaks at an early stage?

◆ Molecular techniques are increasingly identifying the presence of the VT genes in non-O157 strains of *E.coli*. Are these causing disease? What public health action is indicated?

◆ How can we ensure that industry best practice is followed by all visitor farms both large and small?

◆ How long is it justifiable to exclude children aged 6 or 7 years from school as this may deprive them of important educational and social activities?

◆ How can evidence-based public health risk assessment be strengthened?

References

FACE (**Farm and Countryside Education**). 2012. *Preventing or controlling ill health from animal contact at visitor attractions*. http://www.face-online.org.uk/resources/preventing-or-controlling-ill-health-from-animal-contact-at-visitor-attractions-industry-code-of-practice (accessed 8 March 2016).

Health Protection Agency (2011a). *The VTEC support document: background evidence for the public health management of infection with Verotoxigenic Escherichia coli (VTEC)*. https://www.gov.uk/government/uploads/system/uploads/attachment_data/file/323397/VTEC_Support.pdf (accessed 8 March 2016).

Health Protection Agency (2011b). *The management of acute bloody diarrhoea potentially caused by vero cytotoxin producing Escherichia coli in children*. https://www.gov.uk/government/publications/acute-bloody-diarrhoea-potentially-caused-by-vero-cytotoxin-producing-escherichia-coli-managing-cases-in-children (accessed 8 March 2016).

Gov.UK. 2010. *Independent Investigation Committee 2010. Review of the major outbreak of E. coli O157 in Surrey, 2009*. https://www.gov.uk/government/uploads/system/uploads/attachment_data/file/342361/Review_of_major_outbreak_of_e_coli_o157_in_surrey_2009.pdf (accessed 8 March 2016).

Pritchard GC, R Smith, J Ellis-Iversen, T Cheasty, GA Willshaw G.A. 2009. Verocytotoxigenic *Escherichia coli* O157 in animals on public amenity premises in England and Wales, 1997 to 2007. *Veterinary Record,* 164 (18): 545–549.

Further reading

Health Protection Agency 2011. *VTEC Operational Manual*. https://www.gov.uk/government/uploads/system/uploads/attachment_data/file/323416/VTEC_operational_manual.pdf (accessed 18 December 2015).

Pennington, TH. 2009. *Report of the Public Inquiry into the September 2005 Outbreak of E.coli O157 in South Wales*. http://www.ecoliinquirywales.org (accessed 8 June 2016).

Pennington, TH. 2014. *E. coli* O157 outbreaks in the United Kingdom: past, present, and future. *Infection and Drug Resistance,* 19(7): 211–22.

Public Health England. 2013a. *Epidemiology of VTEC in England and Wales*. https://www.gov.uk/government/publications/escherichia-coli-e-coli-o157-annual-totals/escherichia-coli-e-coli-o157-annual-totals-in-england-and-wales (accessed 8 March 2016).

Public Health England. 2013b. *Verocytotoxin-producing Escherichia coli Enhanced surveillance questionnaire*. https://www.gov.uk/government/publications/vero-cytotoxin-producing-escherichia-coli-questionnaire (accessed 8 March 2016).

Public Health England. 2014. *Avoiding infection on farm visits: Advice for the public*. https://www.gov.uk/government/publications/farm-visits-avoiding-infection (accessed 8 March 2016).

Chapter 6

Hepatitis B

Rita Huyton, Sam Ghebrehewet, and David Baxter

OVERVIEW

....

After reading this chapter the reader will be familiar with the:

• the epidemiology and signs and symptoms of hepatitis B,
• the difference between acute and chronic hepatitis B,
• the public health response to single cases of acute and chronic infection, and
• the public health response to a potential cluster of hepatitis B.

Terms

Prophylaxis Protection from infection.
Post-exposure prophylaxis Protection from infection after exposure.
Asymptomatic The absence of signs of infection.
Carrier A person who is carrying an infectious organism but is well (asymptomatic). Carriers are able to infect others.
Inoculation injury An injury that exposes an individual to the blood or body fluids of another individual via a break in the skin such as a needle stick, bite, or scratch. The term includes mucocutaneous exposure, i.e. splashes to the eyes, mucosa, or non-intact skin.
(See further list of terms in the Glossary.)

6.1 Background facts of Hepatitis B

◆ Hepatitis refers to a disease of the liver, i.e. inflammation of the liver.

◆ Hepatitis is often caused by a viral infection (e.g. hepatitis A virus, hepatitis B virus, hepatitis C virus or hepatitis E virus).

◆ There are two distinct outcomes of hepatitis B infection. The acute phase, which occurs in the first six months. If the case does not develop immunity during this time, the virus will persist; this is referred to as chronic hepatitis B.

◆ The average incubation period for hepatitis B infection is 12 weeks (6–24 weeks).

◆ In the UK, acute infectious hepatitis is notifiable by the registered medical practitioner. Diagnostic laboratories are also required to report acute and chronic infection with hepatitis A, B, C, D (delta), and E (see Appendices 4 and 5) .

6.1.1 Clinical signs and symptoms of hepatitis infection

6.1.1.1 Acute phase

Early symptoms (known as prodromal) These may be very mild and similar to a flu-like illness. Some people also develop a transient rash and aching joints (arthropathy).

Typical symptoms Typical symptoms of acute infection present usually after 12 weeks. They may include:

- nausea, vomiting, diarrhoea, abdominal pain, fever,
- jaundice—yellowing of the skin, mucous membranes and whites of the eyes; sometimes accompanied by dark urine and pale stools, and
- abnormal liver enzymes—detected by a blood test.

Severe symptoms

- Less than 1% of people with acute hepatitis B will develop a severe life-threatening form of hepatitis called fulminant hepatitis.

The severity of symptoms varies. Those who experience no symptoms are described as asymptomatic. Children and immunosuppressed adults are most likely to be asymptomatic (CDC 2008; WHO 2002; Colliers et al. 2011).

The likelihood of progressing to chronic infection is inversely related to age: see Table 6.1.

Chronic phase Late features may include:

- liver cirrhosis (scarring of the liver), approximately 20%,
- hepatocellular carcinoma (liver cancer), approximately 5%, and
- end-stage liver disease in 15–40% of cases.

These symptoms develop slowly, typically over a 30–50 year period. Those who acquired their infection in childhood have the worst outcomes as do those co-infected with another virus such as the hepatitis C virus or superinfected with the hepatitis D virus.

The majority of people with chronic hepatitis are asymptomatic but able to infect others. They are referred to as chronic carriers and can remain infectious indefinitely (source: WHO 2002).

6.1.2 **Epidemiology of the infection**

The World Health Organization estimates that more than one-third of the world's population has been infected with the hepatitis B virus and approximately 5% of the global population are chronic carriers. The virus is thought to cause more than one million deaths a year (WHO 2002).

Regions of high endemicity include: all of Africa, some parts of South America, Alaska, northern Canada, parts of Greenland, Eastern Europe, the eastern Mediterranean area, South-East

Table 6.1 Features of hepatitis B virus (HBV) infection

Who develops clinical illness (jaundice)	Age <5 yrs: <10% Age ≥5 yrs: 30–50%
Who develops chronic infection	Age <1yr: >90% Age 1–5 yrs: 25–50% Children >5 yrs and adults: <5%
Case fatality with acute infection	0.5–1%
Premature mortality from chronic liver disease	15–25%

Source: data from World Health Organisation. Global Alert and Response (GAR): Hepatitis B (Geneva, Switzerland: WHO, 2001), Copyright © 2001 World Health Organization, http://www.who.int/csr/disease/hepatitis/whocdscsrncs20011/en/, accessed 03 Feb. 2015; Centers for Diseases Control and Prevention (CDC). Recommendations for Identification and Public Health Management of Persons with Chronic Hepatitis B Virus Infection. Morbidity and Mortality Weekly Report (MMWR), Volume 57(RR08), pp. 1–20, Copyright © 2008 CDC, http://www.cdc.gov/mmwrhtml/preview/mmwrhtml/rr5708a1.htm

Asia, China, and some Pacific Islands. In most of these areas, 5–15% of the population are chronic carriers.

The UK is a low prevalence country (<2% of the population are carriers). In England, London has the highest incidence of acute cases: 1.2 cases per 100,000 population (Public Health England 2014).

Hepatitis B is a vaccine-preventable infection. In the UK there is a targeted vaccination programme aimed at those in risk groups (Public Health England 2013). Examples of risk groups are:

- healthcare workers,
- foster parents,
- custodial inmates,
- sex workers,
- laboratory staff,
- individuals with chronic renal failure, and
- individuals with learning disabilities living in institutional settings.

6.1.3 **Risk factors for transmission of infection**

Humans are the only reservoir. Infectious individuals carry the virus in their blood. The virus is transmitted by exposure to blood. Some body fluids are also infectious, especially semen and vaginal secretions. Hepatitis B is highly infectious, particularly where there are high levels of virus in the blood, as evidenced for example by the detectable Hepatitis B e antigen in blood. Hepatitis B is estimated to be 100 times more infectious than HIV. It can be transmitted by various bloodborne routes.

- High risk factors for acquiring infection include:
  - blood (and serum-derived fluids)—via transfusion, blood products, inoculation injuries, needle-sharing, acupuncture, tattooing, haemodialysis, surgical/dental procedures,
  - sexual—between sexual partners, semen and vaginal fluids are infective, and
  - perinatal transmission is common in hyperendemic areas (South-East Asia, Western Pacific region, sub-Saharan Africa).
- Other risk factors include:
  - horizontal transmission within households—mainly through sharing of personal hygiene products such as razors, tweezers, nail clippers, and toothbrushes. (Source: WHO 2002; Colliers 2011).

6.2 **What's the story?**

- A junior doctor from a local general hospital has notified a case of acute hepatitis B. The case is a 34-year-old male with a history of tiredness for two weeks followed by jaundice, which began one week ago. The patient's condition is now improving.
- Blood samples indicate abnormal liver enzymes and markers of hepatitis B infection.
- After reviewing this case's history and laboratory results, you will need to decide whether the findings are consistent with acute hepatitis B infection.

6.2.1 **Key scenario information**

When a person has hepatitis B, markers of the infection will be detected in that person's blood. Markers consist of antigens (Ag) and antibodies (anti-) (Table 6.2 and Table 6.3).

Table 6.2 Hepatitis B virus markers

Type of marker[1]	Name	Abbreviation	Phase present in		Comment
			Acute	Chronic	
Antigen	Hepatitis B surface antigen	HBsAg	√	√	
Antigen	Hepatitis Be antigen	HBeAg	√	√	indicates v ral replication and high infectivity
Antibody IgG	Hepatitis B surface antibody	anti-HBs	n/a	n/a	indicates immunity either from past infection or vaccination
Antibody IgG	Hepatitis B e antibody (anti-HBe)	anti-HBe	√	√	indicates low infectivity and possible convalescence
Antibody IgM	Hepatitis B core antibody	anti-HBc IgM	√	√ low levels	indicates acute infection low levels can also indicate an exacerbation of chronic infection.
Antibody IgM and IgG (total/combined)	Hepatitis B core antibody	anti-HBc total/ combined	√	√	can also be detected in those that have cleared the infection and have immunity

Source: data from World Health Organisation. Global Alert and Response (GAR): Hepatitis B (Geneva, Switzerland: WHO, 2001), Copyright © 2001 World Health Organization, http://www.who.int/csr/disease/hepatitis/whocdscsrncs2001 1/en/, accessed 03 Feb. 2015.

[1]The markers are complex to interpret and must be considered in relation to each other. At the point of notification sometimes only the HBsAg result is available.

Markers should be interpreted in conjunction with: the clinical presentation for this illness, past medical history, past blood tests, country of origin, travel history and other risk factors.

Seek further guidance from the Health Protection Consultant or Consultant Virologist in the laboratory before deciding if this case is truly a case of acute or chronic infection.

6.2.2 **Top tips**

The following information should be provided by the person making the notification:

◆ patient's demographic details, patient's occupation,

◆ GP details; country of origin/travel history,

◆ admission details (place, time, consultant); basic clinical details including onset date of signs and symptoms,

◆ relevant laboratory test results—past and current,

◆ past medical history; any known risk factors,

◆ if the patient going to be sent home, and

◆ contact details for the patient; and information on sexual/household contacts if possible.

This information is important for deciding on, and undertaking, the necessary public health actions. Be prepared to prompt the person making the notification for the information you need!

Table 6.3 Interpretation of hepatitis B virus markers

Interpretation of the hepatitis B panel

Tests	Results	Interpretation
HBsAg	negative	susceptible
anti-HBc	negative	
anti-HBs	negative	
HBsAg	negative	immune due to natural infection
anti-HBc	positive	
anti-HBs	positive	
HBsAg	negative	immune due to hepatitis B vaccination
anti-HBc	negative	
anti-HBs	positive	
HBsAg	positive	acutely infected
anti-HBc	positive	
IgM anti-HBc	positive	
anti-HBc	negative	
HBsAg	positive	chronically infected
anti-HBc	positive	
IgM anti-HBc	negative	
anti-HBs	negative	
HBsAg	negative	four interpretations possible*
anti-HBc	positive	
anti-HBs	negative	

* (1) May be recovering from acute hepatitis B infection. (2) May be susceptible with a false-positive anti-hepatitis antibody. (3) May be an undetectable level of HBsAg present in the serum and the person is actually a carrier. (4) May be immune and test is not sensitive enough to detect low level of anti-hepatitis B surface antigen in serum.

Adapted from Centers for Diseases Control and Prevention (CDC). A Comprehensive Immunization Strategy to Eliminate Transmission of Hepatitis B Virus Infection in the United States: Recommendations of the Advisory Committee on Immunization Practices (ACIP) Part II: Immunization of Adults. Morbidity and Mortality Weekly Report (MMWR), Volume 55(RR16), pp. 1–25, Copyright © 2006 CDC, http://www.cdc.gov/mmwr/preview/mmwrhtml/rr5516a1.htm

Often when a notification of hepatitis B is made the patient is not in hospital. The person making the notification may not be able to provide the required information. In these situations local procedures must be followed for contacting the patient.

Note: Ensure the responsible clinician has informed the patient of their diagnosis before contact is initiated.

6.2.3 **What immediate action(s) would you take?**

◆ The immediate priorities are to:
  • protect those already exposed, and
  • prevent further spread.

6.2.3.1 Protect those already exposed

The first priority is to protect those already exposed. These will include contacts in the last six months such as sexual partners and household contacts.

6.2.3.2 Prevent further spread

The second priority is to prevent further transmission. Once the case has been informed of their diagnosis an important public health measure is to give advice on preventing transmission. This includes: safer sex and not sharing personal toiletries that may pierce the skin/mucosa such as razors, toothbrushes, nail clippers or scissors. Also consider:

- Is the case a healthcare worker?
- Is the case an injecting drug user?
- Does the case participate in contact sports?
- Are there any other specific risk factors?

Advice on prevention specific to each situation may be required. Initial advice can be given verbally by the health protection practitioner or the doctor/nurse looking after the patient.

6.2.4 **Key scenario information**

People who should be classed as high-priority contacts include:

- sexual partners in the last seven days (unprotected sex),
- anyone who has had direct blood to blood exposure or an inoculation injury with the case in the last seven days—consider contact sports, injuries, assault, and
- anyone who has shared injecting equipment with the case in the last seven days.

Medium priority contacts include:

- as above but exposure occurred over a week ago.

Low priority contacts are:

- household contacts in the last six months.

Those who are not at risk include:

- social contacts,
- work colleagues, and
- classmates.

6.2.4.1 Required actions

High-priority contacts Arrange for the contact to receive hepatitis B immunoglobulin (HBIG). This is most effective within 48hrs of exposure but can be given up to seven days afterwards. In the UK, designated NHS laboratories hold stocks of HBIG. HBIG can be requested by health protection practitioners both in and out of office hours.

At the same time as receiving the HBIG, the first dose of an accelerated schedule of hepatitis B vaccine should be given. The vaccine and HBIG should be administered at different body sites. The vaccine is most effective if given within 48hrs of exposure; if outside the 48hrs, the vaccine should still be given.

GP practices and hospital A&E departments can administer the HBIG and vaccine. Ensure arrangements are made for the contact to receive the rest of the accelerated course of vaccine from their GP.

Medium-priority contacts Arrange for the contacts to receive an accelerated course of hepatitis B vaccine (0, 1, and 2 months schedule). Ideally the first dose should be given within 48hrs but can be given at any time.

Low-priority contacts Arrange for the contacts to receive an accelerated course of hepatitis B vaccine.

All contacts All contacts should have a blood test to check if they have or have had hepatitis B infection. The blood test can be taken at the same time as vaccination/HBIG is given. This blood sample should be stored for two years in case further comparative testing is required.

♦ Giving of prophylaxis should not be delayed by waiting for the blood test result.

♦ Contacts should be offered further blood tests at three and six months because hepatitis B has a long incubation period.

♦ Those receiving the accelerated course of vaccine will require a booster vaccine at 12 months if at ongoing risk.

6.3 Scenario update # 1

♦ The case lives with his girlfriend; she is pregnant.

♦ They have had unprotected sex in the last seven days.

♦ His girlfriend had a blood test for hepatitis B in the antenatal clinic 6 months ago: the result was negative.

6.3.1 Key scenario information

6.3.1.1 Hepatitis B prophylaxis with immunoglobulin, HBIG

HBIG is usually used in combination with hep B vaccine to confer immunity in the following groups.

1. Accidental exposure by blood or other material containing HBsAg through:
   • percutaneous inoculation (needle stick/sharps, bites, scratches),
   • contamination of mucous membranes (spillage into the eye or mouth), or
   • contamination of non-intact skin (open wounds, dermatitis, or eczema).

2. Newborns:
   • newborns of hepatitis B surface antigen positive mothers who are HBeAg positive or anti-HBe antibody negative,
   • mothers who have had acute hepatitis B during the pregnancy, and
   • newborns with a birth weight of 1500g or less, regardless of e-antigen status of the HBsAg positive mother.

3. Sexual contacts (unprotected sex):
   • of individuals with acute hepatitis B who are seen within one week of last contact should be offered HBIG and vaccine, and
   • of individuals with newly diagnosed chronic hepatitis B should be offered vaccine. HBIG may be given in addition if contact occurred in the past seven days.

Other exposed contacts require vaccine only (HPA 2008; PHE 2013).

6.3.2 What further action(s) would you take?

The case's girlfriend should be managed as a high-priority contact. Both hepatitis B vaccine and HBIG are indicated in pregnancy, in the event of a high-risk exposure.

Although his girlfriend was tested for hepatitis B six months ago, she should be tested again because she has recently had a high-risk exposure.

If she tests positive for hepatitis B, the course of vaccine will not provide any benefit and should be discontinued. The health protection team would need to ensure her GP and midwife are informed of the test result. She should be referred to the local screening and immunization team so that the baby can be given vaccination (and HBIG if required) at birth. The child will need the full accelerated course of vaccine and booster vaccination and blood test at 12 months.

If his girlfriend's test result indicates she is not currently infected or had no past infection, she should continue with the accelerated course of vaccine (0-, 1-, and 2-month schedule) and receive a booster at 12 months if at ongoing risk.

The couple should be advised to practise safer sex until the case is no longer infectious, i.e. clears the infection.

Hepatitis B has a long incubation period; the girlfriend should be offered further blood tests at three and six months after exposure.

Note: In the UK, antenatal screening for hepatitis B and HIV is offered to all pregnant women.

6.4 Scenario update # 2

- ◆ The case's teenage nephew has been living with him for the last three months.
- ◆ Two weeks ago his nephew moved back to his parents' home.
- ◆ The case thinks his nephew has used his razor but does not know when.
- ◆ He does not want his nephew to know he has hepatitis B.

6.4.1 Key scenario information

- ◆ The nephew should be managed as a low-priority contact.
- ◆ The risk to the nephew is low but not negligible.
- ◆ Offer the case support and time to think about the situation. Involve the GP or other local health professionals, i.e. community infection prevention and control nurses.
- ◆ The health protection practitioner must consider the protection of the nephew as well as the wishes of the case. Following discussion with the Health Protection Consultant it may be appropriate to write to the nephew's GP advising testing and vaccination. The case details must not be disclosed. The case should always be informed in advance that this will happen.

6.5 Scenario update # 3

- ◆ The case works as a paramedic.
- ◆ What advice would you give about him returning to work?

6.5.1 Key scenario information

The case should be advised to talk to his occupational health department before returning to work.

There are restrictions for some healthcare workers with hepatitis B who carry out exposure-prone procedures. This will depend on their level of infectivity (Department of Health 2000, 2005, 2007).

6.5.2 **Tools of the trade**

Hepatitis B vaccination, response, and boosters

◆ Antibody (anti-HBs) level following vaccination:
  - <10mIU/ml: non response
  - ≥10mIU/ml: protective

Note: No data to support need for booster doses in immunocompetent individuals who have responded to primary course with ≥10mIU/ml (European Consensus Group on Hepatitis B Immunity 2000).

◆ Hepatitis B is a vaccine-preventable disease. Hepatitis B vaccine produces response in 85–90% of people. Poor response is mostly associated with: age over 40 years; obesity; smoking; and alcoholism.

◆ Immunosuppressed individuals or those on renal dialysis may respond less well, and may require larger or more doses of vaccine.

◆ Response to vaccination can take up to six months to confer adequate protection in some individuals.

◆ Vaccination is ineffective for patients with acute or chronic hepatitis B and those with past resolved hepatitis B.

6.5.3 **What further information do you need?**

The health protection practitioner should initiate the collection of more detailed information to ensure all contacts have been identified and to ascertain a likely source for the infection. This is important to prevent further cases. Although sexual transmission is the most common source of exposure, all possible sources should be considered.

Further action is required depending on what infection sources are identified. For example: if a likely source is a tattoo parlour the local authority environmental health officers should be requested to inspect the premises. Similarly, if a likely source is identified to be healthcare premises (e.g., a local dental practice), local community infection prevention and control nurses should be informed as they may need to undertake a review of the infection prevention and control practice of the relevant dental practice.

In addition to investigating sources, the health protection practitioner should recommend that the case:

◆ is tested for other hepatitis viruses and HIV,

◆ is offered a referral to the sexual health clinic if indicated, and

◆ is referred to hepatitis services for ongoing management of his condition.

This is also an opportunity to answer any questions the case has about preventing transmission, i.e. cleaning up blood from cuts at home. It is good practice to ensure the case has access to written information to refer to.

6.6 **What if ... ?**

6.6.1 **The case had chronic hepatitis B?**

◆ With cases of chronic hepatitis B there is no defined incubation period, so it is not possible to identify a source. The collection of detailed information is of limited value and therefore, not required.

◆ The management of cases and contacts is the same as for acute hepatitis B but this should be done by the patient's own doctor without direct input from health protection practitioners. Local procedures vary but this is usually initiated by the health protection team providing written guidance to the patient's doctor/appropriate clinician or by providing information on the lab report.

◆ The written guidance should include recommendations to ensure the case receives other relevant vaccines that are recommended for at-risk individuals (e.g. hepatitis A and annual influenza vaccinations). Patients with chronic liver disease are at risk of complications from these infections.

6.6.2 The case is part of a cluster/outbreak of acute hepatitis B?

Clusters/outbreaks of acute hepatitis B are rare but have been reported in residential institutions and health and social care settings. Standard infection prevention and control precautions are sufficient to prevent the spread of the hepatitis B virus. A cluster/outbreak usually indicates a breakdown in basic infection prevention and control measures. Contaminated blood glucose monitoring equipment is one recognized source of transmission (MHRA 2006).

6.6.3 How would you respond to a cluster or an outbreak of hepatitis B in a given setting?

◆ Obtain detailed information on the cases.

◆ Confirm the standard laboratory results and request genotype and sequence data. These are specialized tests that can indicate how closely related viruses are. This can help to differentiate an outbreak from a coincidental cluster. Further action should not be delayed whilst waiting for these results.

◆ Identify potentially exposed persons and arrange for testing.

◆ Convene an outbreak control team (OCT) meeting.

◆ Amongst other interventions, the OCT may consider implementing the following actions:
  • Request the infection prevention and control team to visit the relevant premises urgently and make an initial assessment.
  • Ensure any recommendations of the infection prevention and control team are implemented without delay.
  • Consider if adequate measures are now in place to ensure the safety of patients and staff.
  • Consider the need for a more detailed infection prevention and control audit, and consider inviting external experts to contribute.
  • Provide written information for patients, relatives, and staff.
  • Prepare a media holding statement.

◆ After the initial response other issues to consider include: ensuring confidentiality of the cases is maintained; maintaining staff training; reviewing the governance arrangements within the relevant organization; considering escalation of the incident to commissioners and regulators if indicated.

6.4 The unanswered question(s) around hepatitis B infection

◆ Given that the UK is a very low-incidence country, and acute cases predominantly occur in high-risk and ethnic minority groups, what is the best strategy for preventing acute cases and reducing prevalence of hepatitis B in the UK?

- How successful is the current UK vaccination policy (antenatal screening and vaccination of infants born to positive mothers and selective vaccination of high-risk groups)?
- Would adopting universal hepatitis B vaccination (e.g. vaccination of adolescents and/or vaccination of infants) be cost effective given the low incidence of hepatitis B in the UK?

6.5 Lessons learned

- It is important to actively follow up contacts of acute hepatitis B; transmission can be prevented by the timely administration of immunoglobulin and vaccination.
- Substantial numbers of individuals with hepatitis B have no symptoms; they are not aware they are carrying the virus and can be infectious indefinitely.
- Sexual contacts and those who have a high-risk exposure (blood to blood) are most at risk of acquiring the infection.
- The UK is a low-prevalence country—however, hepatitis B rates are higher in inner city areas and in ethnic groups from countries of high prevalence. Therefore, local strategies need to reflect the local epidemiology of hepatitis B infection.

6.6 Further thinking

- How can we encourage more at-risk people to be tested for hepatitis B?
- What are the roles of different professionals and organizations in the public health management of hepatitis B infection?
- How can we ensure health promotion messages on safer sex are effective?
- Given the high turnover, what can be done to improve hepatitis B vaccination uptake in prisoners?
- What can be done to improve awareness of hepatitis B in the general population?

References

Centers for Diseases Control and Prevention (CDC). 2006. A comprehensive immunization strategy to eliminate transmission of hepatitis b virus infection in the United States: recommendations of the Advisory Committee on Immunization Practices (ACIP) Part II: Immunization of adults. *Morbidity and Mortality Weekly Report (MMWR)*, **55**(RR16): 1–25. http://www.cdc.gov/mmwr/preview/mmwrhtml/rr5516a1.htm (accessed 8 March 2016).

Centers for Diseases Control and Prevention (CDC). 2008. Recommendations for identification and public health management of persons with chronic hepatitis B virus infection. *Morbidity and Mortality Weekly Report (MMWR)*, **57**(RR08): 1–20. http://www.cdc.gov/mmwr/preview/mmwrhtml/rr5708a1.htm (accessed 8 March 2016).

Colliers L, P Kellam, J Oxford. 2011. *Human Virology*. 4th Edition. Oxford: Oxford University Press.

Department of Health. 2000. *Hepatitis B Infected Health Care Workers. Guidance on Implementation of Health Service Circular 2000/020*. http://webarchive.nationalarchives.gov.uk/20130107105354/http://www.dh.gov.uk/prod_consum_dh/groups/dh_digitalassets/@dh/@en/documents/digitalasset/dh_4057538.pdf (accessed 8 March 2016).

Department of Health. 2005. *HIV Infected Health Care Workers: Guidance on Management and Patient Notification*. http://webarchive.nationalarchives.gov.uk/20130107105354/http:/www.dh.gov.uk/prod_consum_dh/groups/dh_digitalassets/@dh/@en/documents/digitalasset/dh_4116416.pdf (accessed 8 March 2016).

Department of Health. 2007. *Hepatitis B Infected Healthcare Workers and Antiviral Therapy*. http:// webarchive.nationalarchives.gov.uk/20130107105354/http://www.dh.gov.uk/prod_consum_dh/groups/ dh_digitalassets/documents/digitalasset/dh_073133.pdf (accessed 8 March 2016).

European Consensus Group on Hepatitis B Immunity. 2000. Are booster immunisations needed for lifelong hepatitis B immunity? *Lancet*, **355**(9203): 561–65. http://www.thelancet.com/pdfs/journals/ lancet/PIIS0140-6736(99)07239-6.pdf (accessed 8 March 2016).

HPA (Health Protection Agency). 2008. *Immunoglobulin Handbook. Chapter 6 – Hepatitis B*. https:// www.gov.uk/government/uploads/system/uploads/attachment_data/file/327768/Hepatitis_B_ immunoglobulin_Oct_2008.pdf (accessed 8 March 2016).

MHRA (Medicines and Healthcare Products Regulatory Agency). 2006. *Medical Safety Alert. Lancing Devices Used in Nursing Homes and Care Homes—correction to list of disposable single-use lancing devices*. https://www.gov.uk/drug-device-alerts/medical-device-alert-lancing-devices-used-in-nursing-homes-and-care-homes-correction-to-list-of-disposable-single-use-lancing-devices (accessed 8 March 2016).

Public Health England. 2013. *Immunisation against Infectious Disease - The Green Book*. https://www. gov.uk/government/collections/immunisation-against-infectious-disease-the-green-book (accessed 8 March 2016).

Public Health England. 2014. Acute Hepatitis B (England): Annual Report for 2013. *Health Protection Weekly Report*, **18**(33). https://www.gov.uk/government/uploads/system/uploads/attachment_data/file/ 348576/hpr3314_hbv13.pdf (accessed 8 March 2016).

World Health Organization. 2002. *Emergencies preparedness, response. Disease: Hepatitis B*. http://www. who.int/csr/disease/hepatitis/whocdscsrlyo20022/en/ (accessed 8 March 2016).

Chapter 7

Hospital multi-resistant infections

David Harvey and Andrea Ledgerton

OVERVIEW

After reading this chapter the reader will be familiar with:

- an outbreak of multi-resistant bacterial infection in a neonatal unit,
- the public health response to a hospital outbreak caused by a multi-drug-resistant organism,
- the importance of linking clinical findings, the epidemiology, and laboratory results to control the outbreak, and
- the challenges in managing a hospital outbreak caused by a multi-drug-resistant organism.

Terms

Neonate (neonatal) Defined as the period within the first four weeks of birth.
Bacteraemia The presence of bacteria in the blood, detected by a positive blood culture.
Colonization Isolation of the outbreak bacteria from a non-sterile site (skin, nose, rectum, etc.).
Gram negative bacteria (Gr–ve): Bacteria giving a pink colour on Gram staining such as *E.coli*, *Klebsiella pneumoniae*, and *Pseudomonas aeruginosa*.
(See further list of terms in the Glossary.)

7.1 Background facts: hospital multi-resistant infections

◆ Neonates are at considerable risk of infection for the following reasons:

- prematurity and reduced immunity,
- use of invasive devices (e.g. arterial lines, urinary catheters), and
- vulnerability to environmental organisms.

◆ Outbreaks of infection caused by Gr–ve bacteria are not uncommon in neonatal units.

◆ Infection may arise from the neonate's own bacteria (endogenous infection) or be acquired from another source (exogenous infection). In an outbreak, the source may be a neonate, the environment, equipment, or a member of staff or visitor.

◆ Bacteria will take 24hrs to grow and a further 24hrs (sometimes longer) for identification and antimicrobial sensitivity.

◆ Bacterial typing is usually performed in a reference laboratory, and may take several weeks for the final result (see Chapter 4).

7.1.1 **Clinical features and investigation of neonatal infections**

Diagnosing infection in neonates is often difficult as signs are often non-specific (e.g. poor feeding, jaundice and absence of fever). Samples for culture should always include blood, cerebrospinal fluid (CSF), and urine. Samples should be sent from other clinical sites as indicated. General indicators of infection, such as C-reactive protein (CRP) are useful indicators.

Getting adequate samples for the laboratory may be difficult: poor venous access may pick up skin contaminants, urine samples may be contaminated with bacteria from stool. Bacteria which are often not clinically significant in older patients may be pathogenic in neonates (e.g. *Pseudomonas aeruginosa*, *Klebsiella spp.*, *Serratia spp.*). Babies of less than 32 weeks' gestation are extremely vulnerable to infection. Low birth weight of less than 1500g is also associated with high risk.

7.1.2 **Key scenario information**

- Neonatal infections may be early onset, occurring within 48hrs of birth, or late onset >48hrs after birth (Anthony et al. 2013).
- Most early onset infections are derived from the mother's bacterial vaginal flora, an important example being Group B streptococcus infection.
- Neonatal infection outbreaks are usually late onset infections because of the time required for initial colonisation by an outbreak organism.
- Late onset neonatal sepsis in the UK affects 2–3/1000 babies (Vergnano et al. 2011).
- Whilst Gram-positive bacteria (mainly coagulase negative staphylococci), account for most cases of late onset sepsis, these tend to be easier to treat and rarely cause outbreaks.
- Gr–ve bacteria cause approximately 20–40% of all late onset sepsis, with *Klebsiella spp.* responsible for most neonatal outbreaks (Depani et al. 2011).
- Approximately 15% of UK neonatal units have been investigated for a 'recent' infection prevention and control issue, and 12% per year temporarily close for this reason (Francis et al. 2012).
- The source of infection may be the environment, another neonate, contaminated water or equipment, or a staff member/visitor.
- Transmission from the reservoir may be from staff hands/gloves, a shared piece of equipment, etc.
- Contaminated breast milk and the thawing of frozen breast milk has been implicated in outbreaks, especially with *Pseudomonas aeruginosa* (Sanchez-Carrillo et al. 2009; Mammina et al. 2008).

7.2 **What's the story?**

A local hospital infection control doctor (ICD) has a provisional identification of an extended-spectrum beta-lactamase (ESBL) in a blood culture on the neonatal unit. The following summary has been received from the ICD:

- Problem: ESBL Klebsiella pneumoniae (*K. pneumoniae*); testing sensitive to ciprofloxacin, gentamicin, and piperacillin-tazobactam.
- Total number affected = 14 babies: 10 on screening swabs alone; 4 in clinical sites (3 eye swabs; 1 blood culture with presumptive identification, awaiting confirmation tomorrow).

- No. of affected babies currently on unit = 7.
- Source of outbreak likely to be twins who had already been transferred to another neonatal unit and had admission screening swabs that detected ESBL *K. pneumoniae*.

7.2.1 **Key scenario information**

- Most ESBLs are resistant to co-amoxiclav, cephalosporins, ciprofloxacin, with ~80% sensitive to gentamicin. Regarding piperacillin-tazobactam, susceptibility is variable and laboratory results potentially unreliable (Smith and Benjamin 2011).
- Meropenem is the usual empiric drug of choice if infection with ESBL is suspected whilst awaiting laboratory results. Most neonatal units use gentamicin in their empiric antibiotic regimens to cover for Gr –ve sepsis.

7.2.2 **Top tips**

In the absence of typing results, the microbiologist should be able to suggest whether it is likely that cases are linked based on the species characteristics of the organism, the antibiotic susceptibility patterns (antibiogram), and the epidemiology of cases.

7.2.3 **What immediate action(s) would you take?**

- Gather information about the person, time and space epidemiology.
- Assess whether this is an outbreak.
- "A general definition of an outbreak is an observed number of cases greater than that expected for a defined place and time period, or two or more cases with a common exposure (see Chapter 20)." Ensure sample has been sent for typing and consider results if available.
- Clarify whether an incident meeting has been called and the Director of Infection Prevention and Control (DIPC) has been informed.
- Consider which baby groups (intensive care/high dependency/nursery) may require screening.
- Consider which sites (nasal, perineal) may require screening.
- Liaise with the laboratory to expedite results of the samples.
- Instigate initial discussions with relevant professionals as to whether the unit should be closed to new admissions to inform the outbreak control team (OCT).

7.2.4 **Top tips**

The infection control team will be gathering information specifically to ask about:
- the person, time and space epidemiology:
  - Which babies are affected?
  - How long have they been in the unit?
  - When was the ESBL detected in each case?
  - Where and from which body site?
  - What is the relationship between cases and the location of cots?
  - Timeline of admission and samples.

This preliminary information is important to help to determine if this is an outbreak and what measures need to be taken (e.g. holding an OCT).

7.3 **Scenario update # 1**

The ICD identifies that the strains look sufficiently similar to call this an outbreak pending typing results. The typing will take two to three weeks. Two incident meetings have taken place already, with the DIPC chairing. In attendance were the neonatal lead consultant, neonatal lead nurse, lead infection control nurse, and the ICD. From the meetings the following actions have already been agreed:

◆ heightened hand hygiene (staff and visitors),

◆ additional environmental cleans,

◆ aprons and gloves to be used for all babies on the unit,

◆ ESBL-positive babies to be cohorted where possible,

◆ admission, weekly, and discharge screening for ESBL carriage,

◆ environmental sampling of equipment/fixtures for ESBLs,

◆ offer extra shifts to neonatal staff to increase staffing levels in accordance with network staffing guidance,

◆ adhere to visiting policy of strictly two people per space,

◆ medical staff to inform parents if their baby is ESBL positive,

◆ infection control team to provide an ESBL leaflet for parents,

◆ infection control team to provide written information for staff and drop-in sessions,

◆ review antibiotic policy and prescribing practices in order to optimize treatment and reduce selection pressure, and

◆ review use of reusable equipment and consider changing to single use.

7.3.1 **Tools of the trade**

7.3.1.1 OCT

Multi-agency OCT should be considered at this stage to support the investigation. Membership will vary depending on the incident but should include public health, local authority, and communications teams (see Chapter 20).

7.3.1.2 Screening

Many neonatal units perform admission screening for organisms which pose a risk for cross-infection. There is no set formula, however, in terms of what sites to screen or what organisms to look for.

Most units will screen for MRSA at birth. Gr–ve bacteria are also often screened for. This is to look for organisms with specific resistance profiles such as resistance to gentamicin, or specific resistance mechanisms such as ESBL or carbapenemase-producing enterobacteriaceae (CPE). Other organisms that can be screened for include *Pseudomonas* and *Candida spp*.

During outbreaks, extra screens for the organism in question should be considered. For Gr –ve bacteria this is usually admission, weekly, and discharge screens. Rectal swabs and endotracheal aspirates are the sites of choice (Anthony et al. 2013).

7.3.2 **What further action(s) would you take?**

The OCT reviews the steps and evidence with the ICD. There is evidence of:

◆ a likely source (twin babies),

◆ transmission, and

◆ invasive infection, notably bloodstream infection.

There is evidence of an appropriate response including:

◆ screening,

◆ cohorting and source isolation,

◆ enhanced cleaning, and

◆ communication strategy.

There is evidence of appropriate engagement and leadership involving the DIPC and the lead nurses and doctors from the neonatal unit with the infection control team.

The OCT discusses unit closure as a measure to protect future admissions from potential harm. Evidence so far suggests closure is not required given appropriate steps have been taken to protect the safety of current and future admission. It is important to remain vigilant in the unit and await typing results to confirm an outbreak strain.

7.4 Scenario update # 2

One week later you receive a further update:

◆ Still three ESBL positive babies on the unit, one on the high dependency unit (HDU) and two in the nursery.

◆ One new ESBL case with bacteraemia in intensive care having 1:1 nursing.

◆ Infection control nurse has contacted a neighbouring unit with regard to cleaning cot spaces with a chlorine-releasing disinfectant. The unit has concerns about using a chlorine-based product whilst the baby is in the incubator. The neonatal network is being contacted to canvas views about the impact of closure on surrounding neonatal units.

◆ The unit is continuing with heightened infection control measures.

◆ All updated information will be cascaded to staff verbally and in writing.

7.4.1 What further action(s) would you take?

There is evidence of further clinical infection and confusion over cleaning and decontamination. The aim of the next OCT should be to:

◆ assess potential source of spread in the new case,

◆ review effectiveness of measures,

◆ address further measures required,

◆ offer expert advice on areas of contention, and

◆ review whether the unit should still be open to new admissions.

Public health attendance at these OCTs is vital.

7.4.2 Tools of the trade

Within most public health networks, a range of subject experts can be contacted to address specific issues. To address issues around safe cleaning of cots, seek advice from experts in this area.

7.4.3 Key scenario information

High cot-occupancy rates, inadequate spacing between cots, and low nurse-to-baby ratios promote errors and reduce the time for good infection prevention practices. In an outbreak situation, units should review the recommended guidelines for these and ensure they are working to them.

Generally, recommendations are for 1:1 care by nurses qualified for intensive care patients, 2:1 for high dependency, and 4:1 for low dependency. Cot spacing should allow room for two parents, staff to undertake sterile procedures, and equipment such as monitors and ventilators (Anthony et al. 2013).

7.5 Scenario update # 3

◆ The OCT is satisfied that the outbreak is being taken seriously and that expected measures are being implemented. However, given the new bacteraemia the OCT discusses whether unit closure is required.

7.5.1 What further information do you need about the bacteraemia?

◆ When and where did the baby with the bacteraemia acquire the ESBL? This is important to establish whether the unit is seeing new transmission or whether this is invasive disease in a baby already colonized.

◆ Were there any additional risk factors? This will help inform whether the unit is putting babies at risk due to poor practices or whether there was an element of unavoidable progression to invasive disease.

By reviewing the timeline and location of babies, the OCT establishes that:

◆ The baby with the recent bacteraemia had most likely acquired the organism 12 days earlier from a colonised baby in an adjacent cot.

Subsequent bacteraemia was more likely in the baby due to:

◆ prior ceftriaxone for meningitis (i.e. antibiotic selection pressure),

◆ extreme prematurity (26-week gestation), and

◆ ongoing unavoidable use of intravenous devices.

In summary, the bacteraemia does not represent a new risk, and does not represent failure of the mitigating actions. Therefore unit closure based on the bacteraemia is not warranted.

7.5.2 Tools of the trade

If an outbreak continues despite implementing all reasonable measures then consider inviting an external expert panel to visit and give advice. This may be made up of national or regional leads and experts in the appropriate fields.

7.5.3 Top tips

As well as giving advice, seek evidence that the advice is being followed, such as audits of the measures.

7.6 Scenario update # 4

◆ Typing results confirm all the *K. pneumoniae* had the same variable number tandem repeat (VNTR) profile. This strongly indicates cross-transmission. No more new cases were found and, after four more weeks, all the known colonized babies have been discharged.

7.6.1 When would you consider the outbreak over?

The assessment should be based on:

◆ whether there is an ongoing risk,

◆ whether the number of cases has declined, and

◆ whether the probable source has been identified and withdrawn.

In the given scenario, the main 'reservoir' of organisms would have been the babies' gastrointestinal tracts. It would be prudent to continue screening for three to four weeks after the date of last exposure, i.e. date of discharge of the last case. This is because it can take several weeks to detect a transmission. At that point the outbreak could be called over.

7.6.2 Key scenario information

Expert advice from the reference laboratory performing the test may be required in interpreting typing results. The different typing methods have different degrees of discrimination, often depending on the organism in question (Sabat et al. 2013).

7.7 What if ... ?

7.7.1 The first indication of the outbreak was late on a Friday afternoon?

◆ The hospital has a responsibility to provide a safe environment and care, and should have operational plans to respond with appropriately experienced infection control personnel to advise 24/7.

◆ The relevant public health body should be informed.

7.7.2 In the week before the outbreak was detected, two babies had been transferred to the regional neonatal unit, and three had been discharged to three different district hospitals?

◆ Neonatal units share information and transfer babies within neonatal networks of linked units. Public health has a responsibility to work across boundaries, as do hospital infection control teams.

◆ Given that there is a real possibility of a multi-unit or regional outbreak, then there is a pressing need for public health to assume overarching responsibility and coordination, working in collaboration with individual hospitals and interacting with the neonatal network.

◆ Furthermore, national reference services, such as organism typing, might need alerting with view to prioritizing and investigating samples from the affected units.

7.7.3 The isolate was resistant to all antibiotics except chloramphenicol?

◆ This would suggest an untreatable or near untreatable Gr –ve bacteria. It is likely to be a CPE, but more information on the resistance mechanism is needed.

◆ The principles of control would be the same given that the mode of transmission is the same. However, there would be a lower threshold for unit closure if CPE were involved.

◆ The difference here is the consequence of clinical infection, which may be more severe, with a higher probability of death. Because of this, early public health engagement is warranted to ensure all avenues of prevention and control are discussed and implemented as rapidly and effectively as possible.

7.8 **The unanswered question(s) around neonatal outbreaks**

◆ Screening—although admission and weekly screening are often employed, it is not known whether this is a clinically effective practice. Research is required to determine what screening regime for which organisms is most beneficial. With growing resistance problems, it is likely that proactive screening programmes will prove worthwhile.

◆ The role of the environment as a reservoir for Gr –ve bacteria needs exploring. Whilst it is recognized that organisms can survive on various surfaces and live for prolonged periods in taps and sinks, the clinical effectiveness of filters on taps and various deep-cleaning agents needs further research to identify interventions that lead to reduction of clinical Gr –ve bacteria infections.

7.9 **Lessons learned**

◆ By the time an invasive Gr–ve infection occurs, spread with several additional babies already colonized is likely.

◆ Although further clinical infection might occur after introduction of control measures, this may represent the sequelae of transmission that occurred before implementation of control measures.

◆ Whilst there is no clear evidence on the value of routine screening, first principles suggest it is a useful intervention to track movement and spread of organisms. When it is employed as an outbreak control measure, it gives near real-time information on transmission events.

◆ Audit neonatal surveillance protocols.

◆ It is important to ensure appropriate engagement of senior management for the successful implementation of changes in practice and allocation of additional resource.

7.10 **Further thinking**

◆ What more could we do more to prevent hospital/healthcare associated outbreaks?

◆ How could we embed surveillance and outbreak investigation into the working of the neonatal unit?

◆ What new strategies could be introduced to improve infection control in the neonatal unit, including environmental cleaning, reusable versus single-use equipment?

References

Anthony M, A Bedford-Russell, T Cooper, et al. 2013. Managing and preventing outbreaks of Gram-negative infections in UK neonatal units. *Archives of Disease in Childhood. Fetal and Neonatal Edition,* **98**: F549–F553.

Depani SJ, S Ladhani, PT Heath, et al. 2011. The contribution of infections to neonatal deaths in England and Wales. *Pediatric Infectious Disease Journal,* **30**(4): 345–47.

Francis S, H Khan, M Sharland, N Kennea. 2012. Infection control in United Kingdom neonatal units: variance in practice and the need for an evidence base. *Journal of Infection Prevention,* **13**(5): 158–62.

Mammina C, P Di Carlo, D Cipolla, et al. 2008. Nosocomial colonisation due to imipenem-resistant *Pseduomonas aeruginosa* epidemiology linked to breast milk feeding in a neonatal care unit. *Acta Pharmacologica Sinica,* **29**: 1486–92.

Sabat AJ, A Budimir, D Nashev, et al. 2013. Overview of molecular typing methods for outbreak detection and epidemiological surveillance. *Eurosurveillance*, **18**(4): pii = 20380. http://www.eurosurveillance.org/ViewArticle.aspx?ArticleId=20380 (Accessed 8 March 2016).

Sanchez-Carrillo C, B Padilla, M Marín, et al. 2009. Contaminated feeding bottles: the source of an outbreak of *Pseudomonas aeruginosa* infections in a neonatal intensive care unit. *American Journal of Infection Control*, **37**: 150–54.

Smith P, D Benjamin. 2011. Choosing the right empirical antibiotics for neonates. *Archives of Disease in Childhood. Fetal and Neonatal Edition*, **96**: F2–F3.

Vergnano S, E Menson, N Kennea, et al. 2011. Neonatal infections in England: the NeonIN surveillance network. *Archives of Disease in Childhood. Fetal and Neonatal Edition*, **96**(1): F9–F14.

Further reading

Carlet J, V Jarlier, S Harbarth, et al. 2012. Ready for a world without antibiotics? The Pensières Antibiotic Resistance Call to Action. *Antimicrobial Resistance and Infection Control*, **1**:11. https://aricjournal.biomedcentral.com/articles/10.1186/2047-2994-1-11 (accessed 8 March 2016).

European Centre for Disease Prevention and Control. 2014. *Technical Report. Systematic Review of the Effectiveness of Infection Control Measures to Prevent the Transmission of Carbapenemase-producing Enterobacteriaceae through Cross-border Transfer of Patients*. Stockholm: ECDPC. http://ecdc.europa.eu/en/publications/Publications/CPE-systematic-review-effectiveness-infection-control-measures-to-prevent-transmission-2014.pdf (accessed 8 March 2016).

Fraise AP, C Bradley (eds). 2009. *Ayliffe's Control of Healthcare-Associated Infection*. 5th edition. Abingdon: CRC Press.

Hawkey P, D Lewis (eds). 2003. *Medical Bacteriology A Practical Approach*. 2nd edition. Oxford: Oxford University Press.

Mehtar, S. 2010. *Understanding Infection Prevention and Control*. Claremont: Juta and Company.

Regulation and Quality Improvement Authority. 2012. *Independent review of incidents of Pseudomonas aeruginosa infection in neonatal units in northern Ireland*. Final report. http://www.rqia.org.uk/cms_resources/Pseudomonas%20Review%20Phase%20II%20Final%20Report.pdf (accessed 8 March 2016).

Richards C, J Alonso–Echanove, Y Caicedo, et al. 2004. *Klebsiella pneumoniae* bloodstream infections among neonates in a high-risk nursery in Cali, Colombia. *Infection Control and Hospital Epidemiology*, **25**: 221–25.

Sydnori ER, TM Perli. 2011. Hospital epidemiology and infection control in acute-care settings. *Clinical Microbiology Reviews*, **24**: 141–73.

Tacconelli E, MA Cataldo, SJ Dancer, et al. 2014. ESCMID guidelines for the management of the infection control measures to reduce transmission of multidrug-resistant Gram-negative bacteria in hospitalised patients. *Clinical Microbiology and Infection*, **20**: 1–55.

Velasco C, J Rodriguez-Bano, L Garcia, et al. 2009. Eradication of an extensive outbreak in a neonatal unit caused by two sequential *Klebsiella pneumoniae* clones harbouring related plasmids encoding an extended-spectrum beta-lactamase. *Journal of Hospital Infection*, **73**: 157–63.

Voelz A, A Muller, J Gillen, et al. 2010. Outbreaks of *Serratia marcescens* in neonatal and pediatric intensive care units: clinical aspects, risk factors and management. *International Journal of Hygiene and Environmental Health*, **213**: 79–87.

Chapter 8

Influenza

Joanna Cartwright, Anjila Shah,
and Sam Ghebrehewet

OVERVIEW

After reading this chapter the reader familiar with:

- the management of a single case of influenza-like illness (ILI) in the community,
- the use of antivirals for the prophylaxis and treatment of influenza,
- the key public health interventions to prevent spread of ILI in the community, and
- the public health response to clusters and outbreaks of ILI in community settings (e.g. care homes).

Terms

Influenza like illness (ILI) Sudden onset of fever (>38 °C) with cough or sore throat. This is a medical diagnosis made on the presenting symptoms. There are many viruses which can cause ILI.

Influenza illness An acute viral respiratory illness due to infection with the influenza virus.

Post-exposure prophylaxis Protection from infection after exposure.

Antigenic drift The mechanism by which viruses accumulate mutations within the genes that code for antibody binding sites on viruses leading to new progeny viruses that are less likely to be recognised by the same antibodies, i.e., antigenically different.

Antigenic shift A sudden, major change in the influenza virus Haemagglutinin and/ or Neuraminidase surface proteins, resulting in a new influenza virus subtype causing an epidemic or pandemic due to a lack of immunity to the new strain in the human population.

Pandemic An epidemic occurring worldwide, or over a very wide area, crossing international boundaries and usually affecting a large number of people.

(See further list of terms in the Glossary.)

8.1 Background facts: Influenza

Influenza (flu) is an acute viral respiratory illness due to infection with the influenza virus. Transmission is by droplets, aerosol, or through direct contact with respiratory secretions of someone with the infection. The usual incubation period is one to four days. Infection can be passed from person-to-person from the day before symptoms begin to 10 days after symptoms start.

Influenza viruses cause two different epidemiological patterns of infection in humans: yearly epidemics (seasonal flu) and periodic pandemics. Pandemics occur when a virus with a major change in antigenicity infects a host population that is not immune to the new strain, which then spreads easily.

Influenza viruses are divided into subtypes based on two proteins on the surface of the virus: the haemagglutinin (H) and the neuraminidase (N). There are 18 different haemagglutinin subtypes (H1 to H18) and 11 different neuraminidase subtypes (N1 to N11). Changes in these proteins allow the virus to evade the host's immune system. Minor changes, described as antigenic drift, occur progressively from season to season. Antigenic shift occurs periodically, resulting in major changes and the emergence of a new subtype.

There are three types of influenza virus: A, B, and C. Influenza A is the commonest cause of outbreaks and pandemics. Influenza B tend to cause less severe disease than influenza A and smaller outbreaks affecting mainly children. Influenza C is common but rarely causes significant morbidity.

Many other viruses can cause an influenza-like illness: acute viral respiratory infections include *Respiratory syncytial virus, Parainfluenza, Rhinovirus, Human metapneumovirus and Coronavirus OC43*; bacterial infections include *Streptococcus pneumoniae, Haemophilus influenzae, Chlamydophila pneumoniae*, and *Bordetella pertussis*. In the absence of a laboratory confirmed diagnosis the illness is referred to as influenza-like illness (ILI).

8.1.1 Clinical aspects of influenza infection

A significant proportion of infections (30–50%) are asymptomatic (Wilde et al. 1999). Complications include viral pneumonia, secondary bacterial pneumonia, sinus infection, ear infection (otitis media) particularly in children, and worsening of pre-existing chronic health conditions such as asthma or heart failure.

8.1.2 Epidemiology of the infection

Since 1900, there have been four pandemics, in 1918, 1957, 1968, and 2009. In the UK most seasonal cases occur between late December and March, although sporadic cases can occur at any time of year.

Influenza affects all age groups, with the highest incidence in children, but the most serious complications, leading to hospitalization, and deaths in the elderly. Between 3000 and 30,000 excess winter deaths per year are attributed to influenza in the UK (Donaldson et al. 2010).

8.1.3 Influenza surveillance

The WHO's Global Influenza Programme (GIP) collects and analyses virological and epidemiological influenza surveillance data from around the world. The regular sharing of quality influenza surveillance and monitoring data by countries allows WHO to:

- provide countries, with worldwide information about influenza transmission, allowing national policy makers to prepare for coming seasons,
- describe critical features of current influenza epidemiology, including risk groups, transmission characteristics, and impact,
- monitor global trends in influenza transmission, and
- support the selection of influenza strains for vaccine production.

In England, influenza surveillance is carried out by Public Health England (PHE) (PHE 2015a). Additional information for England is provided by the Royal College of General Practitioners (RCGP), for Scotland by Health Protection Scotland, for Wales by Public Health Wales, and for Northern Ireland by the Public Health Agency. Several sources of data, including data from primary care surveillance, virological surveillance, information on outbreaks, and hospital surveillance schemes are used. During the influenza season, weekly national influenza reports and graphs are produced.

Every year, when surveillance data indicates that there is a substantial likelihood that people present-ing with ILI are infected with an influenza virus, the four UK Chief Medical Officers (CMOs) issue similar letters to healthcare professionals including medical directors of hospitals and GPs. The CMOs advise GPs and relevant healthcare professionals that they may prescribe antiviral medicines for the prophylaxis and treatment of influenza for people at risk at NHS expense.

8.2 What's the story?

◆ After visiting a care home, a local GP reports a case of ILI to public health at the beginning of January. The case is an ill 70-year-old with chronic heart disease. The patient has acute respiratory illness, which may be influenza. The GP is requesting advice, since the care home staff are anxious and asking the GP what actions they should take?

8.2.1 What immediate action(s) would you take?

◆ The immediate advice and action will depend on several factors. Ascertain the following about the case, residents, and staff to facilitate decision making:

- Clinical details about the patient, onset of symptoms and vaccination status; what sample, if any, has been taken? Is the patient in a single room?
- Details of other residents in the home with an ILI; total number of residents in the home and vaccination status.
- Details of staff with symptoms of ILI; total number of staff in the home and vaccination status.
- Is there any evidence to indicate that influenza is circulating in the community?

8.2.2 Key scenario information

People at risk of severe influenza (PHE 2014) are:

◆ aged 65 years and older,
◆ pregnant,

or those who suffer from:

◆ chronic disease (respiratory, heart, kidney, liver, neurological disease, and diabetes), and
◆ immunosuppression, including HIV.

In the UK, influenza vaccination is offered to these groups on an annual basis. The vaccine is also recommended for people living in a long-stay residential care home or other facility, main carers for elderly or disabled persons, and health and social care workers with direct patient contact.

In 2012 the Joint Committee on Vaccination and Immunisation (JCVI) recommended that the seasonal influenza (flu) programme should be extended in the UK to all children aged between 2 years and less than 17 years. The phased introduction of the childhood flu programme began in 2013 (PHE 2014).

8.3 Scenario update # 1

◆ The GP rings back with the information requested. Symptom onset was 24 hours ago and the patient is vaccinated against seasonal influenza. The GP has taken a nasopharyngeal swab for laboratory conformation. The case lives in a single room with ensuite toilet. There are 30 other residents and ten staff members in the home; no other residents or staff are ill with an ILI, and all residents are vaccinated; very few staff have had flu vaccination.

8.3.1 **Tools of the trade**

Not everyone who has symptoms of influenza requires testing. A confirmatory test informs management for patients in hospital; patients who are at risk of complications; and cases which occur when influenza has not yet been reported in the community.

Testing should be in liaison with a local virologist/microbiologist.

In order to confirm the diagnosis of influenza, a nose or throat swab with fluid from respiratory secretions can be taken in viral transport medium for molecular testing by polymerase chain reaction (PCR).

In the UK, specialist laboratories can also carry out strain typing and testing for antiviral resistance.

8.3.2 **What further action(s) would you take?**

◆ In this case the person has an ILI and falls into an at-risk group, with presentation within 24 hours of symptom onset. If surveillance indicators suggest influenza is circulating in the community, the likelihood of an ILI being due to influenza virus is high.

◆ Advice should be given regarding simple infection control measures to stop further spread of infection, i.e. isolation in a single room until a minimum of five days after the onset of symptoms, using tissues to cover the mouth and nose when he coughs or sneezes, putting used tissues in a bin as soon as possible ('Catch it, bin it, kill it'). Respiratory hygiene, including regular handwashing with soap and water, as well as regularly cleaning surfaces, such as door handles, to get rid of the virus, is also indicated.

◆ Daily surveillance should be undertaken for any new cases.

◆ The GP and care home staff should be reminded that vaccination against influenza is recommended for health and social care workers who could pass on the infection to vulnerable people.

8.3.3 **Key scenario information**

National institute of Health and Care Excellence (NICE) has produced guidance on the treatment (NICE 2009) and prophylaxis (NICE 2008) of influenza with antivirals.

8.3.3.1 Treatment

The antiviral drugs Oseltamivir and Zanamivir are recommended for the treatment of influenza in adults and children if the national surveillance schemes indicate that influenza virus A or B is circulating, the person is in an at-risk group, and can start treatment within 48 hours (or within 36 hours for Zanamivir) of the onset of symptoms.

8.3.3.2 Prophylaxis

The antiviral drugs Oseltamivir and Zanamivir are recommended for the prophylaxis of influenza in adults and children if the national surveillance schemes indicate that influenza virus A or B is circulating, the person is in an 'at-risk' group, and can start prophylaxis within 48 hours (or within 36 hours for Zanamivir) of exposure.

Note: for community settings, such as care homes, prophylaxis and treatment with antivirals may be indicated even if guidance has not been issued by the four CMOs, but this will need to be discussed with national experts and agreed with relevant Department of Health bodies.

8.4 Scenario update # 2

◆ Three days later the care home reports that three other residents in the same home have developed respiratory symptoms. The infection control nurse is concerned that there may be an outbreak of acute respiratory illness at the home.

8.4.1 What further information do you need?

◆ Have the three new symptomatic residents been assessed by their GP and what is the diagnosis?
◆ What are the onset dates of these three cases?
◆ How closely do the residents of the home mix?
◆ What is the result of the nasopharyngeal swab taken from the first case three days ago?
◆ Is there enough information to determine whether this is an outbreak or not?

8.4.2 Key scenario information

Two or more cases (as defined below) arising within the same 48-hour period OR three or more cases arising within the same 72-hour period, which meet the same clinical case definition and where an epidemiological link can be established are considered an outbreak.

Signs and symptoms may include:

◆ oral temperature of 37.8° or more,

AND

◆ new onset or acute worsening of one or more respiratory symptoms: cough (with or without sputum), hoarseness, nasal discharge or congestion, shortness of breath, sore throat, wheezing, sneezing, chest pain,

OR in older people

◆ an acute deterioration in physical or mental ability without other known cause; temperature in the elderly may not be raised.

8.4.3 Tools of the trade

8.4.3.1 Epidemiological investigation

Place (where and what the nature of contact between individuals), person (basic information about cases, details of signs and symptoms), time (date of onset, timeline of illness).

8.4.3.2 Microbiological investigation

Confirmation of the responsible organism should be done as soon as possible. Nose/throat swab in virus transport medium should be taken from up to five cases with the most recent onset of symptoms.

8.4.3.3 Environmental investigations

Key to defining context, layout of the home, spread of infection, the interconnectedness between different areas in the home.

8.5 Scenario update # 3

◆ GP has assessed all three cases as having ILI. The first swab taken three days ago has been reported as influenza A. The onset for one case was 24 hours ago and two cases 12 hours ago. All 30 residents mix freely within the home and share common living areas.

8.5.1 **What further action(s) would you take?**

◆ Given the information elicited, this is an outbreak. A decision should be made whether an Outbreak Control Team (OCT) should be convened or not.

8.5.2 **Top tips**

◆ The decision regarding the need and urgency to convene an OCT should be guided by the risk assessment: e.g. severity, spread (large number of cases, contacts), intervention needed (number of residents needing treatment or prophylaxis, need for coordination of actions of various agencies), and context.

◆ Some outbreaks may be managed without the need to convene an OCT, particularly if there are a number of ILI outbreaks in nearby care homes. Alternatively, one OCT may oversee all outbreaks in care homes. Not convening an OCT does not mean that no public health actions are required.

◆ If convened, the OCT will decide on outbreak control measures to be implemented. These would include implementing enhanced infection control measures for health and care settings, and influenza-specific measures, including the use of antivirals for the prophylaxis and treatment of contacts and cases.

◆ The OCT will ensure adequate resources are available to undertake outbreak management.

◆ The OCT will agree a communications strategy for informing the public and key stakeholders.

◆ The OCT will decide when the outbreak can be considered over.

8.5.3 **Key scenario information**

Infection control measures

◆ Measures to reduce exposure include:
  • closing home to new admissions,
  • isolation of ill residents,
  • segregation of staff to care for affected or unaffected residents,
  • excluding symptomatic staff for five days, and
  • restrictions on visitors.

◆ Hand hygiene respiratory etiquette and appropriate use of personal protective equipment.

◆ Regular cleaning and appropriate waste disposal.

Influenza specific outbreak control measures (in accordance with NICE and PHE guidance)

◆ Treatment of all symptomatic patients and prophylaxis for asymptomatic patients as appropriate with antivirals is recommended for all at-risk patients, where antivirals can be started within 48 hours (36 hours with Zanimivir) of onset of symptoms or exposure unless contraindicated (NICE 2009).

◆ Prophylaxis for care home staff with patient contact and in at risk groups needs to be arranged.

Note: Previous influenza immunization does not preclude post-exposure prophylaxis (PHE 2015b).

8.6 **Scenario update # 4**

◆ The media have found out about the outbreak. The press are suggesting that there is severe illness in the care home and an epidemic of influenza in the area and are asking what is being done about it.

8.6.1 **How would you respond to the media enquiry?**

◆ Review the press statement already prepared by the OCT.

◆ In liaison with public relations and communications staff of all relevant agencies, ensure the key messages include:

- information about the number of cases in the care home without disclosing any confidential information,
- a brief outline of public health actions already taken,
- information for relative and visitors about the risk of catching influenza,
- information about the importance of influenza vaccination for at-risk groups and health and social care staff,
- information to the general public who may have symptoms of flu not to visit places such as care homes or hospitals,
- information about the importance of maintaining good respiratory and hand hygiene, and
- information regarding influenza activity in the community added as appropriate.

8.7 **What if ... ?**

8.7.1 **The cases were from a school/college/university?**

College/university residential settings will need to be considered individually. Those who share a dormitory or sitting room are likely to be considered household contacts, and prophylaxis needs to be considered for those in high-risk groups. If the setting is for those with special educational needs, it is important to consider wider prophylaxis and treatment with antivirals in a timely manner.

8.7.2 **The cases are from a boarding school with special needs pupils?**

These educational settings will be managed in the same way as care homes with elderly and at-risk residents. It is important to consider implementing public health measures promptly including prophylaxis and treatment with antivirals as soon as an outbreak of ILI is confirmed.

8.7.3 **The cases were in a hospital ward?**

The ward would need to be closed to admissions, prophylaxis prescribed for all exposed patients, staff vaccination reviewed, stringent exclusion of sick staff, isolation or cohorting of sick patients, and strict adherence to droplet precautions for nursing sick patients.

8.7.4 **A hospital patient diagnosed with influenza is to be discharged to a care home?**

Patients admitted to hospital from care homes who are diagnosed with influenza may remain infectious to others even after discharge from hospital, and infection control measures are indicated throughout this time.

Patients may be discharged from hospital at any point when the following criteria are satisfied (PHE 2015c):

- In the view of the treating clinical staff, the patient has clinically recovered sufficiently to be discharged to the care home. Note that there is no requirement for the resolution of all symptoms or a minimum period of antiviral therapy.
- Antiviral and other appropriate treatment will be completed after discharge.
- Appropriate infection control measures to prevent transmission of infection, including single-room dwelling or cohorting, will be continued outside hospital until a minimum of five days after the onset of symptoms.
- The discharge is planned in accordance with local hospital policy.

8.8 Lessons learned

- Influenza-like illness can be caused by many different viruses, only one of which is influenza virus.
- Infection control measures, including prophylaxis and treatment with antivirals, are the mainstay of reducing transmission in outbreaks and their impact should not be underestimated, especially in the elderly or frail individuals.
- Responding to an outbreak requires early intervention and close and effective multi-agency working based on existing agreed arrangements.
- Influenza-like illness may occur in fully vaccinated communities.

8.9 Further thinking

- What can be done to strengthen the evidence for the use of antivirals in cases of influenza and in contacts of people with influenza in care homes?
- What can be done to improve timely implementation of control measures such as prescribing antivirals to close contacts in care home settings (both within and out-of-hours) where residents are registered with multiple GP practices?
- What can be done to strengthen the evidence base for flu vaccination, and improve uptake of vaccination in at-risk groups and healthcare workers?
- What are the roles of different professionals and organizations in the public health management of influenza outbreaks?

References

Donaldson LJ, PD Rutter, BM Ellis, et al. 2010. English mortality from A/H1N1 comparisons with recent flu mortality. *BMJ*, **340**: c612.

NICE. 2008. *Technology Appraisal Guidance 158. Oseltamivir, amantadine (review) and zanamivir for the prophylaxis of influenza.* http://publications.nice.org.uk/oseltamivir-amantadine-review-and-zanamivir-for-the-prophylaxis-of-influenza-ta158 (accessed 8 March 2016).

NICE. 2009. *Technology Appraisal Guidance 168 Amantadine, Oseltamivir and Zanamivir for the Treatment of Influenza.* http://publications.nice.org.uk/amantadine-oseltamivir-and-zanamivir-for-the-treatment-of-influenza-ta168 (accessed 8 March 2016).

Public Health England (PHE). 2014. *Influenza: Immunisation against infectious disease - The Green Book, Chapter 19.* https://www.gov.uk/government/publications/influenza-the-green-book-chapter-19 (accessed 8 March 2016).

PHE. 2015a. *Weekly national flu reports.* www.gov.uk/government/statistics/weekly-national-flu-reports (accessed 8 March 2016).

PHE. 2015b. *Managing Outbreaks of Acute Respiratory Illness in Care Homes: Information and Advice for Health Protection Units.* https://www.gov.uk/government/publications/acute-respiratory-disease-managing-outbreaks-in-care-homes (accessed 8 March 2016).

PHE. 2015c. *Supplementary guidance for health protection teams involved in prevention and control of influenza and other respiratory viral infections among care home residents.* https://www.gov.uk/government/uploads/system/uploads/attachment_data/file/400455/Care_homes_suppl_PHE.pdf (accessed 8 March 2016).

Wilde JA, JA McMillan, J Serwint, et al. 1999. Effectiveness of influenza vaccine in health care professionals: a randomised trial. *JAMA*, **281**:908–13.

Further reading

Hawker J, N Begg, I Blair, et al (eds). 2012. *Communicable Disease Control and Health Protection Handbook.* 3rd edition. London: John Wiley & Sons.

Heymann, LD (ed). 2014. *Control of Communicable Diseases Manual.* 20th edition. Washington, DC: American Public Health Association.

Chapter 9

Legionnaires' disease

Nick Phin, Falguni Naik, Elaine Stanford, and Sam Ghebrehewet

OVERVIEW

After reading this chapter the reader will be familiar with:

- the background information and epidemiology of Legionnaire's disease,
- the surveillance of Legionnaires' disease,
- the public health response to a single case, and
- the details of investigation and control of clusters and outbreaks of Legionnaires' disease.

Terms

Legionellosis Collective term for syndromes caused by infection with Legionella.
Pontiac fever Mild non-pneumonic, self-limiting influenza-like illness caused by Legionella infection.
Urinary antigen test Testing urine for Legionella surface antigen, specific to *L. pneumophila* serogroup 1.
(See further list of terms in the Glossary.)

9.1 Background facts: Legionnaires' disease

- Legionnaires' disease is the name given to an uncommon but potentially fatal pneumonia, often associated with generalized sepsis. It is caused by bacteria of the genus *Legionella*. Legionnaires' disease was named after an outbreak at a 1976 American Legion's convention, where the disease was first recognized.

- The term used to describe any Legionella infection is Legionellosis. Any of the different species of Legionella can cause the pneumonic illness, Legionnaires' disease, or a mild, non-fatal, self-limiting illness without pneumonia called Pontiac fever.

- Over 60 different species of Legionella have been identified, all with the potential to cause human infection; although approximately 95% of confirmed human infections are caused by *Legionella pneumophila* (Gomes-Valero et al. 2014). Other species, such as *L. longbeachae*, *L. bozmanii*, and *L. macdidii* rarely infect humans due to their varying virulence and distribution in the environment.

- There are 15 distinct serogroups of *L. pneumophila*; over 80% of cases tested are found to be infected by *L. pneumophila* serogroup 1 (Helbig et al. 2002). Serogroups can be further divided into subgroups and genetic sequence types.

- Legionnaires' disease is not spread from person-to-person.

- Transmission is by inhalation of droplets or aerosols of water containing Legionella bacteria, although *L. longbeachae* is found in soil and compost and thought to cause infection by aspiration of particles dispersed through the handling of soil/compost.
- The incubation period is usually 2–10 days (median 6–7). Evidence from point source outbreaks, however, suggests this can extend to 19–21 days.
- Legionnaires' disease is a notifiable disease in many countries, including the United Kingdom.
- Initial diagnosis is made by testing urine for the presence of excreted bacterial surface antigens. The majority of commercial assays are specific for *L. pneumophila* serogroup 1 and may not detect infection caused by other species or serogroups.

9.1.1 Clinical signs and symptoms of Legionnaires' disease

- The early features are non-specific influenza-like symptoms which could apply to a range of illnesses.
- Late features include pneumonia, confusion, renal failure, and generalized sepsis.

9.1.2 Key scenario information

9.1.2.1 Case definition: confirmed case of Legionnaires' disease

A clinical or radiological diagnosis of pneumonia with laboratory evidence of one or more of the following:

- isolation (culture) of *Legionella* species from clinical specimens,
- presence of *L. pneumophila* urinary antigen determined using validated reagents/kits,
- detection of *Legionella spp.* nucleic acid (e.g. by PCR) in a clinical specimen, and/or
- positive direct fluorescence (DFA) on a clinical specimen using validated *L. pneumophila* monoclonal antibodies (also referred to as a positive result by direct immunofluorescence (DIF).

9.1.3 Epidemiology of Legionnaires' disease

- Legionnaires' disease mainly occurs in people over 50 years of age although individuals with underlying risk factors of any age are susceptible.
- The overall rate of infection is highest in the 60–69 years age group. Male cases predominate, with a 3:1 male:female ratio (Naik et al. 2008).
- Of the 331 confirmed cases of Legionnaires' disease reported in England and Wales during 2014, 186 (56.2%) were community acquired, 139 (42.0%) were from travel abroad, and six (1.8%) were linked to a healthcare facility (Naik and Dabrera 2015).
- The case fatality rate for Legionnaires' disease is generally 8–12% but can be higher depending on factors such as late diagnosis, inappropriate antibiotic treatment and comorbidities (Bartram et al. 2007).
- Cases of Legionnaires' disease are usually sporadic but outbreaks can occur when man-made water systems such as evaporative cooling systems (cooling towers), hot and cold water systems, and spa pools become contaminated with Legionella bacteria. Any system where contaminated water can be aerosolized has the potential to transmit Legionella and cause outbreaks.
- Incidence of Legionnaires' disease is thought to be affected by atmospheric temperature and relative humidity, with higher incidence seen during warmer and damper months.

9.1.4 **Risk factors for infection**

◆ Risk factors include smoking, diabetes, chronic heart disease, pulmonary comorbidities (such as asthma, chronic obstructive airways disease) and immunosuppression (i.e. transplant patients, those on long-term steroids and cancer patients).

◆ Occupational and recreational risks can come from exposure to uncontrolled water systems. For example:

  • evaporative cooling systems (cooling towers): large towers in rural locations and smaller units fixed to buildings in urban and rural areas,

  • hot and cold water systems, including taps, toilets, showers, hoses, sprinklers and fountains/water features in domestic, leisure, work and public buildings and institutions, and

  • spa pools.

9.2 **What's the story?**

◆ A hospital clinician has identified a case of community-acquired pneumonia (CAP) in a 65-year-old man, Case A, with a three-day history of fever, lethargy, chest pain, and increasing shortness of breath.

◆ A Legionella urinary antigen test was positive.

◆ Sputum samples have been sent to the laboratory for culture and nucleic acid detection.

◆ The patient is receiving antibiotic therapy in accordance with national guidelines and public health personnel have been notified.

9.2.1 **Key scenario information**

Testing for Legionella infection should be considered for all patients with severe CAP, particularly those with risk factors or recent history of travel. All CAP patients need testing during an outbreak.

Legionella-positive urine samples should be sent to the national reference laboratory for confirmation.

Urinary-antigen-positive patients should have lower respiratory samples, such as sputum or bronchioalveolar washings (lavage) (BAL) cultured and typed to enable identification of the source.

9.2.2 **What immediate action(s) would you take?**

◆ As a notifiable disease, Legionnaires' disease must be reported to the appropriate public health bodies, which in the UK is the local authority or health protection team, and the enhanced surveillance form completed and sent to the national surveillance centre, and the following risk assessment undertaken.

  • Details of the case's activities in the two weeks prior to onset of symptoms must be collected as soon as possible. If the case is too ill to provide details, a close family member or a friend can be interviewed.

  • Identify all potential sources of infection in the environment that the patient may have been exposed to in the 14 days prior to onset (e.g. a cooling tower near the patient's home or workplace or leisure centre frequented by the patient).

  • Assess which possible sources pose the greatest risk to the public (e.g. a cooling tower known to have had a prohibition order in its recent history or a large spa pool on display in a busy shopping centre). Arrange for local environmental health officers (EHOs) to follow up on any sites highlighted.

9.2.3 **Top tips**

The following information is essential to guide and prioritize investigations:

◆ **Accurate date of onset of symptoms.**

◆ **Comprehensive 14-day history of activities and travel.**

◆ **Accurate travel details:** if the case spent one or more nights of the incubation period away from home, the names and addresses of the accommodation sites, and dates of stay. All travel-associated cases of Legionnaires' disease are reported to the European Legionnaires' Disease Surveillance Network (ELDSNet). ELDSNet identify clusters (where two or more confirmed cases have been associated with the same accommodation site within two years).

◆ **Hospital details:** if a case spent one or more nights of the incubation period in a hospital or healthcare facility, the dates of stay, ward names, and any changes in rooms/beds. Rapid investigation of hospitals associated with a case of Legionnaires' disease is essential, to rule it out as a source of infection as other vulnerable patients could be at risk.

Be prepared to question the person being interviewed for clear, accurate and detailed case history! The time and care taken in obtaining this information will help to rapidly focus the public health investigation towards the most likely source.

9.3 **Scenario update # 1**

The preliminary 14-day history indicated that Case A was exposed to the following sites/activities:

◆ gardening at home,

◆ attended a members only golf club with a sprinkler system,

◆ visited a garden centre with water features, and

◆ attended a hospital outpatient appointment.

L. pneumophila serogroup 1 was isolated from the sputum sample.

Based on the preliminary information, the hospital and garden centre pose a potential risk to a large proportion of the public and, to a lesser extent, so does the golf club, although access is restricted to members and employees. The patient's home may also have possible sources of exposure.

9.3.1 **What further action(s) would you take?**

◆ Determine whether there are any other current or previous cases of Legionnaires' disease associated with, or close to, the hospital or garden centre.

◆ Review the hospital risk assessments, water management plans, and maintenance records.

◆ Arrange for EHOs to undertake an initial assessment of the garden centre and review its risk assessment and maintenance records.

9.3.2 **Top tip**

Environmental sampling should only be carried out if concerns are raised during the initial site visit and/or from the maintenance records.

9.4 **Scenario update # 2**

◆ There have been no other cases associated with the hospital and the hospital water maintenance records are satisfactory.

- The garden centre is large, close to the town centre, with a number of small water displays and sprinklers which are only used during the warm dry months. There have been no previously associated cases. However, there was a case (Case Y) four months earlier in a local resident living 2.5 km away.
- Case A lives in a terraced house with his son, who is fit and well with no underlying conditions or risk factors.

9.4.1 Key scenario information

A possible source is any unit, system, or installation that is capable of producing aerosols.

Possible sources identified in the 14-day patient history are reviewed to determine the most likely source of infection, and should provide a framework to guide the investigation. The cases can also be categorized according to the most likely exposure as follows:

- **Healthcare-associated or nosocomial**: includes hospital or care accommodation stays or outpatient/clinic appointments.
- **Travel-associated**: includes overnight stays in any commercial accommodation site or vessel in any country.
- **Community-acquired**: where a community/domestic source has been identified or appears most likely, with or without evidence of travel or nosocomial exposure.

Most cases will, however, have multiple potential sources (and may fit into multiple categories above); each should be considered individually according to likely risk to the public, and investigated appropriately.

9.4.2 What further information do you need?

- Details of Case Y. For example: What was the category of exposure i.e., did the case travel or was the source considered to be in the community? Was the local area investigated? Was a source identified?
- Exclude possible sources in the surrounding areas between the garden centre and the previous case.
- When were the sprinklers at the garden centre last used? How are the sprinklers and water features stored and maintained?

9.5 Scenario update # 3

- A second case (Case B) who lives in close proximity to the garden centre which is in the opposite side of town to Case Y is identified, but was abroad for some of their incubation period. The local area was not investigated as there were no other cases in close proximity and the case was abroad for some of the incubation period (refer to 9.8.1).
- There are two cooling towers near Case B.
- The sprinklers at the garden centre have not been used in the last six weeks and, according to the EHOs' assessment, are well maintained.
- The case finding exercise identifies a third case (Case C) who works in close proximity to Cases A and B and has links to the golf club.
- At this stage the hospital and the garden centre have not raised any additional concerns and do not require further actions. The cooling towers and golf club need further investigation.

9.5.1 **What further action(s) would you take?**

◆ Obtain details of Case C, i.e. when did the case experience onset of symptoms? Was the golf club investigated? Was a source identified?

◆ Request the EHOs carry out a brief reconnaissance of the two local cooling towers.

9.5.2 **Tools of the trade**

To determine whether two or more cases are associated, investigations need to be carried out in three separate areas:

◆ **Epidemiological investigation**: is there a link in time and place between the case(s) and the potential exposure.
  • Two or more cases in close proximity, i.e. within approximately 6 km. This is based on a large outbreak in Pas-de-Calais, where dispersion of aerosols extended over at least 6 km from the source (Nguyen et al. 2006).
  • Two or more cases within sufficient proximity in time (i.e. dates of onset within six months).

◆ **Microbiological investigation**: respiratory samples from every case are essential so that an isolate can be grown and the strain identified using nucleic acid techniques such as polymerase chain reaction (PCR) to determine the sequence based typing of the strain.

Typing data can then be used to compare cases' strains with each other to indicate whether they are likely to have a common source.
  The patient strains can also be compared against environmental strains from potential sources. Indistinguishable clinical and environmental strains provide strong evidence for the source of infection.

◆ **Environmental investigation**: sampling should be undertaken before any remedial actions are taken. Environmental samples can be isolated and typed in the same way as clinical samples. The sequence based typing of the environmental strain can then be compared to determine if it matches the clinical strain.

9.6 **Scenario update # 4**

◆ The two cooling towers were found to be well managed; their maintenance records are up to date and showed the last sample tested for Legionella to be negative.

◆ Case B is positive by urinary antigen and culture and PCR identified the infecting strain as, *L. pneumophila* serogroup 1 subgroup Benidorm, sequence type 117. Case B did not attend any healthcare facilities. The case works full time at the local bakery and spends every Saturday and Sunday afternoon at the same golf club as Cases A and C. The golf club has not been investigated further.

◆ Case C is a 57-year-old male diagnosed with community acquired Legionnaires' disease with onset of symptoms four days prior to Case A.

9.6.1 **What further action(s) would you take?**

◆ Following confirmation of the second case and the case finding exercise identifying Case C with a link to the golf club; the golf club should be investigated by the EHOs and an Incident Control Team (ICT) convened. The investigation involves a site inspection and a review of maintenance records and water monitoring regimes.

♦ If the review and/or inspection raises concerns, sampling of all possible sources should be carried out, including: the site water system and its components, i.e. taps, showerheads, air conditioning units, on-site leisure facilities (e.g. swimming and spa pools), ground irrigation systems and surrounding cooling towers.

9.7 Scenario update # 5

♦ The results from Case A are positive for *L. pneumophila* serogroup 1 subgroup Benidorm, sequence type 117—the same strain that infected Case B.

♦ Case C was infected by *L. pneumophila* but no respiratory sample was available for strain typing; however, due to the epidemiological link of Case C with Cases A and B, it is still investigated as part of the cluster.

♦ Preliminary results from water samples taken from the golf club showers are positive for *Legionella species*.

♦ The media are now aware of the cases and suggest the golf club is responsible for infecting more than a dozen people with a 'killer bug'. They have just contacted your department asking what is being done about it.

9.7.1 How would you respond to the media enquiry?

♦ The ICT should release a pre-prepared (reactive) press statement.

♦ Give only confirmed information.

♦ Respect patient confidentiality.

♦ Stick to the facts—do not speculate!

♦ Relay the following key messages in every press release:
- there is no person-to-person transmission,
- explanation of the usual mode of infection, and
- general symptoms with advice to seek medical attention if concerned.

9.7.2 Top tips

It is best practice to only have one nominated individual directly communicating with the media or, if multiple agencies are collaborating, one joint statement should be agreed and released.

In speaking to the media, be prepared! Have the agreed case numbers and accurate details on investigations and actions. Stick to the facts.

9.8 What if ... ?

9.8.1 Case A had been abroad during the incubation period?

♦ If a case stayed one or more nights in any accommodation site other than their home during the incubation period, the accommodation must be considered a possible source and travel details recorded.

♦ Accurate history must be obtained regarding the name and address of the site(s) where the case stayed, exact travel dates and information about exposure to any other possible exposure whilst travelling. Details of the accommodation sites and travel dates are reported to the European Legionnaires Disease Surveillance Network (ELDSNet) who monitor travel associated cases of Legionnaires' disease across member states.

9.8.1.1 Key scenario information

◆ Most European countries are members of ELDSNet and are required to report all travel-associated cases of Legionnaires' disease to the scheme and adhere to the European guidelines (ECDC 2012).

European guidelines

◆ **Single case:** a document produced by ELDSNet outlining good practice for minimizing the risk of Legionella infection is issued to the owners of every commercial accommodation site associated with one case of Legionnaires' disease over a two year period.

◆ **Cluster/outbreaks:** an accommodation site associated with two or more cases of Legionnaires' within two years must be inspected and a risk assessment and environmental investigation carried out, followed by the implementation of control measures.

9.8.2 There were other Legionella risk factors in the hospital?

Consider the following possibilities: the hospital at which Case A had an appointment was associated with previous cases of Legionnaires' disease; or Case A had been an inpatient; or the hospital maintenance records had anomalies indicating an increased risk of exposure to Legionella? (**Note:** These guidelines apply to all healthcare facilities and not exclusively to hospitals.)

◆ The hospital infection control lead should be notified immediately and encouraged to convene an ICT.

◆ Review potential risk to vulnerable patients and implement emergency remedial measures. These might include temporary measures such as fitting filters to showers and taps and restricting the use of water outlets that tested positive.

◆ The hospital risk assessment and control procedures should be reviewed, and arrangements made for environmental samples to be tested by an accredited laboratory. Sampling of areas causing greatest concern should be arranged (e.g. areas occupied by the most vulnerable, areas with previous positive water samples, ward occupied by the current case).

◆ Ensure actions are taken to isolate and remedy areas that test positive for Legionella.

9.9 The unanswered question(s) around Legionnaires' disease

◆ The epidemiology of Legionnaires' disease suggests a high proportion of under-reporting. *Legionella spp.* are known to be the causative agent in many cases of severe CAP. An estimated 2–5% of CAP cases are due to Legionella infection, which is about ten times higher than numbers recorded by well-established surveillance systems (Ishiguro et al. 2013). Therefore, the true burden of infection attributed to the organism is not known.

◆ Differences have been observed in the population profile and prevalence of the strains of Legionella commonly isolated from environmental samples compared to clinical samples. The prevalence of some strains known to cause infection in humans differs greatly from the prevalence of the same strain in the environment. This could be due to different species colonizing only very specific niches or disparities in the virulence of the strains.

9.10 Lessons learned

◆ The symptoms of Legionnaires' disease are similar to those of many other respiratory diseases and often reported as community-acquired pneumonia of undetermined source.

◆ Legionnaires' disease is not spread through person-to-person transmission. Each case arises from direct exposure to contaminated aerosol/droplets. The source of infection should be identified if possible, as every case could potentially signal the start of a large point source outbreak.

◆ The only way to prevent incidents of Legionnaires' disease is through the implementation of stringent measures in the control and management of water systems.

9.11 **Further thinking**

◆ How can we reduce or prevent future clusters/outbreaks of Legionnaires' disease?

◆ What can be done to improve timeliness of diagnosis of Legionnaires' disease?

◆ What are the roles of different professionals and organizations in the public management of Legionnaires' disease?

References

Bartram J, Y Chartier, JV Lee, et al. 2007. *Legionella and the Prevention of Legionellosis.* Geneva: World Health Organization.

ECDC. 2012. *European Legionnaires' Disease Surveillance Network (ELDSNet): Operating procedures.* European Centre for Disease Prevention and Control. 1–23.

Gomez-Valero L, C Rusniok, M Rolando, et al. 2014. Comparative analyses of Legionella species identifies genetic features of strains causing Legionnaires' disease. *Genome Biology,* **15**(11): 505.

Helbig JH, S Bernander, M Castellani Pastoris, et al. 2002. Pan-European study on culture-proven Legionnaires' disease: distribution of Legionella pneumophila serogroups and monoclonal subgroups. *European Journal of Clinical Microbiology & Infectious Diseases,* **21**(10): 710–16.

Ishiguro T, N Takayanagi, S Yamaguchi. 2013. Etiology and factors contributing to the severity and mortality of community-acquired pneumonia. *Internal Medicine (Tokyo, Japan),* **52**(3): 317–24.

Naik FC, KD Ricketts, TG Harrison, CA Joseph. 2008. Legionnaires' Disease in England and Wales 1999–2005. *Health Protection Report,* **2**(49).

Nguyen TM, D Ilef, S Jarraud, et al. 2006. A community-wide outbreak of legionnaires disease linked to industrial cooling towers—how far can contaminated aerosols spread? *Infect Diseases,* **193**(1): 102–11.

Naik FC, G Dabrera. 2015. *Legionnaires' Disease in England and Wales 2014.* London: Public Health England. PHE publications gateway number: 2015145.

Further reading

Hawker J, N Begg, I Blair, R Reintjes, et al. (eds). 2012. *Communicable Disease Control and Health Protection Handbook,* 3rd edition. London: John Wiley & Sons.

Heymann LD (ed.). 2014. *Control of Communicable Diseases Manual.* 20th edition. Washington, DC: American Public Health Association.

HSE (**Health and Safety Executive**). 2013. *Approved Code of Practice (L8)—The Control of Legionella Bacteria in Water Systems.* pp. 1–28. http://www.hse.gov.uk/pubns/books/l8.htm (accessed 8 June 2016).

Paranthaman K, FC Naik. 2015. *Guidance on the Control and Prevention of Legionnaires' disease in England. Technical Paper 1—Disease Surveillance.* London: Public Health England, pp. 1–28.

Lee JV, C Joseph. 2002. Guidelines for investigating single cases of Legionnaires' disease. *Communicable Disease and Public Health/PHLS,* **5**(2): 157–62.

Lim WS, SV Baudouin, RC George, et al. 2009. British Thoracic Society guidelines for the management of community acquired pneumonia in adults: update 2009. *Thorax,* **64**(Suppl. III): iii1–iii55.

Chapter 10

Measles

David Baxter, Gill Marsh, and Sam Ghebrehewet

OVERVIEW

After reading this chapter the reader will be familiar with:

- the epidemiology and clinical features of measles,
- the public health response to a single case of measles,
- the investigation and control of clusters and outbreaks of measles, and
- the public health response to an outbreak of measles in a school; and an exposure to measles in a healthcare setting.

Terms

Ro (Basic reproductive number) Is the average number of new cases generated by one infectious case (secondary cases) over the course of its infectious period, in an entirely susceptible population (Heffernan et al. 2005).

Index case The first case to come to the attention of the investigator; not always the primary case.

Primary case The case that introduced the disease into the group or population.

Post Exposure Prophylaxis (PEP) Drugs/vaccines/immunoglobulins offered to provide protection from infection or illness after exposure.

Herd protection Occurs when a high percentage of the population is immune (by vaccination or prior infection/disease), which makes it difficult for a disease to spread as there are very few unprotected people. This provides a degree of protection to individuals without individual immunity.

(See further list of terms in the Glossary.)

10.1 Background facts: measles

- Measles is a systemic viral infection caused by an RNA virus from the Paramyxovirus family.
- It is a human-only pathogen—primates may be infected in a laboratory situation but they are unable to sustain transmission to a human host.
- The source of infection is a human with acute measles—there is no carrier state.
- The incubation period: 7–14 days (average 10–12 days).
- Measles is infectious from the onset of symptoms (typically four days before the appearance of rash) to four days after the appearance of rash.

- Measles is spread by airborne or droplet transmission or direct contact with respiratory secretions. The virus can survive in the air or on inanimate objects (synonym fomites) for up to two hours (Centers for Disease Prevention and Control 2015).
- It is one of the most highly infectious communicable diseases with basic reproductive number (Ro) of 11-18 (Anderson and May 1992). Contact of 15 minutes or more in the same room as someone with measles is sufficient to be deemed a significant exposure and to transmit infection (Public Health England 2014a).
- Measles is a notifiable disease in the UK.

10.1.1 Clinical signs and symptoms of measles

- Early or **prodromal symptoms** which *may* include:
  - high fever,
  - coryzal symptoms (cough, cold, or runny nose),
  - red and watery eyes or conjunctivitis, and
  - Koplik spots (small red spots with bluish-white centres) inside the mouth.
- Later symptoms
  - characteristic red/brown blotchy maculopapular (non-vesicular) rash (appears 3–4 days after first symptoms).
- The typical distinctive rash is non-itchy, starts on the face and upper neck, then spreads, across the trunk and limbs, eventually reaching the hands and feet. As measles is now a rare illness, the rash is commonly confused with other viral infections, leading to an incorrect suspicion of measles.
- The most common complications of measles infection are otitis media (7–9% of cases), diarrhoea (8%), pneumonia (1–6%), and convulsions (0.5%).
- Other, rarer, complications include: post-infectious encephalitis (1 in 1000); and subacute sclerosing panencephalitis, a progressive and uniformly fatal nervous system infection due to persistent measles virus infection (Public Health England 2013).
- Complications are more common and more severe in poorly nourished and/or chronically ill children, including those who are immunosuppressed. Death occurs in one in 5000 cases in the UK and is higher in children under 1 year of age, lower in children aged 1–9 years and rises again in teenagers and adults.

10.1.2 Epidemiology of the infection

- Measles is vaccine-preventable. A single measles vaccine was introduced in the UK in 1968, with the combined measles–mumps–rubella (MMR) vaccine introduced from 1988.
- Coverage with single measles vaccine was poor and although numbers of cases fell, the circulation of measles was not interrupted. However post-1988, uptake of MMR quickly increased and soon reached in excess of 90% coverage. Consequently, the numbers of measles notifications fell to very low levels.
- Unfortunately, controversy about potential links between the MMR vaccine and autism in the late 1990s, which were later proved unfounded (Farrington et al. 2001; Taylor et al. 1999), decreased confidence in the vaccine, and uptake in the UK reduced from 92% in 1996 to 80% in 2003 (Public Health England 2014b). Consequently, in the UK, laboratory-confirmed cases

of measles have increased in recent years and outbreaks of measles continue to occur (e.g. large outbreaks have occurred between 2010–2014 in Liverpool, the North East, and South Wales).

10.2 **What's the story?**

♦ An 11-year-old child is admitted to the paediatric ward with a high fever and a maculopapular rash. The rash started on the face 24 hours earlier and gradually spread over the body.

♦ The child has been notified as a suspected case of measles. He had been coughing and generally unwell before he developed a pyrexia of 39° C and a rash.

10.2.1 **What immediate action(s) would you take?**

♦ Undertake a risk assessment of the suspected case to ascertain the case confidence, i.e. whether the case is possible, probable, or confirmed.

♦ Ascertain as much information as possible from the notifying clinician in order to classify the case confidence.

♦ The public health actions required will depend on the case confidence.

♦ In the UK, public health action is only required for probable or confirmed cases.

10.2.2 **Key scenario information**

10.2.2.1 Measles case confidence

Due to its high infectivity, public health follow-up should begin before laboratory confirmation. Case classification and risk assessment are based on both clinical and epidemiological factors.

10.2.2.2 Suspected case of measles

1. Any individual in whom a clinician suspects measles.
2. Any individual with a fever *and* a maculopapular rash *and* at least one of the following: cough, coryza or conjunctivitis.

Suspected cases should be further classified as probable or possible, based on an assessment of epidemiological factors:

♦ Epidemiological link—a person with clinically diagnosed measles who has been in contact with a laboratory confirmed case within the incubation period. Other factors that may suggest an epidemiological link are:

• travel to an area where measles is endemic or there is a current outbreak, and/or

• membership of a group known to have poor MMR vaccine uptake (e.g. Traveller or Steiner communities).

Consequently:

♦ *No* epidemiological factors or link—the case is deemed *Possible.*

♦ *With* epidemiological factors or link—the case is deemed *Probable.*

10.2.2.3 'Confirmed' case of measles:

Diagnosis is proven by laboratory testing.

10.2.3 **Top tips**

Obtain the following from the notifying clinician, the case and/or the parent/guardian in order to assess the case confidence.

10.2.3.1 Caller's details

◆ name, address, designation, and contact number
◆ when and where the case was clinically assessed.

10.2.3.2 Demographic details

◆ name, DOB, sex, ethnicity, and NHS number,
◆ address, including postcode,
◆ current address if not the home address,
◆ contact phone number and parent/guardian details if case is a child,
◆ school/nursery/university,
◆ occupation and workplace (if relevant), and
◆ GP name and address and phone number.

10.2.3.3 Clinical/epidemiological assessment

◆ clinical history (including onset dates for prodrome, rash and diagnosis),
◆ vaccination history (MMR, MR or single measles and number of doses),
◆ contact with a confirmed or suspected case,
◆ UK and non-UK travel in previous four weeks,
◆ member of, or contact with a high-risk population (e.g. international students, Steiner, Traveller family), and
◆ mode of transport to health appointment.

The above information is important for deciding on, and undertaking, the necessary public health actions.

10.3 **Scenario update # 1**

◆ Following a discussion with the notifying clinician, it is clear that the symptoms and presentation meet the clinical case definition of suspected measles.
◆ The mother of the suspected case informed the notifying clinician that the family had just returned from a holiday in East Africa.
◆ The mother also confirmed that:
  • There was an ongoing measles outbreak in the area where they stayed in East Africa.
  • Her son had received all recommended immunizations with the exception of MMR.

10.3.1 **What further action(s) would you take?**

Given that the child's symptoms meet the clinical case definition, and their history of travel to an area with an ongoing measles outbreak, the child will be classified as a probable case. The following public health action will, therefore, be required:

◆ Identify all close contacts of the patient as soon as possible.
◆ Identify vulnerable contacts:
  • infants,
  • pregnant women, and
  • immuno-compromised individuals.

- Determine the significance of the exposure and assess individual contacts, including health care worker (HCW) and healthy contacts' susceptibility to measles infection.
- Consider the need for and arrange any post-exposure prophylaxis (PEP) with MMR or Human Normal Immunoglobulin (HNIG) as appropriate. MMR prophylactic vaccination should be given within 72hrs and HNIG as soon as possible and no later than six days after exposure.

10.3.2 **Key scenario information**

The priorities for contact tracing are:

1. **Immunocompromised contacts** are at risk of severe disease and cannot receive live MMR vaccine.
2. **Vulnerable immunocompetent contacts**—pregnant women and infants who are below the age of routine immunization—are susceptible to severe disease.
3. **Health care worker contacts**—may act as a source of transmission to vulnerable individuals. HCWs should be excluded from work from the fifth day after exposure unless they can demonstrate protection, i.e. two doses of MMR or serologically measles IgG +ve. If susceptible they should receive a dose of MMR as soon as possible after exposure and should remain excluded until 21 days post-exposure or be symptom free and measles IgG +ve at least 14 days after MMR vaccination.
4. **Healthy contacts**—may benefit from post-exposure vaccination within 72hrs of contact if they are unimmunized or incompletely immunized against measles. Vaccination is still worthwhile after this time for prospective protection.

10.3.2.1 Has there been a significant exposure?

The exposure is deemed significant if:

- a probable or confirmed case was infectious at the time of the contact- (four days before to four days after onset of rash), **AND**
- there has been face-to-face contact for any duration, and either
- a healthy immunocompetent individual has been in a room with the case for 15 minutes or more or
- an immunocompromised individual has been in a room with the case for any duration (Health Protection Agency 2010) or entered the room within two hours of an infected individual leaving a room (Centers for Disease Control and Prevention 2014).

10.4 **Scenario update # 2**

- Information from the mother indicated that the child was in year 6 at a local primary school before he became unwell with cold-like symptoms and a cough.
- The child was sent home unwell from school, and two days later he developed a rash.
- Information from the local hospital indicated he was in the A&E waiting room for 45 minutes before being triaged and transferred to an enclosed isolation room on the paediatric ward.

10.4.1 **What further action(s) would you take?**

- The child will have been infectious for two days whilst at school, so contact tracing should also include pupils and staff.
- Following a thorough risk assessment, an action plan for school contacts will need to be considered (e.g. an offer of MMR catch-up vaccination for the whole school population or concentrate solely on any vulnerable contacts).

◆ The action plan should include a communication strategy. Information should be provided to all parents as soon as possible (normally through sending out letters), so that those at risk are reminded of the symptoms to look out for and unimmunized or incompletely immunized individuals can seek vaccination. In addition, any new cases will be more likely to seek early medical attention. It is also paramount to alert relevant local healthcare facilities to the risk of measles.

◆ The hospital should undertake contact tracing of any vulnerable contacts (patients, visitors, and staff, including non-clinical staff) who may have had significant exposure to the case

10.4.2 **Key scenario information**

Children in the UK are offered two doses of MMR vaccination before starting school. Two doses of MMR are effective in protecting against measles, mumps, and rubella infections. Therefore, measles immunity can be assumed in an individual who has received two (documented) doses of a measles containing vaccine or is measles IgG +ve. If MMR vaccine uptake is good in a school (95% or above), introduction of measles is unlikely to result in an outbreak, as sufficient children will be immune to provide herd protection to protect the unimmunized.

10.4.3 **Top tips**

10.4.3.1 Is the contact susceptible to measles?

Assessing an individual's susceptibility to measles depends on various factors:

◆ **Date of birth/age**: due to changes in measles epidemiology overtime and introduction of measles vaccination.

◆ **Past history of infection**: natural infection confers lifelong protection.

◆ **The individual's vaccination history**: a single dose of measles-containing vaccine is known to be at least 90–95% effective in protecting against clinical measles (Demicheli 2012). A second dose gives protection to almost all who were unprotected after the first dose.

◆ **Maternal history of infection/vaccination for an infant**: a full-term infant under three months will have passive immunity from its mother if she has had measles infection. Passive protection from maternal vaccination, however, cannot be guaranteed (Health Protection Agency 2009).

◆ **Past medical history**: individuals who are immunosuppressed may still be at risk despite previous immunization or natural infection (HPA 2009; PHE 2013).

Remember that there is a need to act quickly and prioritize the most important public health actions—MMR prophylactic vaccination within 72 hours, and HNIG as soon as possible, and no later than six days after exposure, to susceptible individuals deemed at high risk following exposure to measles.

10.5 **Scenario update # 3**

◆ The diagnosis of the 11-year-old child is now confirmed by the laboratory as measles virus of the same strain type as the one circulating in East Africa.

◆ Three more probable measles cases were notified from the same school—one from the same class as the 11-year-old and the other two from the same school but in different year groups.

◆ In addition, the local hospital confirmed that a 7-month-old baby presented at the same A&E recently with a clinical presentation of measles, no foreign or UK travel, and no links to high-risk populations.

◆ Further investigation reveals that the baby had been in A&E on the same day and time as the confirmed case. The baby was with his aunt and 11-year-old cousin, who had broken his arm, and had been in the waiting room for approximately 20 minutes with the case. The baby had not previously been highlighted as a contact, as contact tracing had focused on patients.

10.5.1 What further action(s) would you take?

◆ As the diagnosis is confirmed, an alert should be sent to all local healthcare providers and public health teams.

◆ The four new cases should be followed up individually by contact tracing and arranging PEP as appropriate.

◆ The school is now experiencing an outbreak of measles (two or more probable or confirmed cases of measles with an epidemiological link). It would be necessary to establish a multiagency Outbreak Control Team (OCT) to jointly plan and implement the public health response (PHE 2014c). The OCT may consider various measures to control spread of the outbreak depending on local circumstances, including:

  • offering a school-based immunization programme

  • offering a wider catch-up immunization programme across the locality (school or community based)

  • considering media issues and developing a communication strategy.

◆ The notification of the baby with probable measles indicates nosocomial (healthcare setting) spread, and infection control advice should be reiterated.

◆ Individuals with rash or any prodromal symptoms should be triaged to ensure that suspected measles cases are nursed in isolation facilities.

10.5.2 Top Tips

Local knowledge (e.g. of MMR uptake rates) will help risk assessment of the situation. Coordinated partnership working between local authority public health teams, screening and immunization teams and health protection teams is paramount in order to ascertain MMR uptake data for the relevant age group and, if possible, the relevant school. This will enable assessment of the likely impact of the first or subsequent cases attending that setting whilst infectious and help determine the scale of response required.

10.6 Scenario update # 4

◆ There are now 11 confirmed cases and 19 probable cases, four weeks after the first case was notified.

  • five confirmed and four probable from the same school where the first case attended,

  • two confirmed and eight probable from a nursery, one of whom is the sibling of a confirmed case from the first case's school, and

  • three confirmed cases who attended A&E at the same time as the first case and seven secondary cases, three of whom have attended the local high school whilst infectious.

◆ The 24-year-old mother of the 7-month-old baby infected in A&E is currently in the Intensive Care Unit (ICU) with probable measles meningitis and secondary pneumonia. She is ventilated and her prognosis is poor.

◆ Concern about the outbreak is spreading in the community and the media have found out there is a seriously ill patient in the ICU whose baby was infected whilst at the local hospital.

10.6.1 **How would you respond to the community concern and media enquiry?**

◆ Update the holding press statement with the aim of releasing it once agreed by partners, i.e. in liaison with public relations/communications staff.

◆ Use this opportunity to share relevant information and provide public health advice for both healthcare professionals and the general public.

◆ Press/media statement may include the following:

• Appropriate measures (immunoglobulin and vaccination) are being implemented to protect those at higher risk.

• Local professionals (health protection, public health, NHS, local authority, local health education, etc.) are working collaboratively to manage and control the outbreak.

• Parents of children under 16 and young adults under age 25 should check they are appropriately immunized against measles with MMR, and arrange to be immediately immunized if not.

• Advise that people should ring before attending a healthcare facility if they think they have symptoms suggestive of measles, especially if they have a rash or have been in contact with someone with measles, and that they should remind staff on their arrival.

10.6.2 **Top tips**

It is good practice for the OCT and any other relevant agencies to have a nominated spokesperson to deal with media enquiries.

The spokesperson should be prepared with key messages and have checked that all the relevant information is correct and up to date.

Ensure that any information shared includes advice that would enable the public to recognize early signs and symptoms of measles infection.

Communicate only OCT-agreed information, stick to the facts, and don't get drawn into speculation(s).

Respect confidentiality: don't give away any identifiable patient information.

10.7 **What if ... ?**

10.7.1 **The case had been infectious whilst on the plane?**

◆ Contact tracing of individuals who were on the plane would have to take place. The relevant measles guidance would need to be followed (Health Protection Agency 2012).

◆ It is likely international liaison would be necessary.

10.7.2 **The cases were from a nursery?**

◆ The initial response would be the same as to a case in a school.

◆ As MMR immunization (2 doses) is not routinely completed before three years four months to five years of age, it is likely there are more susceptible contacts, more PEP will be required, and ongoing spread is more likely.

10.8 **Lessons learned**

◆ Measles is infectious before the onset of the rash and these early prodromal symptoms can be mistaken for other viral illnesses.

◆ Two doses of MMR vaccine are extremely effective at providing long-term protection against measles. It is, however, important that a high percentage of the population are vaccinated with two doses (95% or above) to provide herd protection to vulnerable individuals who cannot be vaccinated (e.g. babies and immunosuppressed individuals).

◆ Herd protection is very useful but has limitations in its application.

◆ Measles is very infectious and spreads quickly within susceptible populations, and the need for prompt action cannot be overemphasized.

◆ Healthcare facilities can lead to ongoing transmission to vulnerable individuals if infection control and isolation procedures are not rigidly adhered to, and high staff vaccination uptake rates are not maintained.

10.9 **Further thinking**

◆ How can we reduce or prevent future measles disease clusters/outbreaks?

◆ What can be done to improve early reporting of highly infectious diseases such as measles?

◆ How can we use immunization uptake data to predict clusters or outbreaks?

◆ What can be done to optimize triaging and immediate isolation of suspected measles cases, and high consequence infectious diseases in healthcare settings, such as walk-in centres, GP in and out-of-hours services, and A&E departments?

◆ What can be done proactively to protect the health of immunosuppressed individuals for the future?

References

Anderson R, R May. 1992. *Infectious Diseases in Humans. Dynamics and Control.* Oxford: Oxford University Press.

CDC. 2014. *Transmission of Measles.* http://www.cdc.gov/measles/about/transmission.html (accessed 8 March 2016).

CDC. 2015. *Measles—Q&A about Disease & Vaccine.* http://www.cdc.gov/vaccines/vpd-vac/measles/faqs-dis-vac-risks.htm (accessed 8 March 2016).

Demicheli VR, A Rivetti, MG Debalini, et al. 2012. Vaccines for measles, mumps and rubella in children. *Cochrane Database of Systematic Reviews* 2: CD004407. doi:10.1002/14651858.CD004407

Farrington P, E Miller, B Taylor. 2001. MMR and autism: further evidence against a causal association. *Vaccine*, 19(27): 3632–35.

Health Protection Agency. 2009. *Measles: post-exposure prophylaxis.* https://www.gov.uk/government/publications/measles-post-exposure-prophylaxis (accessed 8 March 2016).

Health Protection Agency. 2010. *National Measles Guidelines.* https://www.gov.uk/government/publications/national-measles-guidelines (accessed 8 March 2016).

Health Protection Agency. 2012. *Measles: guidance for HPA staff on international travel and travel by air.* https://www.gov.uk/government/uploads/system/uploads/attachment_data/file/394754/Measles_guidance_for_HPA_staff_on_international_travel_and_travel_by_air.pdf (accessed 8 March 2016).

Heffernan J, R Smith, L Wahl. 2005. Perspectives on the basic reproductive ratio. *Interface*, 12(104): 281–93.

Public Health England (PHE). 2013. *Measles: Immunisation against infectious disease - The Green Book, Chapter 21.* https://www.gov.uk/government/publications/measles-the-green-book-chapter-21 (accessed 8 March 2016).

PHE. 2014a. *Measles: Symptoms, Diagnosis, Complications and Treatment (factsheet).* https://www.gov.uk/government/publications/measles-symptoms-diagnosis-complications-treatment/measles-symptoms-diagnosis-complications-and-treatment-factsheet (accessed 2 February 2015).

PHE. 2014b. *Completed primary courses at 2 years of age: England and Wales.* https://www.gov.uk/government/publications/completed-primary-courses-at-2-years-of-age-england-and-wales (accessed 8 March 2016).

PHE. 2014c. *Communicable disease outbreak management: operational guidance.* https://www.gov.uk/government/publications/communicable-disease-outbreak-management-operational-guidance (accessed 8 March 2016).

Taylor B, E Miller, CP Farrington et al. 1999. Autism and measles, mumps, and rubella vaccine: no epidemiological evidence for a causal association. *Lancet,* **353**(9169): 2026–29.

Further reading

Hawker J, N Begg, I Blair et al. 2012. *Communicable Disease Control and Health Protection Handbook.* 3rd edition. London: John Wiley & Sons.

Heymann LD (ed). 2014. *Control of Communicable Diseases Manual.* 20th edition. Washington, DC: American Public Health Association.

PHE. 2014d. *Evaluation of vaccine uptake during the 2013 MMR catch-up campaign in England.* https://www.gov.uk/government/publications/evaluation-of-vaccine-uptake-during-the-2013-mmr-catch-up-campaign-in-england (accessed 8 March 2016).

Chapter 11

Meningitis and meningococcal disease

Sam Ghebrehewet, David Conrad, and Gill Marsh

OVERVIEW

After reading this chapter the reader will be familiar with:

- the epidemiology and clinical features of meningitis caused by *Neisseria meningitidis*, which can also result in other invasive illnesses (meningococcal disease, e.g. meningococcal septicaemia),
- the public health response to a single case of meningococcal disease,
- the investigation and control of clusters and outbreaks of meningococcal disease in an educational setting, and
- the response to cases of meningococcal disease in different circumstances/situations that require different public health actions.

Terms

Meningitis Inflammation of the meninges, a fine membrane covering the brain and spinal cord.

Gram-negative diplococcus Is a round bacterium that typically presents in the form of two joined cells (e.g. Gram-negative *Neisseria meningitidis*).

Droplet precautions The use of personal protective equipment (PPE) to prevent transmission of droplet infections. This includes face mask, gloves, and apron for contact with the patient or their environment. Eye protection should also be worn for aerosol-generating procedures.

Close contact In a case of meningococcal disease, close contact is defined as a contact in a household type setting during the seven days before onset of illness.

(See further list of terms in the Glossary.)

11.1 Background facts: meningitis and meningococcal disease

- Relatively common causes of meningitis include viruses (e.g. herpes simplex) and *Neisseria meningitidis* bacteria (also known as *meningococci*).
- Other bacterial causes of meningitis include *Haemophilus influenzae* type B (HiB), *Streptococcus pneumoniae*, *Listeria monocytogenes*, and *Escherichia coli*.
- Infection caused by *Neisseria meningitidis* (or *meningococci*) is described as meningococcal disease. Invasive meningococcal disease includes both meningitis and septicaemia.
- There are approximately 3400 cases of bacterial meningitis and septicaemia each year in the UK: 10% result in death and 15% of survivors will have long-term effects (e.g. brain damage, deafness and multiple amputations) (Viner et al. 2012).

- Meningitis or other invasive diseases caused by either HiB or *meningococci* are of public health significance and cases require public health follow-up to facilitate communicable disease control. No public health action is required for other forms of meningitis.

- The average incubation period for meningococcal disease is three to five days, but it could be as long as ten days.

- It is transmitted via aerosol, droplets, or direct contact with respiratory secretions.

- Acute meningitis is a notifiable disease in England under the Health Protection (Notification) Regulations, 2010 (see Appendix 4).

11.1.1 Clinical signs and symptoms of meningococcal disease

- Early symptoms (some non-specific) include:
  - headache,
  - drowsiness,
  - neck stiffness,
  - pyrexia (fever),
  - photophobia (intolerance to light),
  - non-blanching rash (does not disappear when pressed under a clear drinking glass),
  - vomiting, and
  - muscle and joint pain.
- Late features may include:
  - confusion,
  - convulsions, and
  - coma.
- Signs of septicaemia (sepsis) include:
  - cold hands and feet,
  - leg pains,
  - abnormal skin colour, and
  - haemorrhagic rash (bleeding under the skin).

11.1.2 Epidemiology of the infection

- The majority of meningococcal disease occurs in children younger than 5 years, with a peak incidence in those under 1 year of age, and a smaller secondary peak at 15–19 years of age (PHE 2013a).

- Most cases of meningococcal disease occur sporadically, with less than 5% of cases occurring in clusters. Outbreaks are rare but are more likely to occur amongst teenagers and young adults in schools, universities, and other educational and community settings such as nurseries.

- Meningococcal disease shows marked seasonal variation, with a peak in winter.

- Based on outer cell membrane and capsular polysaccharide antigens, meningococci are divided into distinct serogroups and the most common serogroups that cause disease worldwide are groups A, B, C, W135, X and Y (PHE 2012).

- Prior to the introduction of the Men C vaccine (1999), most disease in the UK was caused by serogroups B and C. The number of cases caused by serogroup C, however, has reduced significantly in all age groups since routine Men C vaccination was introduced. Serogroup B now accounts for 85–90% of all cases of meningococcal disease in infants and toddlers and 67% of all disease in England and Wales (PHE 2015).

11.1.3 **Risk factors for infection**

- Most cases of meningococcal infection are acquired through exposure to an asymptomatic carrier. *N. meningitidis* inhabits the mucosal membrane of the nose and throat, where it usually causes no harm. Up to 11% of a population may be asymptomatic carriers of the bacteria (Christensen et al. 2010).
- Specific risk factors for meningoccocal infection include:
  - smoking,
  - mucosal lesions,
  - concomitant respiratory infections,
  - age—the disease mainly affects young children, but is also common in older children and young adults,
  - living in closed or semi-closed communities (e.g. halls of residence), and
  - underlying health condition (e.g. asplenia/splenic dysfunction).

11.2 **What's the story?**

- A local hospital paediatrician has notified a case of an 11-month-old infant who has been unwell for three days with fever, drowsiness, refusing to feed, and a non-blanching rash.
- The paediatrician in consultation with a Health Protection Practitioner agrees this is a case of 'probable meningococcal septicaemia'.
- Samples have been taken from the infant and laboratory investigation to confirm the diagnosis is under way.
- The infant is being treated with antibiotics.

11.2.1 **Tools of the trade**

If meningococcal disease is suspected, samples of blood and/or cerebrospinal fluid (CSF) will usually be taken from the patient and sent for testing.

If *N. meningitidis* bacteria are present, they can be cultured or their DNA detected by polymerase chain reaction (PCR) testing. As well as confirming their presence, this is important for identifying the specific serogroup of the bacteria causing the infection.

To confirm a case, *N. meningitidis* must be isolated or DNA identified, from a part of the body which is normally sterile (e.g. blood or CSF), or a throat or eye swab of a clinical case.

11.2.2 **Top tips**

The following information should be provided by the professional making the notification:

- patient and GP details,
- admission details (place, time, consultant),

- basic clinical details including date of onset of signs and symptoms,
- relevant laboratory tests carried out and available results,
- whether the person was vaccinated against meningococcal disease,
- whether the patient was given penicillin before being admitted to hospital,
- current antibiotic treatment,
- if the case attends an educational establishment or child minder, and
- information on contacts.

This information is important for deciding on, and undertaking, the necessary public health actions.

11.2.3 **What immediate action(s) would you take?**

- The immediate action required will depend on whether the case is 'possible', 'probable', or 'confirmed'.

11.2.4 **Key scenario information**

Notified cases of meningococcal disease are classed as 'possible', 'probable', or 'confirmed', depending on the level of certainty in the diagnosis.

A case is *possible* when an alternative diagnosis is considered to be at least as likely (e.g. a viral infection may be considered equally, or more, likely).

A case is *probable* when alternative diagnoses are considered to be less likely, based on clinical symptoms and clinical opinion.

In *confirmed* cases the diagnosis has been proven by laboratory testing.

The classification of the case is based on discussions and agreement between the treating clinician and the Health Protection team with input from the microbiologist where appropriate.

- In the UK, public health action is only required for probable or confirmed cases of meningococcal disease (PHE 2012).
- As it has been agreed this is a probable case the following actions are required.
    - (a) Identify close contacts of the patient as soon as possible (see Box 11.1).
    - (b) Ensure close contacts receive the necessary prophylaxis as soon as possible (ideally within 24hrs, although there is some benefit in giving prophylaxis to contacts up to four weeks after the onset of symptoms in the case). The main aim of this is to reduce the number of secondary cases of meningococcal disease by reducing carriage, and thus transmission, of pathogenic strains of *N. meningitidis*.
    - (c) Ensure the case receives antibiotics that will also eliminate carriage (see Box 11.2).
    - (d) Arrange information for other relevant contacts of the case who do not require prophylaxis (including any worried well). For example, send a letter to nursery/school contacts.
    - (e) Arrange vaccination for the case, with their GP, where necessary. This is not urgent and is to protect against future infection for A, B, C, W135, and Y. This will depend on laboratory results, previous vaccination history, and underlying health conditions.
    - (f) Consider post-exposure vaccination of contacts depending on type of *meningococcus* (can be arranged up to four weeks after case onset).
- Groups A, Y, and W135—offer immunization to all close contacts.
- Group C—offer immunization unless they have completed immunization in the last 12 months.

- Group B: after a single case of invasive Group B meningococcal disease Men B vaccine should not routinely be offered to contacts (Ladhani et al. 2014). Ensure contacts born after 1 May 2015 are immunized as per the routine schedule.

   g) Regardless of the type of meningococcus in the index case recommend that any at-risk household contacts (asplenia, splenic dysfunction, or known complement deficiency) have received or are offered both the MenACWY conjugate vaccine and Men B vaccine.

Box 11.1 Close contacts at risk of meningitis and meningococcal infection

Close contacts include:

- those who have stayed overnight in the same house with the case in the seven days before the onset of initial symptoms,
- university students sharing a kitchen in a hall of residence,
- Boy/girlfriends, intimate kissing (not kissing on the cheek), and
- anyone who gave direct mouth-to-mouth resuscitation or those who had exposure to respiratory secretions of the patient into their conjunctivas or mucosal surfaces.

Those requiring additional consideration:

- child-minding contacts.

Those who won't normally be considered as close contacts, and do not routinely require prophylaxis include:

- playgroup/party/nursery/school/work contacts,
- those who sat in a car/plane with the case, and
- contacts of contacts.

Box 11.2 Antibiotics effective in reducing carriage of meningitis and meningococcal infection

The following antibiotics are effective in reducing carriage (reducing the risk of invasive disease for about 1 month):

- ciprofloxacin (a single dose and the treatment of choice, for contacts of all ages including pregnant women, unless contraindicated),
- rifampicin (two-day course), and
- ceftriaxone (has to be given by injection) (PHE 2012).

Ceftriaxone is often used to treat cases and will eradicate carriage. Cefotaxime is sometimes used to treat infection; however, it is not known if this is effective at reducing carriage. Therefore, cases treated with cefotaxime will also require prophylactic antibiotics.

11.3 **Scenario update # 1**

- Later in the day, the child deteriorates and has a respiratory arrest. The consultant paediatrician and an anaesthetist intubate (insert a tube to maintain an open airway) the child.
- Nursing staff who were in the room at the time (but did not assist with the intubation) request antibiotics to protect themselves. One of these staff is pregnant.

11.3.1 **What further action(s) would you take?**

- Only healthcare workers (HCWs) who have been exposed to visible respiratory droplets require prophylaxis. In this situation, therefore, only the consultant paediatrician and the anaesthetist may have been exposed and should be recommended prophylaxis if they have not used appropriate personal protective equipment (PPE). This is the employer's responsibility, usually via occupational health.
- All the remaining HCWs, including the pregnant woman, should be given information on meningococcal disease and reassurance. The Meningitis Now website is a useful resource https://www.meningitisnow.org/.

11.4 **Scenario update # 2**

- Unfortunately, the infant didn't survive.
- The laboratory result was reported as Group B *N. meningitidis*.
- Ten days after the death of the patient, a further case of meningitis has been reported from a local nursery.
- The infant who died had attended the same nursery two days per week. The nursery staff and parents are anxious and asking what actions they should take.

11.4.1 **Key scenario information**

- After one case in most settings, the risk of another case is always raised.
- Although the absolute risk to contacts is low, the risk to those living in the same household as the case is higher in the first 48hrs after presentation of the case (invasive disease develops in 1 in 300 of household contacts) and returns to background risk levels after four weeks (PHE 2012).
- Outside the household setting, the highest absolute risks are seen in the preschool setting and the lowest in the secondary school setting. In preschool, the risk is thought to be 1 in 1500 (Hastings et al. 1997). Preschool-aged children generally have less immunity to *meningococcus*.
- Children in the preschool age group are commonly colonized with *Neisseria lactamica*, which is believed to confer protection. Therefore, prophylaxis with antibiotics would also eradicate *Neisseria lactamica*, losing this protection.
- In the UK prophylaxis is not offered after a single case of meningococcal disease in an educational setting, but information is given to appropriate contacts.

11.4.2 **What further information do you need?**

- What is the diagnosis of the second case (possible, probable or confirmed meningococcal meningitis?). This is important in determining whether these two cases represent a true cluster. Cluster refers to two or more probable or confirmed cases with an epidemiological link which warrants further investigation.

- Check the dates of onset of illness in the two cases and nursery attendance in the seven days before.
- Clarify if there are any other links between the two cases.
- How many children attend the nursery and how closely do they mix?

11.4.3 **Tools of the trade**

11.4.3.1 Epidemiological investigation

This should include:

1. **Place**: where and what was the nature of contact between suspected cases/individuals?
2. **Person**: basic information about the individual (age, sex, etc.) and details of the individual including signs and symptoms, history of activity/movement in the period of interest.
3. **Time**: date of onset, timeline of illness, date and time of contact with other cases or individuals of interest.

11.4.3.2 Microbiological investigation

It is important to consider all relevant tests (nasopharyngeal swab, cerebrospinal fluid (CSF), PCR, and blood cultures), as identification of an isolate would help to prove or reject a link between cases.

11.4.3.3 Environmental investigation

This is key to defining and determining the context of the source or spread of the infection. In this case, the nursery class sizes, room arrangements, including the interrelation between classes, and the history of daily child and staff activity, would help to identify significant contacts.

11.5 **Scenario update # 3**

- The first case last attended nursery on 3 April and became unwell the same day.
- The second case has clinical signs of meningitis and Gram-negative *diplococci* (suggestive of *N. meningitidis*) have been grown from the sample of CSF. The date of onset was 13 April.
- Although the parents of the two cases know each other, they were not in social contact outside the setting of the nursery.
- The nursery has a total of 24 children divided into three classes: Babies (n = 6), Toddlers (n = 8), and Preschool (n = 10). Both cases were in the Babies class. All children who arrive early in the morning stay in the Toddlers classroom until 9am when they go to their separate classes. On sunny days the children may also play in the garden together, sharing toys, and this has occurred on several occasions in the last month.
- There is still no information whether the second case has Group B meningococcal disease.

11.5.1 **What further action(s) would you take?**

- All appropriate public health action would be undertaken for the new case as for the first.
- Although there is no laboratory confirmation of a link, it is reasonable and appropriate to presume that the second case is linked to the first on the basis that:
  - the second case has clinical symptoms of meningitis,
  - Gram-negative *diplococci* have been identified from CSF from the second case, and this makes *N. meningitidis as* most likely cause, although it cannot be confirmed until the organism is isolated. Please note, PHE guidance (PHE 2012) would deem this as a confirmed case,

- the second child developed symptoms ten days after the first, and
- the nursery provides a confirmed epidemiological link.

◆ The next step is to undertake a public health risk assessment in order to identify any high-risk group(s).

◆ As there are now two linked (one probable and one confirmed) cases from the same educational establishment this would be deemed a cluster. It would be useful to consider establishing an Incident or Outbreak Control Team (OCT) in order to coordinate a multi-agency approach.

◆ Depending on the quality and completeness of the information obtained for undertaking the risk assessment, the experience and judgement of the individual in charge of the situation, or the views of the OCT, one of the following options may be considered appropriate.

  - Option 1: providing chemoprophylaxis for the whole nursery, including staff, if the mixing between the Babies, Toddlers, and Preschool classes is considered significant.
  - Option 2: limiting chemoprophylaxis to the Babies' class and staff only, if the mixing between the different nursery classes is considered minimum and insignificant.
  - Option 3: providing chemoprophylaxis with Men B vaccination for the whole nursery, including staff, if the mixing between the Babies, Toddlers, and Preschool classes is considered significant.
  - Option 4: limiting chemoprophylaxis and Men B vaccination to the Babies class and staff only, if the mixing between the different nursery classes is considered minimum and insignificant.

11.5.2 **Key scenario information**

There are both pros and cons to be considered when deciding who should receive prophylaxis and vaccination.

Over-treatment may clear carriage of protective strains, expose people to unnecessary side effects, and increase the potential of inducing antibiotic resistance.

On the other hand, limiting chemoprophylaxis and vaccination to the most at-risk individuals may cause considerable anxiety, particularly among parents of children not receiving antibiotics in a nursery or school outbreak.

◆ Whichever option is chosen, further information should be provided to all parents as soon as possible (normally via letter), so that those at risk are reminded of the symptoms to look out for and any new cases will be more likely to seek early medical attention.

◆ A holding press statement should be prepared for use as required.

11.5.3 **Top tips**

Remember that there is a need to act quickly and prioritize the most important public health actions—prophylaxis should ideally be given within 24hrs to those who are considered to be at high risk. Early consultation with national experts to discuss the risk assessment, available options and priority actions is essential. For vaccine recommendations see Table 11.1.

11.6 **Scenario update # 4**

◆ The media have found out about the story. The press are suggesting that there is an epidemic of meningitis in the area and they have just contacted your department asking what is being done about it.

11.6.1 **How would you respond to the media enquiry?**

◆ Prepare a press statement in liaison with public relations/communications staff.

◆ Give only confirmed information.

◆ Respect confidentiality—do not give any identifiable patient information.

◆ Stick to the facts—do not speculate.

◆ Give key messages:
  - The risk of transmission to contacts is low.
  - Antibiotics and vaccination are being given only to children/staff at higher risk.
  - It is important to avoid causing alarm.

11.6.2 **Top tips**

Before speaking to the media, make sure that you are the appropriate person to do so—your department may have a nominated media/communications officer whose role is to deal with the media.

If you are nominated to speak to the media, make sure that you are prepared with your key messages and have checked that all the relevant information is correct and up to date.

11.7 **What if ... ?**

11.7.1 **There were further cases of meningococcal disease from the same nursery?**

◆ It is important to determine if the cases are all of the same strain and the likely exposure setting of the cases is the nursery. However, if one is a confirmed case and others probable, with typing unknown as yet, they are treated as linked.

◆ If there is no evidence the cases are of different strains, at least one is confirmed, and exposure setting is likely to be the nursery, an Outbreak Control Team will definitely need to be convened, if this was not done previously, and all public health interventions implemented as soon as possible.

◆ Option 1 is now likely to be the immediate action, i.e. providing chemoprophylaxis for the whole nursery (n = 24), including staff, followed by consideration of option 3 or 4 (Men B vaccination), which is less urgent.

11.7.2 **The cases were from a school/college/university?**

◆ The same response to that of a nursery case will be followed.

◆ Guidance recommends that in college/university halls of residence those who share a kitchen are considered as close contacts (PHE 2012). However, living arrangements are often fluid and residential places will need to be considered on individual case circumstances.

11.7.3 **The cases were from a community?**

◆ It is much more difficult to determine a community outbreak of meningococcal disease.

◆ Seek expert input (Consultant Regional Epidemiologist in the UK) early in order to determine the case definition in terms of place, person, and time, the geographical boundary of the denominator population, and the background incidence rate (from surveillance data base) for a defined time period (usually a year), defined population and geographical area.

◆ In the UK a community meningococcal disease incidence rate of higher than 40/100,000 can be used to indicate an outbreak (PHE 2013a).

11.7.4 The cases were infected with *Haemophilus influenzae* Type B (HiB) instead of *N. meningitidis*?

◆ Infection with *Haemophilus influenzae* Type B can present as meningitis (60%), epiglottitis (15%), bacteraemia (10%); other complications include pneumonia, pericarditis, cellulitis, joint and bone pains.

◆ The principle of chemoprophylaxis for close contacts is similar to meningococcal disease but there are important differences (PHE 2013b) (see 'HiB SIMCARD' p. 314)

11.8 Unanswered questions around meningococcal disease

◆ Although the absolute risk of meningococcal disease is low, we still do not know if the balance of risks and benefits is favourable to widespread prophylaxis. This would require a further evidence base such as a cluster-randomized trial, i.e. a trial in which schools rather than individuals would be randomly allocated to the intervention or control group. In general, UK guidelines on public health management of meningococcal disease are based on observational studies and there are still some grey areas that require judgement. Therefore, when in doubt, early consultation with national PHE experts is essential.

11.9 Lessons learned

◆ The early features of meningococcal disease are non-specific and can be misdiagnosed by healthcare professionals. The disease progresses rapidly and the classical features occur late or near death.

◆ Although the absolute risk to contacts is low, the risk to those living in the same household as the case is higher in the first 48hrs after presentation.

◆ Clusters in educational settings are rare, but when they occur they cause considerable public anxiety, and the value of communicating information early with concerned pupils, parents/guardians, and staff should not be underestimated.

11.10 Further thinking

◆ In addition to promoting immunization against meningococcal disease, what can be done to reduce or prevent future meningococcal disease clusters/outbreaks?

◆ How can we use vaccination uptake rates and surveillance data to predict clusters or outbreaks?

◆ What are the roles of different professionals and organizations in the public health management of meningococcal disease?

◆ How can evidence-based public health risk assessment be strengthened?

References

Christensen H, M May, L Bowen, et al. 2010 Meningococcal carriage by age: a systematic review and meta-analysis. *Lancet Infectious Diseases*, 10(12): 853–61. doi: 10.1016/S1473-3099(10)70251–6

Hastings L, J Stuart, N Andrews et al. 1997. A retrospective survey of clusters of meningococcal disease in England and Wales, 1993 to 1995: estimated risks of further cases in household and educational settings. *Communicable Disease Report: CDR Review*, 7(13): R195–R200.

Ladhani SN, R Cordery, S Mandal et al. 2014. *Preventing secondary cases of invasive meningococcal capsular group B (MenB) disease: benefits of offering vaccination in addition to antibiotic chemoprophylaxis to close contacts of cases in the household, educational setting, clusters and the wider community.* Version 1.1. https://www.gov.uk/government/publications/invasive-meningococcus-capsular-group-b-menb-preventing-secondary-cases (accessed 8 March 2016).

PHE. 2012. *Guidelines for public health management of meningococcal disease in the UK.* https://www.gov.uk/government/publications/meningococcal-disease-guidance-on-public-health-management (accessed 8 March 2016).

PHE. 2013a. *Meningococcal: Immunisation against infectious disease - The Green Book, Chapter 22,* https://www.gov.uk/government/publications/meningococcal-the-green-book-chapter-22 (accessed 8 March 2016).

PHE. 2013b. *Haemophilus influenzae type b (Hib): revised recommendations for the prevention of secondary cases.* https://www.gov.uk/government/publications/haemophilus-influenzae-type-b-hib-revised-recommendations-for-the-prevention-of-secondary-cases (accessed 8 March 2016).

PHE. 2015. Invasive meningococcal disease (laboratory reports in England): 2013/2014 annual data by epidemiological year. *Health Protection Weekly Report: Infection Report*, 9(3). https://www.gov.uk/government/uploads/system/uploads/attachment_data/file/397913/hpr0315_imd.pdf (accessed 8 March 2016).

Viner MR, R Booy, H Johnson et al. 2012. Outcomes of invasive meningococcal serogroup B disease in children and adolescents (MOSAIC): a case-control study. *Lancet Neurology*, 11(9): 774–83.

Further reading

Cartwright VAK, D Hunt, A Fox. 1995. Chemoprophylaxis fails to prevent a second case of meningococcal disease in a day nursery. *Communicable Disease Report: CDR Review*, 5(13): R199.

Chatt C, R Gajraj, J Hawker, et al. 2014. Four-month outbreak of invasive meningococcal disease caused by a rare serogroup B strain, identified through the use of molecular PorA subtyping, England, 2013. *Eurosurveillance*, 19(44).

Hawker J, N Begg, I Blair, et al. (eds). 2012. *Communicable Disease Control and Health Protection Handbook*, 3rd edition. London: John Wiley & Sons.

Heymann LD (ed). 2014. *Control of Communicable Diseases Manual.* 20th edition. Washington, DC: American Public Health Association.

Stewart A, N Coetzee, E Knapper, et al. 2013. Public health action and mass chemoprophylaxis in response to a small meningococcal infection outbreak at a nursery in the West Midlands, England. *Perspectives in Public Health*, 133(2): 104–109.

Universities UK. 2004. *Managing meningococcal disease (septicaemia or meningitis) in higher education institutions.* http://www.universitiesuk.ac.uk/highereducation/Pages/MeningitisGuidelines.aspx (accessed 8 March 2016).

Table 11.1 Vaccine recommendations following cases of probable or confirmed invasive meningococcal disease

Table 11.1 Vaccine recommendations in response to cases of probable or confirmed invasive meningococcal disease

Confirmed Serogroup	Any serogroup/probable cases	Group C	Group A, Y or W135	Men B
Index Case	Recommend MenC containing conjugate vaccine to unimmunized index cases <25 years old. Recommended Men B vaccine for all unimmunized or partially immunized individuals under age 2 who were born after 1 May 2015. Unimmunized, or incompletely immunized for age cases in a risk group for meningococcal disease (e.g. asplenia, complement deficiency) should be offered, or complete the recommended immunization course of MenACWY and Men B conjugate vaccines.	A booster dose of Men C containing conjugate vaccine is required for previously immunized cases.	Unimmunized, or incompletely immunized for age, index cases in a risk group for meningococcal disease (e.g. asplenia, complement deficiency) should be offered, or complete the recommended immunization course of MenACWY conjugate vaccine. Those who received the vaccine more than 12 months previously should receive an extra dose of MenACWY conjugate vaccine.	Unimmunized, or incompletely immunized for age, index cases under age 2 years, born after 1 May 2015, or of any age who are in a risk group for meningococcal disease (e.g. asplenia, complement deficiency) should be offered, or complete the recommended immunization course of Men B vaccine (Bexsero®).
Close Contacts	Recommend MenC containing conjugate vaccine to unimmunized close contacts < 25 years old. Recommended Men B vaccine for all unimmunized or partially immunized individuals under age 2 who were born after 1 May 2015. Unimmunized, or incompletely immunized for age contacts in a risk group for meningococcal disease (e.g. asplenia, complement deficiency) should be offered, or complete the recommended immunization course of MenACWY and Men B conjugate vaccines.	Those unimmunized or partially immunized should complete the course with MenC containing vaccine. Contacts who were only immunized in infancy and those who completed the recommended immunization course (including the 12-month booster or the Men ACWY adolescent booster) more than one year before should be offered an extra dose of MenC containing vaccine.	Recommend appropriate course of Men ACWY conjugate vaccine (up to 4 weeks after) to close contacts of any age. For probable cases with A, W135 or Y cultured from nasopharyngeal swab, the quadrivalent conjugate vaccine should be offered to close contacts of any age.	Offer or complete recommended course of Men B vaccine for unimmunized or incompletely immunized contacts under age 2 born after 1 May 2015. After a single case Men B vaccine should **not** be routinely offered to other household contacts. If a second MenB case occurs in the same family, Men B vaccine should be offered for all household contacts even if the interval between the two cases is >30 days.

(Continued)

Table 11.1 Continued

Confirmed Serogroup	Any serogroup/probable cases	Group C	Group A, Y or W135	Men B
Educational Setting Contacts: **One case**	Recommend MenC containing conjugate vaccine for all unimmunized individuals <25 years old. Recommended Men B vaccine for all unimmunized or partially immunized individuals under age 2 who were born after 1 May 2015. Recommended that unimmunized, or incompletely immunized for age individuals in a risk group for meningococcal disease (e.g. asplenia, complement deficiency) receive the recommended immunization course of MenACWY and Men B conjugate vaccines.	Recommend MenC containing conjugate vaccine for all unimmunized individuals <25 years old i.e., as part of the routine immunization programme.	Men ACWY vaccine should not be routinely offered to contacts after a single case of confirmed group ACW or Y disease in an educational setting. It is recommended that unimmunized, or incompletely immunized for age, individuals in a risk group for meningococcal disease (e.g. asplenia, complement deficiency) should complete the recommended immunization course of MenACWY conjugate vaccine.	Men B vaccine should not be routinely offered to contacts after a single case of confirmed or probable Group B disease in an educational setting unless it is recommended as part of routine immunization schedule to individuals under age 2 who were born after 1 May 2015 and are unimmunized or incompletely immunized. It is also recommended that unimmunized, or incompletely immunized for age, individuals in a risk group for meningococcal disease (e.g. asplenia, complement deficiency) should complete the recommended immunization course of Men B conjugate vaccine.
Educational Setting contacts: **Cluster**	Recommend MenC containing conjugate vaccine for all unimmunized individuals <25 years old. Recommended Men B vaccine for all unimmunized or partially immunized individuals under age 2 who were born after 1 May 2015. Recommended that unimmunized, or incompletely immunized for age individuals in a risk-group for meningococcal disease (e.g. asplenia, complement deficiency) receive the recommended immunization course of MenACWY and Men B conjugate vaccines.	MenC containing conjugate vaccine should be offered to all previously unimmunized individuals who were offered antibiotics. If the cluster involves MenC conjugate vaccine failures, further investigation may be required.	Men ACWY conjugate vaccine should be offered to all individuals of any age who were offered antibiotics.	Following confirmation of a Men B cluster, Men B vaccine should be offered to the same group that would receive antibiotic chemoprophylaxis as soon as practically possible unless they are fully immunized against MenB.

Chapter 12

Tuberculosis

Musarrat Afza, Marko Petrovic,
and Sam Ghebrehewet

OVERVIEW

After reading this chapter the reader will be familiar with:

- the clinical presentation, risk factors and brief epidemiology of tuberculosis (TB),
- the public health response to a single case of TB in the community,
- the public health response to one or more cases of TB in an educational setting, and
- the investigation and control of TB in the healthcare or occupational setting.

Terms

Mycobacterium tuberculosis (MTB) complex Organisms causing latent TB infection (LTBI) and TB disease. The important members of the complex are *Mycobacterium tuberculosis* (causes most TB disease), *M. bovis*, and *M. africanum*.

Mycobacteria other than tuberculosis Do not belong to the MTB complex; also referred to as 'environmental' or 'atypical' mycobacteria. They may cause disease that clinically resembles TB, but that is not usually transmissible person-to-person.

Sputum-smear-positive TB (sometimes called 'open' or 'infectious' TB) Pulmonary TB in which mycobacteria are present in a smear of sputum examined under a microscope usually stained with Ziehl-Neelsen stain to look for acid and alcohol fast bacilli (AAFB/AFB).

Active TB Disease caused by a member of the MTB complex family; it is determined by positive smear or culture from any part of the body or when there is sufficient radiographic, clinical, or laboratory evidence to support a diagnosis for which treatment is indicated.

Latent TB infection (LTBI) Individuals with evidence of infection with MTB complex but without symptoms or signs of disease. Such individuals may be at risk of progressing to active TB disease and may be offered treatment.

Culture Growing mycobacteria in the laboratory from patient specimens. It enables:

- ◆ confirmation of TB disease (culture-confirmed case) (MTB complex),
- ◆ confirmation of the species of mycobacteria,
- ◆ drug sensitivity testing, which will guide appropriate treatment, and
- ◆ strain typing, which helps determine if the isolate is part of a cluster.

BCG (Bacille Calmette-Guèrin) Live TB vaccine.

Tuberculin A reagent which is derived from inactivated TB bacilli and is used to perform the tuberculin skin test (TST or Mantoux test).

Interferon-gamma release assay (IGRA) Test measuring immune reaction to *M. tuberculosis*.

Anti-Tuberculosis Treatment (ATT) The treatment for active TB is usually given in two phases: an initial four-drug course (isoniazid, rifampicin, pyrazinamide, ethambutol) for two months, then isoniazid and rifampicin alone for a further four months or longer. For LTBI the standard treatment is six to nine months.

Chemoprophylaxis Treatment of LTBI to prevent progression to TB disease or isoniazid prophylaxis to prevent disease in exposed children.

Directly observed therapy (DOT) Patient observed taking each and every dose of their TB treatment. Usually applied in the UK only to patients in risk groups (previously non-adherent to treatment, those with multi-drug resistant (MDR) TB).

(See further list of terms in the Glossary.)

12.1 Background facts: tuberculosis

12.1.1 What is tuberculosis?

Tuberculosis (TB) is a communicable disease caused by bacilli belonging to the MTB complex. It can affect any part of the body but most commonly affects the lungs (pulmonary TB). Pulmonary TB can be infectious, while extra-pulmonary TB (e.g. lymph node TB) is not infectious.

TB is spread when patients with pulmonary TB cough, sneeze, sing, or talk, resulting in the production of droplets containing MTB complex bacilli. When droplets are inhaled, TB infection may be established.

TB is usually not easy to catch: only about 30% of exposed individuals become infected. Of these, only 5–10% will develop early disease. In the remaining 90–95%, the infection is contained (latent TB). About 10% of patients in whom the infection is contained will reactivate later in life if their immune system is weakened by a medical condition or certain drug treatments (Chaisson and Nachega 2003).

12.1.2 Epidemiology of TB

Globally in 2013, there were an estimated nine million new cases of TB and 1.5 million deaths from the disease. More than half (56%) of the new cases were in the South-East Asia and Western Pacific Regions and around a quarter of cases were in the African Region (WHO 2014).

In the UK, the incidence of TB is 12.3/100,000 population. Around three-quarters (73%) of TB cases occurred in people born outside the UK, with only 15% diagnosed within two years of entering the UK. TB remains concentrated in the most deprived populations and in large, urban areas with London accounting for the highest proportion of cases in the UK (PHE 2014).

12.1.3 Clinical signs and symptoms of TB

General symptoms of TB include:

- fever,
- night sweats, which can be severe (enough to soak the bedsheets),
- poor appetite and loss of weight, and
- severe tiredness and lack of energy.

Pulmonary TB may also, present with:

◆ cough for more than three weeks,

◆ coughing up phlegm that might be bloody, and

◆ shortness of breath.

Other symptoms of TB depend on which part of the body is affected (e.g. swelling of neck lymph nodes or blood in the urine).

12.1.4 Risk factors for infection and disease

Transmission of TB usually requires close prolonged contact with an infectious case. Risk factors for progression from LTBI to active disease include:

◆ HIV positive,

◆ solid organ transplantation,

◆ blood cancer,

◆ gastrectomy or jejuno-ileal bypass,

◆ chronic kidney failure or on haemodialysis,

◆ treatment with anti-tumour necrosis factor-alpha, steroids, or any other immuno-suppressive drug,

◆ silicosis,

◆ extremes of age: very young children or the elderly,

◆ diabetes,

◆ people who are dependent on drugs or alcohol, and

◆ people with chronic poor health.

12.1.5 Confirming TB diagnosis

Diagnosis is confirmed by culture, histology, or molecular tests on sputum or other clinical samples. Standard culture is slow, taking 6–12 weeks, compared to liquid culture which can take 2–3 weeks. With molecular tests based on targeted amplification using polymerase chain reaction (PCR) of specific fragments of the *M. tuberculosis* genome, results can be obtained within 1–2 days (PHE 2013).

For diagnosing LTBI, tuberculin skin test (TST) or IGRA tests are done for those aged 65 years or younger, followed by assessment of active TB for contacts who test positive (NICE 2016).

In addition to culture or molecular testing on aspirate from lymph nodes or cerebrospinal, peritoneal or pleural fluids, extrapulmonary TB can be confirmed by characteristic histopathological features in a biopsy specimen.

12.2 What's the story? Part I

◆ A college student presented to a local GP with a history of weight loss and intermittent cough for a few months and was prescribed a course of antibiotics twice. When symptoms did not improve, a chest X-ray (CXR) was done which showed cavitation in the lungs.

◆ The case was referred to the local chest physician for further investigation. Pending sputum culture, the consultant decided that TB was the most likely diagnosis as the case was from a high-incidence area, and started a full course of anti-tuberculosis treatment (ATT). The consultant contacted the relevant public health body for advice, due to the possibility of a large number of contacts.

12.2.1 **Tools of the trade**

Determining how infectious the case is likely to be based on:

◆ History of productive cough and presence of high number of AFBs in sputum samples (three early morning sputum samples should be obtained to aid the diagnosis of pulmonary TB).

◆ The CXR appearance, especially the presence of cavities, increases the probability that the case is infectious.

12.2.2 **Top tips**

The following information should be obtained from the TB clinicians:

◆ patient and GP details,

◆ admission details if relevant (place, time, consultant),

◆ clinical details including date of onset of symptoms, especially productive cough,

◆ radiological and laboratory results if available,

◆ history of BCG vaccination,

◆ occupational/school history and date last attended. Check whether the patient was symptomatic whilst at work/nursery/school/college,

◆ history of recent travel to high-incidence TB countries or family origin from a high TB incidence country, and social risk factors for TB disease e.g., current or previous injecting drug use, homelessness, alcohol misuse etc., and

◆ information on household and other contacts.

12.2.3 **What immediate action(s) would you take?**

◆ Check results of the sputum smear or PCR test.

◆ Get a full history from the TB control nurse.

◆ Assess risk of transmission based on how infectious the case is likely to be.

◆ Identify possible contacts of the case.

12.2.4 **Key scenario information**

TB surveillance depends on notification of suspected and culture-confirmed cases. A suspected case is one that, in the absence of culture confirmation, meets the following criteria:

◆ A clinician's judgement that the patient's clinical and/or radiological signs and/or symptoms are compatible with tuberculosis,

AND

◆ A clinician's decision to treat the patient with a full course of anti-tuberculosis therapy.

Note: Two weeks of treatment render most cases of TB non-infectious.

12.2.4.1 The main objectives of TB contact tracing are to:

◆ identify, diagnose and treat individuals infected but without evidence of disease, i.e. LTBI,

◆ identify associated cases of active TB,

◆ detect a source, and

◆ identify candidates for BCG vaccination.

12.2.4.2 Individuals who should be classed as 'close contacts' include:

- people who live in the same household with the case, i.e. those sharing a bedroom, kitchen, bathroom or sitting room with the index case during their potentially infectious period.
- close associates such as boyfriend or girlfriend, and
- frequent visitors to the home of the case.

Usually, the above contacts are classified as close contacts only if they have had a cumulative exposure time of more than 8hrs to a symptomatic TB case, although this is not an absolute rule.

12.2.5 **Top tips**

Screening should be offered to the household/close contacts of any person with pulmonary or laryngeal TB (NICE 2016). Priority should be given to contacts of those index cases who are considered highly infectious or where there are susceptible contacts (e.g. children under 5 or HIV-positive individuals).

12.3 **Scenario update # 1**

- Three consecutive sputum samples were AFB positive.
- Sputum PCR test was positive for TB.
- The student had a productive cough whilst at college. The family moved to the UK from India five years ago.
- They all received BCG vaccination in childhood.
- Two younger teenage siblings and parents were asymptomatic.
- Both parents had normal CXR (TST/IGRA was not done as they were both over 35 years of age and neither were healthcare workers, as per NICE 2011 guidance).

12.3.1 **What further action(s) would you take?**

- Because there is evidence that the case has been attending the college whilst being potentially infectious with TB, an Incident Control Team (ICT) meeting should be convened as soon as possible in order to agree how to proceed with screening at the college (see Chapter 20).
- ICT will need to determine the nature and extent of the incident, and aim to:
  - identify, screen, and offer treatment to potentially source individuals,
  - prevent and control further spread,
  - ensure sufficient resources are available to manage the incident,
  - undertake risk assessment and decide on appropriate contact screening in the college,
  - ensure timely and appropriate communication with students, staff, media, and other stakeholders, as appropriate,
  - manage internal and external communications, and
  - ensure appropriate follow-up of all contacts including monitoring of screening results, and implementation of relevant clinical and public health actions.

12.4 **Scenario update # 2**

- ◆ Culture was positive for *Mycobacterium tuberculosis* after two weeks on rapid liquid culture.
- ◆ The two siblings had a positive IGRA test and were referred for assessment of active TB disease. Their chest X-rays were normal and they were started on treatment for LTBI.
- ◆ The case is responding well to treatment and would be returning to college after two weeks of therapy.

12.4.1 **What further action(s) would you take?**

As the two siblings had LTBI with no evidence of active TB disease, no public health action is indicated in the school they attend.

12.4.2 **Top tips**

It is possible that the head of the school attended by the case's siblings may express concern. These enquiries are normally dealt with by the TB control nurse who would have reassured the school that the siblings pose no risk of transmission of TB in school.

12.4.3 **Key scenario information**

TB risk from contact with an infectious person (Musher 2003):

None known	1 in 100,000
Casual social contact	1 in 100,000
School, workplace	1 in 50 to 1 in 3
Bar, social club	Up to 1 in 10
Dormitory	1 in 5
Home	1 in 3
Nursing home	1 in 20

12.5 **Scenario update #3**

- ◆ There are 2000 students in at the index case's college. The case attended one class of 20 students taught by three lecturers for 30hrs a week.
- ◆ The case did not partake in extracurricular activities and this class did not have significant interaction with other students in the college.

12.5.1 **What further action(s) would you take?**

- ◆ The ICT should consider screening of staff and students attending the same class.
  - • All students and staff under 35 were offered IGRA testing (all tested negative).
  - • Staff over 35 were offered a CXR. (One member of staff born in a country with high TB prevalence had an abnormal CXR and was referred to TB service for further investigations. This person did not have a cough but had enlarged neck lymph glands. The tissue from the glands tested positive for TB on culture, and strain typing was undertaken. The strain type was different from that of the student.)

12.5.2 **Key scenario information**

Public health action is usually undertaken only for cumulative exposure of more than 8hrs, although this is not an absolute threshold and action should depend on local risk assessment. In some cases shorter exposure may prompt public health action in response to a highly infectious case or where contacts are particularly susceptible as in hospital settings.

Screening outside the household should always start with those who have had the greatest exposure to the case in the period during which the case was symptomatic (ripples from 'stone in the pond' principle). Those with lesser degrees of contact should usually only be screened if transmission has been demonstrated amongst those with closer contact. There should be a lower threshold for screening contacts that are more susceptible to TB (NICE 2011, NICE 2016).

The screening will include some or all of the following:

◆ completing a questionnaire that includes questions about symptoms, risk factors, BCG vaccination history, and

◆ TST and/or IGRA blood test and chest X-ray.

12.5.3 **Tools of the trade**

The ICT should consider the findings of the following:

◆ **Epidemiological investigation**: the nature of contact between the case and exposed individuals.

◆ **Microbiological investigation**: consider all sample types (sputum, bronchoalveolar aspirate, biopsy specimens); if further cases are identified, molecular typing or whole genome sequencing may help to support or refute a link.

◆ **Environmental investigation**: the context/setting of the spread of the infection. In this case relevant information includes the size of classroom, amount of ventilation, and presence of air cleaning systems.

12.6 **Scenario update # 4**

◆ No student or staff member appears to have acquired infection from the index case.

12.7 **What's the story? Part II**

◆ A local hospital's microbiologist telephoned local public health body/local health protection team regarding an adult admitted to the intensive care unit (ICU) three days previously, in respiratory failure.

◆ The patient was admitted to a respiratory ward three weeks earlier, after being unwell and pyrexial.

◆ The patient was treated for pneumonia as his CXR showed left-sided shadowing and left-sided pleural effusion.

◆ A sputum sample, which was sent one week ago, was then reported positive for AFB; a full course of ATT was started.

12.7.1 **What immediate action(s) would you take?**

In addition to the information to be gathered on notification of a case (specified in section 12.2.2):

◆ If not already done, recommend isolation of the patient in a single room or negative pressure room, if available.

◆ Instigate contact tracing in the hospital.

12.7.2 **Top tips**

In the hospital setting the infection prevention and control team (IPCT) has a lead role in managing the public health investigation and in ensuring all infection control measures are observed. Health protection professionals will offer support.

12.8 **Scenario Part II update # 1**

The patient had:

◆ a history of inflammatory bowel disease and had been immunosuppressed due to treatment,

◆ a cough for approximately six weeks before admission to hospital,

◆ worked in the family business: a slaughterhouse (abattoir), and

◆ grown up on a local beef cattle farm and consumed unpasteurized milk.

PCR test on sputum was positive for MTB.

Unfortunately, the patient died three days later in the ICU.

12.8.1 **What further action(s) would you take?**

◆ Convene an ICT (see Chapter 20) to lead and oversee the community aspect of public health management of the incident.

◆ Coordinate identification of patients and staff exposed in the ICU and ward through the hospital IPCT.

12.9 **Scenario Part II update # 2**

◆ Culture results confirmed *Mycobacterium bovis* (*M.bovis*) infection.

◆ The patient's spouse (aged 49) and three teenage children were screened. The children tested positive on IGRA and were started on treatment for LTBI. The spouse is currently asymptomatic with non-specific changes on CXR, which is to be repeated at a later date.

◆ The TB control nurse was contacted by several work contacts as they were concerned about catching TB. They wanted to know from where the case had acquired TB. They were particularly concerned as this abattoir took TB-infected cattle for slaughter.

12.9.1 **Key scenario information**

◆ Human infection with *M. bovis* can cause TB that is clinically and pathologically indistinguishable from that caused by *M. tuberculosis*.

◆ *M. bovis* is usually transmitted to humans by infected milk, although it can also spread via aerosol droplets.

◆ In the UK cattle are randomly tested for the disease and immediately culled if infected, but can still be used for human consumption.

◆ In areas of the developing world where pasteurization is not routine, *M. bovis* is a more common cause of human tuberculosis.

◆ Person-to-person spread is possible.

◆ The source may remain unknown.

12.9.2 **What further action(s) would you take?**

◆ The ICT will consider and decide whether or not to instigate wider TB screening of the workplace, extended close and social contacts, and hospital contacts.

12.9.3 **Tools of the trade**

The ICT should consider epidemiological, microbiological and environmental findings as for *Mycobacterium tuberculosis* cases (see section 12.5.3).

In this case, further relevant information includes the size of workspace, and slaughter house practices that result in exposure to bovine TB through aerosol generation.

12.9.4 **Top tips**

It would be useful to prepare a holding press statement in agreement with key stakeholders to ensure that consistent and accurate information is shared with the public.

It would also be useful to nominate the communications lead/spokesperson from the ICT.

12.10 **Scenario Part II update # 3**

◆ Four out of the ten workplace contacts were screened.
◆ Six hospital staff who were exposed during aerosol generating procedures on the patient and five patients were identified for screening.
◆ All four work contacts were asymptomatic and tested negative on IGRA.
◆ The spouse of the case developed clinical TB during follow up for LTBI. She did not work in the family business.
◆ Molecular typing showed that the spouse had an identical strain of bovine TB as the case, suggesting person-to-person transmission in the household setting.
◆ One out of the six hospital staff identified as contacts screened positive for LTBI, and had worked in, and immigrated from, a country with high TB prevalence.
◆ The hospital IPCT concluded that the member of staff who tested positive had TB risk factors independent of this case.
◆ Three out of the five patients identified as close contacts tested negative for TB. Two had died from unrelated reasons.

12.10.1 **What further action(s) would you take?**

The ICT would need to make conclusions after reviewing the whole outbreak.

◆ The ICT considered the results of screening and concluded that there was no evidence of onward transmission from the case to those exposed at the workplace. They decided that contact tracing was not to be extended to the remainder of abattoir workers.
◆ The ICT concluded that the case had reactivation of TB as a result of immunosuppression due to treatment for other conditions. It was considered possible that the case had originally acquired TB infection through the work environment (farmer/abattoir worker).

12.10.2 **Top tips**

Patients whose strain types are genetically indistinguishable may be part of a chain of transmission; this needs epidemiological investigation.

12.11 **Scenario Part II update # 4**

- The media have found out about the story. The press is suggesting that a farmer has acquired TB from cattle. They are concerned about the safety of meat from the infected cattle for human consumption.

12.11.1 **How would you respond to the media enquiry?**

Issue the multi-agency press statement agreed by the ICT, ensuring that there is a lead public relations/communications contact point identified.

- Give only confirmed information.
- Respect confidentiality—don't give away any patient-identifying information.
- Stick to the facts—don't get drawn into speculation!
- Give the following key messages:
  - The risk of transmission of TB from cattle to humans is very low.
  - TB is a treatable disease.
  - Employees in the abattoir are being screened for TB.
  - Meat from TB-infected cattle is safe for human consumption.
  - The Health and Safety Executive (HSE) are reviewing practices in the abattoir.

12.12 **What if ... ?**

12.12.1 **There are further cases of TB identified in the hospital or occupational setting?**

- It is important to determine if the cases were exposed to the index case whilst he was symptomatic and if the strain types are indistinguishable or different. If some/all of the isolates are of the same strain, and the exposure is likely to be the hospital or occupational setting, the ICT needs to be re-convened (as an Outbreak Control Team; see Chapter 20) to consider further public health investigations and extended screening.

12.13 **Lessons learned**

- It is important to adhere to the 'stone-in-the-pond' approach for screening of contacts of a TB case. Wider screening should be limited to a clearly defined group of non-household contacts.
- Inappropriate and unnecessary screening can create wider anxiety as TB diagnosis is still associated with stigma.
- The probability of identifying LTBI that may be unlinked to the cases concerned is high in TB endemic areas/regions, making interpretation of the results difficult.

12.14 **Further thinking**

- What can be done to improve TB prevention and control in the UK?
- How can we reduce or prevent future TB clusters/outbreaks?

◆ Is there a need for a national strategy with regard to identification and treatment of LTBI? If so, how would the strategy ensure the screening of all at-risk individuals, i.e. including those not registered with a GP or who do not have contact with the NHS?

◆ What are the hallmarks of an effective national TB screening programme for visitors/immigrants from TB-endemic areas/countries/regions?

References

Chaisson RE, J Nachega. 2003. Tuberculosis. In *Oxford Textbook of Medicine*, edited by DA Warrell, TM Cox, JD Firth et al. Oxford: Oxford University Press.

NICE (National Institute for Health and Care Excellence). 2011. *Clinical Guideline 117: Tuberculosis: Clinical Diagnosis and Management of Tuberculosis, and Measures for its Prevention and Control.* http://www.nice.org.uk/guidance/cg117 (accessed 8 March 2016).

NICE. 2016. *Tuberculosis NICE Guideline.* https://www.nice.org.uk/guidance/ng33 (accessed 8 March 2016).

Musher D. 2003. How Contagious Are Common Respiratory Tract Infections? *New England Journal of Medicine*, 348: 1256–66.

Public Health England (PHE). 2013. *Position Statement: Direct Molecular Testing for Tuberculosis in England, Scotland and Wales.* https://www.gov.uk/government/uploads/system/uploads/attachment_data/file/326133/Position_statement_Direct_molecular_testing_for_tuberculosis_in_England_Scotland_and_Wales_July_2013.pdf (accessed 8 March 2016).

PHE. 2014. *Tuberculosis in the UK. 2014 Report.* https://www.gov.uk/government/uploads/system/uploads/attachment_data/file/360335/TB_Annual_report__4_0_300914.pdf (accessed 8 March 2016).

World Health Organization (WHO). 2014. *Global Tuberculosis Report.* http://www.who.int/tb/publications/global_report/en/ (accessed 8 March 2016).

Further reading

Davies PDO, SB Gordon, G Davies (eds). 2014. *Clinical Tuberculosis.* 5th edition. London: CRC Press.

Fallahi-Sichani M, JL Flynn, JJ Linderman, et al. 2012. Differential risk of tuberculosis reactivation among anti-TNF therapies is due to drug binding kinetics and permeability. *Journal of Immunology*, 188(7): 3169–78.

Hawker J, N Begg, I Blair, et al. (eds). 2012. *Communicable Disease Control and Health Protection Handbook.* 3rd edition. London: John Wiley & Sons.

Heymann LD (ed). 2014. *Control of Communicable Diseases Manual.* 20th edition. Washington, DC: American Public Health Association.

Interdepartmental Working Group on Tuberculosis. 1998. *The Prevention and Control of Tuberculosis in the United Kingdom: UK Guidance on the Prevention and Control of Transmission of HIV-related Tuberculosis, Drug-resistant, Including Multiple Drug-resistant Tuberculosis.* http://webarchive.nationalarchives.gov.uk/20130107105354/http://www.dh.gov.uk/prod_consum_dh/groups/dh_digitalassets/@dh/@en/documents/digitalasset/dh_4115299.pdf (accessed 8 March 2016).

Public Health England (PHE). 2013. *Tuberculosis: Immunisation against infectious disease - The Green Book, Chapter 32.* https://www.gov.uk/government/publications/tuberculosis-the-green-book-chapter-32 (accessed 8 March 2016).

PHE. 2014. *Bovine Tuberculosis: Guidance on Management of the Public Health Consequences of Tuberculosis in Cattle and Other Animals (England).* https://www.gov.uk/government/uploads/system/uploads/attachment_data/file/359464/Bovine_TB_Guidance_090814_FINAL.pdf (accessed 8 March 2016).

PHE. 2014. *TB Resources.* https://www.gov.uk/government/collections/tuberculosis-and-other-mycobacterial-diseases-diagnosis-screening-management-and-data (accessed 8 March 2016).

Section 3

Emergency preparedness, resilience and response (EPRR), and business continuity case studies and scenarios

Chapter 13

Business continuity: Illustrated by hospital ward closures

Alex G. Stewart, Sam Ghebrehewet, and David Baxter

OVERVIEW

After reading this chapter the reader will be familiar with:

- the process of identifying critical functions and the process of business planning (business continuity plan implementation),
- the interventions and processes that can be implemented to mitigate any impact on business, including multi-agency working (e.g. role of community care),
- the role of robust plans for incident management and business continuity, and
- the management of the situation including communication when things go wrong with the response, or with the size and magnitude of the situation (e.g. norovirus and influenza outbreak).

Terms

Passive surveillance system A surveillance system that relies on the routine reporting of event or disease data by those individuals or organizations involved in the diagnosis or detection (e.g. notifiable diseases surveillance). This system relies on cooperation; provides basic information about an event or diseases; is less expensive; and may suffer from underreporting (see also Chapter 21).

Syndromic surveillance The near real-time collection, analysis, and interpretation of health-related data about clinical pictures to provide early warning for action against public health threats (see also Chapter 21).

Rising tide incidents Emergency increasing from an initial steady state over a period of time.

(See further list of terms in the Glossary.)

13.1 Background facts: business continuity in healthcare

All healthcare organizations need to have robust business continuity plans in place in order to maintain their services to the public and patients and as part of their contractual arrangements as a provider of NHS funded care (NHS England Business Continuity Management Toolkit 2014).

Business continuity planning refers to an organization identifying essential functions, relevant resources, and required facilities (people, premises, information technology, information, stakeholders, and partners) and plans for when such resources are not available.

Every organization can find itself in a situation which challenges its ability to carry out its normal, daily functions. This may be an internal matter (loss of Information Technology (IT) server functionality, illness of key staff) or external (adverse weather stopping essential staff travelling to work, smoke from a fire elsewhere affecting the site).

13.1.1 **Key scenario information**

The aim of a business continuity plan is to embed the concept of business continuity into the organizational culture so that it becomes second nature to everyone (Cerullo and Cerullo 2004). The three principal objectives of an effective business continuity plan are to:

1. prevent or lessen the risk of an incident occurring,

2. reduce the impact of an incident once it has occurred, and

3. cut the time it takes to restore conditions to business as normal. Given that this might not be possible quickly, during the planning and testing stages it is important to prioritize activities, services, and interdependencies so that they can be restored in order of importance.

There are three key components of a business continuity plan:

1. A Business Impact Analysis:

    (a) identifies critical functions the organization must perform to deliver essential activities,

    (b) identifies risks to these functions,

    (c) rates these risks according to probability of occurrence and impact on the organization,

    (d) recommends avoidance, mitigation, or absorption of the risk, and

    (e) identifies ways to avoid or mitigate the risk.

2. A Disaster Contingency Recovery Plan identifies:

    (a) procedures to implement when a disaster occurs,

    (b) primary and alternative team members and their specific duties, including executive management roles,

    (c) notification procedures and alternative meeting site locations,

    (d) work-around processes to keep the function operational while damaged resources are being restored to a 'business as usual' condition,

    (e) a contact list of all personnel and the functions they are qualified to perform,

    (f) all internal and external partners with their primary and alternative contacts, and

    (g) reporting forms (expenses, activities, etc.).

3. Training and Testing includes:

    (a) developing test methods,

    (b) simultaneous testing and training of the disaster recovery team,

    (c) revision of the plan, and

    (d) further testing and training to repeat the cycle. Testing the plan is essential to determining whether or not it is adequate to address critical risks. In addition to ensuring that the disaster recovery team members (both primary and alternatives) know what to do, testing under increasingly realistic conditions helps develop confidence and avoid panic during a disaster event.

13.1.2 **Key points to note in the investigation**

The actual incident that causes the business continuity issue is less relevant at this point than understanding the processes for preparedness, resilience, and response to this and other pressures on the organization.

A major incident requires a structured organizational response. Whereas, a number of years ago, the approach may have been based on developing and implementing a unique and individual management response for each possible incident (e.g. one for transport failure and one for communication failure), the current preferred approach is to use a generic response plan based on a validated decision-making model such as the Integrated Emergency Management Steps (see Figure 3.1 in Chapter 3):

- **Anticipate**: stay alert for new hazards and threats (horizon scanning),
- **Assess**: evaluate identified threats by likelihood of occurrence *vs.* impact if they occur,
- **Prevent**: take necessary steps to stop the threat materializing,
- **Prepare**: plan for possible disruption; practice and review/revise the plans on a regular basis,
- **Respond**: react and counter the immediate consequences of an emergency, and
- **Recover**: manage the long-term consequences of an incident and return to normal as quickly as possible, allowing the full cycle to start again.

Do not plan directly for norovirus or other outbreaks but include them in the generic plan as specific appendices.

13.2 **What's the story?**

- On Friday morning in your local district general hospital (DGH) a patient recovering from a myocardial infarction on an elderly medicine ward developed acute diarrhoea and vomiting.

13.2.1 **Key scenario information**

- Microbiological testing for diarrhoea and vomiting should be part of the hospital's standard response.
- Identification of the onset date and time is important: cases arising after 48hrs after admission are hospital acquired; before that it will be safe to consider them as community acquired, unless further investigation proves otherwise.
- Norovirus can present as suddenly feeling sick followed by forceful vomiting and watery diarrhoea. Some people may also develop:
  - a raised temperature (over 38°C/100.4°F),
  - headaches,
  - painful stomach cramps, and
  - aching limbs.

Symptoms usually appear 1–2 days after exposure, but can start sooner. Most people make a full recovery within a couple of days.

13.2.2 **What immediate action(s) would you expect to be taken?**

The Infection Prevention and Control Nurses (IPCN) were informed (through direct contact from the ward or through surveillance systems in place within the hospital).

The patient was moved into a side room in line with standard infection prevention and control procedures (see Chapter 18), appropriate infection control precautions were implemented, and suitable specimens were taken. Local health protection/public health teams are not informed about this routine situation.

13.2.3 **Key scenario information**

- Recognition and reporting of the case resulted from the hospital passive surveillance system.

- Standard procedures, such as isolation of infectious patients, are part of the prevention step of integrated emergency management.

13.3 Scenario update # 1

- Late the next morning, two further patients, and one member of the domestic staff who cleaned up vomit from the first patient, also reported acute onset diarrhoea and vomiting. The first patient is recovering well.

13.3.1 Key scenario information

Kaplan's criteria (vomiting in >50% of affected persons, mean incubation period of 24–48hrs, and mean duration of illness of 12–60hrs) can be used prior to microbiology results to determine a likely norovirus outbreak. About 30% of norovirus outbreaks do not meet these criteria (Kaplan et al. 1982).

13.3.2 What further action(s) would you expect to be taken?

The working diagnosis by the Infection Prevention and Control Team is that the four people likely suffer from a norovirus infection. The IPCN put the three affected patients into a four-bedded unit (cohorting) and stopped all ward transfers within the hospital and discharges. The staff member was asked to stay off work until 48hrs after their symptoms cleared.

The hospital director on call and Director of Infection Prevention and Control were informed as well as the hospital bed bureau. Decisions were made about prioritization of patients to be admitted and to which ward they would go.

The hospital reviewed their intelligence about diarrhoea and vomiting outbreaks in the wider community as part of their strategic thinking about these cases: could there be 'something going on' in the community?

The hospital also reviewed its business continuity plans, since norovirus can spread easily and there may quickly be more cases within the hospital or an influx of dehydrated patients from the community with similar symptoms.

13.3.3 Key scenario information

- Norovirus is not a notifiable disease unless food poisoning is suspected and reporting is on a voluntary basis. Approximately 3000 people annually are admitted to hospital with norovirus in England; the incidence in the community is about 16.5% of the 17 million cases of infectious intestinal disease in England per year, with some evidence of an increase over the past 10 years (PHE 2012).
- Norovirus is a common hospital-associated infection in the UK with 881 hospital outbreaks in England in 2013 (593 laboratory confirmed), causing the closure of 810 wards.
- Ward closure within three days of the onset of a norovirus outbreak has been shown to reduce both the numbers of bed days lost per outbreak and the duration of outbreaks (Lopman et al. 2004).

13.4 Scenario update # 2

- The ambulance trust indicates they are responding to a high volume of calls across their patch, which covers several other district hospitals as well as the one with norovirus. Many of the calls to the ambulance trust are from relatives of elderly people with vomiting. A nearby hospital has been closed to admissions due to influenza-like illness.

13.4.1 **Key scenario information**

Norovirus often circulates quietly in the community since it is usually a self-limiting illness and, while it may lead to increases in GP appointments, this is not commonly reflected in laboratory reports, as it is not usually tested for in primary care. As a result, laboratory confirmation that the disease is circulating can be limited. Syndromic surveillance is the best way to be alerted to circulating diseases like this that do not warrant detailed investigation nor hospitalization, but which may become a burden on the health services due to the numbers of (1) patients who may become sick enough to justify hospitalization, and (2) staff who may go off sick or stay at home to attend family members.

A norovirus outbreak is unlikely to start as a major incident (for any of the affected organizations), but the potential is evident given the organism's high infectivity. Furthermore, a 'less serious event' may become a major incident if, for example, one of the involved organizations is already experiencing other problems such as significant capacity issues. It is always beneficial to review plans early and prepare in advance.

13.4.2 **What further action(s) would you expect to be taken?**

Advice was given by community IPCNs and public health to care homes on treatment, fluid intake, health care referrals, general infection control, and hygiene.

13.4.3 **What further information do you need?**

The latest infectious intestinal disease activity bulletin, from the local health protection team/field epidemiology service, was issued earlier in the week and noted an increase in (1) diarrhoea and vomiting presentations to GPs, and (2) calls to the national telephone health service.

13.4.4 **Tools of the trade**

Surveillance records provide information routinely, which can be analysed prospectively to identify rising trends, or retrospectively when a particular issues is raised.

Infectious intestinal disease activity bulletin and other bulletins (e.g. covering influenza-like illness) are issued during the relevant season by the local health protection team/field epidemiology service as a guide to public health and clinical professionals to indicate 'rising tide' situations that might develop into problems for acute trusts or primary care providers.

13.5 **Scenario update # 3**

- ◆ The Emergency Department has reported an increase in attendance for diarrhoea and vomiting over the past three weeks.
- ◆ Meanwhile, another ward has been closed following reports of six patients with diarrhoea and/or vomiting.

13.5.1 **What further action(s) would you expect to be taken?**

The Director of Infection Prevention and Control reviewed, with the hospital IPCN team, hospital information on diarrhoea and vomiting cases to identify possible infectious hotspots.

Contingency plans for outbreaks were implemented through the setting up of an Outbreak Control Team (OCT) (see Chapter 20), closure of wards, and cohorting of patients, with samples taken for confirmation of the outbreak.

With four wards closed, the business continuity plan for the hospital was initiated, since the critical functions of the hospital (caring for the sick) were being compromised.

Questions were asked as to why the Director of Infection Prevention and Control or the IPCNs had not been informed of the increase in A&E attendance due to diarrhoea and vomiting, which could have led to earlier isolation of cases.

13.6 Scenario update # 4

◆ On Monday morning, another two wards report diarrhoea and vomiting in three patients and one staff, and four patients and two staff, respectively.

13.6.1 What further action(s) would you expect to be taken?

There is clearly ongoing transmission in the hospital. Think about:

1. apprising/informing partner organizations (GPs and other primary care services, ambulance trust, nearby hospitals, clinical commissioning groups (CCGs) and any other commissioners, such as NHS England or equivalent in the devolved administrations, including those who are responsible for contracting hospital services) of the situation (NHS England 2015), and
2. issuing a media statement since relatives and staff will spread word quickly in the local community. Families should be asked to keep their visitors to a minimum, not to visit if unwell themselves, and to restrict their movement in the hospital building to accessing the relevant wards.

13.6.2 Tools of the trade

The business continuity plan should be generic enough to cover a wide variety of situations, but may include information on particular threats, such as ward closure, that will affect the working of the organization and need specific responses.

The outbreak control plan should cover identification of cases: epidemiology, microbiological and environmental investigations, and the provision of control measures.

13.6.3 Top tips

Use the business continuity plan earlier rather than later; it is always easier to scale back than to catch up. Consider if it is better during planning (rather than during an incident) to identify (1) which services can be stopped or (2) which services the hospital must continue to provide.

Making mutual aid arrangements is part of business continuity planning so that each organization knows what is expected of them and knows how to respond or whether an outside situation may activate their own business continuity plan.

At this stage a number of organizations would be affected by this situation—the hospital (ward closed), the clinical commissioning group, local general practitioners, and the out-of-hours (OOH) primary care provider (who refer patients to the hospital), ambulance service and care homes.

13.7 Scenario update # 5

◆ It became known that there were recent and current outbreaks involving more than 65 patients and staff in eight of the 14 local care and nursing homes—two had stopped all admissions, including from the hospital, thus blocking hospital beds with well patients. The OOH provider reported a 20% increase in acute diarrhoea and vomiting cases across all ages, starting about three weeks previously.

◆ Staffing levels in the hospital dropped significantly: a local school closed due an outbreak of an influenza-like illness; hospital staff were staying off work to care for children and elderly relatives. A few staff appeared to be staying away to avoid contact with norovirus, while others continued to work, even when unwell themselves.

13.7.1 What further action(s) would you expect to be taken?

What is the local plan for escalation? Support (mutual aid) for extra staff may need to be sought through the appropriate NHS mechanism (although, as here, it may not be available, since other organizations are also dealing with similar problems).

Questions need to be asked (and answered) about the ongoing transmission: why are staff coming in to work unwell (not staying away from work for 48hrs after the last bout of diarrhoea or vomiting)? Are infection control measures being followed properly within the hospital? Was there a situation when staff or patients moved between affected wards?

What are the local plans for returning to normal? Why is this important at this time?

13.8 Scenario update # 6

◆ The next week all but one ward (of a total of six affected) reopened, following two complete incubation periods (96hrs) free of new cases, and a deep clean. Staff were back at work. The media hounded the hospital, asking why the incident escalated so far and what was done about planning for such situations.

13.8.1 How would you plan for another critical incident?

A debrief of relevant staff across all involved professions and grades should be held, asking what went well and what could be improved. These observations should be collated, assessed, and woven into a revised plan as appropriate (see Chapter 20).

13.8.2 Top tips

◆ Writing the business continuity plan should include the identification of core business that it is essential to keep running as much as possible (for a hospital, admissions are one such business; others may include emergency operations or deliveries).

◆ Write a holding press statement covering all the issues of the situation (only issue when necessary or if asked).

13.9 What if ... ?

◆ The outbreak was due to invasive group A streptococcus? Or was centred in the neonatal ward due to *Pseudomona aeruginosa*?

◆ The situation was a fire in the electrical supply and the expected return of the electrics keeps being put back by four hours each time a deadline is reached?

◆ Flooding cut the power and the generator ran out of fuel (most hospitals only hold about 8hrs fuel supply)?

- The hospital was caught in the smoke plume from a fire at a nearby chemical works?
- There was a major staff shortage due to circumstances beyond the hospital's control?

The hospital business continuity and major incident plans are relevant to all of these incidents. Amongst other things, the plans should describe and outline:

- how the relevant plans are activated, what escalation system(s) they have in place, and who assumes responsibility at each stage,
- how the organization will respond to a significant incident, in line with the formal organization communications strategy,
- details of the activity with regard to surge capacity planning in order to ensure that critical services are maintained in periods of peak activity,
- how mutual aid from other NHS providers can be requested if a disruptive incident occurs, including information on alternative locations from which the service/activity could be delivered in case of denial of access,
- the recovery and restoration principles and how they will be managed and by whom, and
- how lessons identified from the incident will affect future plans.

Source: NHS England Business Continuity Management Toolkit, 2014.

13.10 **Lessons learned**

- Incidents that lead to a business continuity issue are not always easy to recognize initially. Stay alert!
- Often critical situations arise from a combination of a number of smaller problems that alone do not merit a sustained, coordinated response.
- Every staff member has a part to play in responding to a business continuity situation and should be aware of the important parts of the plan that apply to their role, their team, and department.
- Equally, any staff member, no matter what their position in the organization, may have pertinent observations and ideas about how to improve the planning or response or recovery. Listen to them!
- After any incident, a debrief should be held with all relevant staff to identify lessons, which should be integrated into the relevant plan.
- Anticipation and preparation for future incidents should build on any actual incident or near incident as well as on changing threats identified within and outside the organization.

13.11 **Further thinking**

- What are the limits of capacity, capability, and drivers within the public sector to implement an effective business continuity programme in the face of constant change and ever-reducing resources?
- Why is business continuity often made more complicated and fragmented and not focused on simple methods to keep a business running? There is a constant stream of guidance, standards, etc. being published. Why? Are they necessary?
- Why does a common, known, and predictable virus (norovirus) continue to cause hospital ward closures, regularly causing disruption to critical business in most (small or big, general or specialist) healthcare settings?

References

Cerullo V, MJ Cerullo. 2004. Business continuity planning: a comprehensive approach. *Information Systems Management*, **21**(3): 70–78.

Kaplan JE, R Feldman, DS Campbell, et al. 1982. The frequency of a Norwalk-like pattern of illness in outbreaks of acute gastroenteritis. *American Journal of Public Health*, **72**: 1329–32.

Lopman BA, MH Reacher, IB Vipond, et al. 2004. Epidemiology and cost of nosocomial gastroenteritis, Avon, England, 2002–2003. *Emerging Infectious Diseases*, **10**: 1827–34.

NHS England. 2015. *NHS England Emergency Preparedness, Resilience and Response Framework*. https://www.england.nhs.uk/wp-content/uploads/2015/11/eprr-framework.pdf (accessed 8 March 2016).

NHS England Business Continuity Management Toolkit. 2014. *NHS England Business Continuity Management Toolkit: Guidance*. EPRR Corporate Team. https://www.england.nhs.uk/wp-content/uploads/2014/01/toolkit-cover-doc.pdf (accessed 8 March 2016).

Public Health England (PHE). 2012. *National Resource for Infection Control. Guidelines for the management of norovirus outbreaks in acute and community health and social care settings*. https://www.gov.uk/government/publications/norovirus-managing-outbreaks-in-acute-and-community-health-and-social-care-settings (accessed 8 March 2016).

Further reading

Borodzicz EP. 2005. *Risk, Crisis and Security Management*. London: John Wiley & Sons.

Cabinet Office. 2012. *Business Continuity for Dummies*. London: John Wiley & Sons.

Centre for the Protection of National Infrastructure. n.d. *Business continuity planning*. http://www.cpni.gov.uk/Security-Planning/Business-continuity-plan/ (accessed 8 March 2016).

GovUK. n.d. *Business Continuity Management Toolkit—Gov.UK*. https://www.gov.uk/government/uploads/system/uploads/attachment_data/file/137994/Business_Continuity_Managment_Toolkit.pdf (accessed 8 March 2016).

Harris JP, GK Adak, SJ O'Brien. 2014. To close or not to close? Analysis of 4 years' data from national surveillance of norovirus outbreaks in hospitals in England. *BMJ Open*, **4**(1): e003919. doi:10.1136/bmjopen-2013-003919.

Chapter 14

Fire and fear: Immediate and long-term health aspects

Laura Mitchem, Henrietta Harrison, and Alex G. Stewart

OVERVIEW

....

After reading this chapter the reader will be familiar with:

- the potential impacts of fires on health,
- the multi-agency response to a major incident,
- the factors to consider during the response to a fire, and
- community concerns associated with fires.

Terms

Air Quality Cell (AQC) Multi-agency group convened for major chemical incidents such as fires, explosions, and major chemical releases, which brings together experts in assessing air pollution for chemical incident response.

Controlled burn A restricted or controlled use of water/foam on fires to reduce potential environmental impacts of chemical or contaminated fire-water run-off.

Geographic Information System (GIS) Visualization tools that allow users to create interactive queries, analyse spatial information, edit data in maps, and visually present relationships, patterns, and trends.

Recovery coordinating group (RCG) Multi-agency group which manages return to normality after incident.

Receptors People potentially affected by the incident.

(See further list of terms in the Glossary.)

14.1 Background facts: fire and health

- ◆ Fires can cause significant health concerns within local communities affected by any associated smoke plume.

- ◆ In recent years, there has been an increase in the number of long-burning fires. Fires at waste-processing and recycling facilities, involving a variety of household and commercial waste, can be difficult to control and extinguish and have the capacity to burn for many weeks, generating significant media and public concern and fear associated with their potential to affect public health.

- ◆ The impact of the plume on the health of the community depends on the properties of the chemical species within the plume (e.g. concentration and solubility), plume dispersion (meteorological conditions, topography, etc.), and the duration of exposure of vulnerable people (sensitive receptors; e.g. the elderly, those with pre-existing respiratory and cardiac conditions, children). Smoke will be diluted in the air due to atmospheric dispersion, reducing the concentration of substances within the plume.

◆ The composition of the plume is dependent on a number of factors including the materials involved, and the nature of the fire (temperature, oxygen availability, etc.), making it difficult to predict accurately the substances local sensitive receptors may be exposed to.

◆ A smoke plume typically consists of a mixture of gases, liquid droplets, and solid particles (complex mixture of particle size and type). Irritants and particulate matter are the main health concern.

◆ An overview of common types of fires and resulting products of combustion is detailed below (see Wakefield 2010 for further details).

  • Waste fires: stored waste includes refuse derived fuel, wood chips, and composting materials. Products of combustion are complex, due to the varied nature of the materials involved. A wide range of pollutants can be produced including particulate matter (PM_{10} and $PM_{2.5}$), and organic and inorganic irritant gases (e.g. hydrogen cyanide, nitrogen oxides, ammonia, hydrogen chloride).

  • Tyre fires: ground/chopped tyres can result in a fire that is difficult to extinguish. Products of combustion include large quantities of sulphur dioxide, organic and inorganic irritants, and PM_{10} and $PM_{2.5}$.

  • Warehouse fires: it can be difficult to identify materials involved in a warehouse fire, limiting the ability to provide tailored advice. There may be real concerns about the fibre release from asbestos-containing materials (e.g. roofing tiles and sheets).

  • Moorland/forest/bush fire/health lands: these long-burning fires, which often cover a large area, have caused air quality problems in many countries, often leading to respiratory effects in those exposed. Products of combustion include PM_{10} and $PM_{2.5}$, and respiratory irritants including formaldehyde.

◆ Irritant gases, present in most fires, can cause irritation to the eyes, nose, throat, and lungs, coughing and wheezing, breathlessness, phlegm production, and chest pain. Inorganic irritants include oxides of sulphur and nitrogen, hydrogen chloride, hydrogen bromide.

◆ Fires have the potential to generate high levels of PM_{10} and $PM_{2.5}$, resulting in local, short lived peaks of pollution. Elevated levels of particulate matter are associated with short- and long-term effects on mortality, and increased hospital admissions relating to cardiovascular and pulmonary disease. For susceptible individuals with pre-existing respiratory conditions, particulate air pollution can exacerbate their conditions.

14.2 **What's the story?**

◆ A large fire has broken out at a waste management centre. A plume of thick black smoke is visible at a distance of 10 km, generating significant media interest. Local health protection/public health team have been informed.

◆ There are schools, nursing homes, and residential properties close to the site.

14.2.1 **Key scenario information**

◆ Fires at waste-processing and recycling facilities present many challenges for the fire and rescue service (FRS). Waste is often tightly packed on the site or stored within buildings, making aggressive fire fighting difficult due to limited space between stockpiles and poor access. Water availability and management of large volumes of fire-water run-off can also affect fire-fighting activities, often resulting in the decision to undertake a controlled burn, which may not be in the best interest for public health.

◆ Plumes can be large, visible over long distances, resulting in concern to those living close to the fire, and further afield, generating local and national media attention.

◆ Fires can cause significant health concerns within local communities affected by the smoke plume. Concerns can be associated with:

- impacts on local air quality and health,

- presence of hazardous substances, or

- impacts of fire-water run-off on the environment (e.g. controlled waters) and public health (e.g. water supplies, recreational water use).

◆ Materials involved, predicted duration, plume behaviour, meteorological conditions and locations of sensitive receptors are key information for the initial stage of the response.

14.2.2 **Top tips**

◆ Any smoke can irritate; therefore, individuals are advised to avoid exposure to the plume.

◆ Symptoms of exposure include eye irritation, coughing, wheezing, breathlessness, phlegm production, and chest pain. Smoke can exacerbate existing conditions, and individuals with pre-existing underlying respiratory or heart conditions (e.g. asthma, cardiovascular conditions, chronic obstructive pulmonary disease), children, and the elderly are particularly susceptible.

◆ Most healthy individuals only suffer transient and reversible effects after exposure to low levels of smoke. It is very unlikely that any long-term effects will occur as a result of acute exposure to smoke.

◆ Those with pre-existing conditions should use their inhalers as normal.

◆ Individuals who develop symptoms should seek medical advice.

◆ Coordinated multi-agency communication is key to ensuring those with the potential to be affected are aware of protective actions to minimize their exposure.

14.2.3 **Tools of the trade**

◆ Meteorological Office modelling (CHEMET) to predict area potentially affected by plume,

◆ use of GIS/maps to determine local population and locations of sensitive receptors, and

◆ local knowledge with feedback from the incident.

14.2.4 **What immediate action(s) would you take and what further information do you need?**

◆ Obtain information to undertake the risk assessment (Box 14.1).

◆ Identify those at risk from plume.

◆ Confirm agencies involved and whether a major incident has been declared.

◆ Review contents of media messages issued.

Box 14.1 Acute Incident Checklist: summary of issues to be considered

Incident details:

- name, contact details of notifying organization,
- incident details: type (e.g. fire), location, time started, substance(s) released, affected media (e.g. air, water),
- current incident control measures (e.g. containment, control burn),
- public health messages in place (e.g. shelter/evacuation) and who issued them,
- monitoring or modelling in place, and
- command and control structures in place.

Exposure assessment:

- establish **source** (e.g. fire)—**pathway** (e.g. inhalation)—**receptor** (e.g. public in the affected area)? If incomplete, there is no public health risk,
- details of those exposed (e.g. individuals or communities),
- measures required (e.g. decontamination, hospital assessment, shelter/evacuation),
- wider public health requirements (e.g. public health messages to affected communities), and
- susceptible receptors nearby (e.g. schools, old people's homes, hospitals).

Ongoing investigation and information:

- access specialist chemical public health advice,
- provision of environmental and/or chemical public health advice to appropriate organizations,
- establish actions to be taken by responders,
- assess whether an Air Quality Cell required,
- attend multi-agency meetings,
- confirm lead organization for communications and media messages,
- liaise with NHS and consider alerting GPs, hospitals, etc., and
- ask if other agencies need to be informed (e.g. Food Standard Agency).

Recovery:

- attend Recovery Coordination Group multi-agency meetings until incident stood down,
- make site visit(s),
- assess health impacts and consider long-term surveillance or follow-up,
- continue long-term communications to the public,
- establish whether further environmental sampling required, and
- conduct/participate in internal and external debriefs to identify lessons learnt and improve future response.

14.2.5 **Key scenario information**

Sheltering indoors significantly reduces exposure to smoke, and is considered appropriate for short-lived fires. Shelter messages are usually issued initially by the emergency services.

Go In—Stay In—Tune In!

◆ Go indoors.

◆ Close all windows.

◆ Turn off any mechanical ventilation including air conditioning.

◆ Tune in to local radio/TV.

◆ Check the Internet and social media for news.

◆ Stay in until advised.

14.3 **Scenario update # 1**

◆ The FRS has advised that the warehouse contains 100,000 tonnes of baled waste, including paper and plastics. They are struggling to access the fire due to the large quantities stored within the building, and predict the fire is likely to burn for a number of days, potentially weeks. There are concerns about access to water supplies, and possible contamination of a nearby waterbody. A major incident has been declared.

◆ A Strategic Coordinating Group (SCG) has been established, and Public Health attendance has been requested at a Scientific and Technical Advice Cell (STAC) (Figure 14.1).

14.3.1 **Key scenario information**

14.3.1.1 **Strategic Coordinating Group (SCG)**

The SCG maintains a strategic overview of the operation, and leads the incident response. It focuses on the overall picture rather than detailed tactical or operational decisions, and determines long-term and wider impacts or risks with strategic implications.

Aims include:

◆ agree strategic aims, objectives and priorities,

◆ determine policy, for implementation by the Tactical Coordinating Group (TCG),

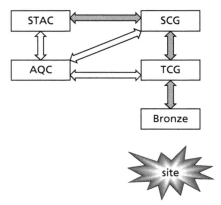

Fig. 14.1 The relationships of the local multi-agency groups convened in an emergency to coordinate the response (see text for abbreviations)

- act as an interface with local and National Government,
- liaise with neighbouring agencies/authorities,
- coordinate communication to the public or allocate appropriate agency to lead on communications,
- ensure regular meetings and availability of situational reports (SitReps), and
- ensure transition from the operational stage to recovery.

Membership varies according to the scale and nature of the incident and should be reviewed throughout. Representatives must have the knowledge, expertise, and authority to identify and commit resources on behalf of their organization.

14.3.1.2 Tactical Coordinating Group (TCG)

The TCG ensures the actions taken at an operational level are coordinated, coherent, and integrated to achieve maximum effectiveness and efficiency.
    Aims include:

- direct tactical operations to ensure a coordinated response,
- determine priorities for allocating available resources,
- plan and coordinate how and when tasks will be undertaken,
- obtain additional resources if required,
- assess significant risks and organize appropriate actions, and
- ensure health and safety of the public and personnel.

Membership varies according to the scale and nature of the incident and normally comprises the most senior operational member of each organization.

14.3.2 Key scenario information

14.3.2.1 Scientific and Technical Advice Cell (STAC)

STAC ensures provision of timely, coordinated scientific and technical advice to the SCG and Recovery Coordinating Group (RCG), often when there are wide health and environmental consequences of the emergency.
    Aims include:

- bring together technical and scientific experts from agencies involved in the response,
- provide a single point of advice to the SCG on scientific, technical, environmental, and public health consequences of the incident, and
- develop public health advice and formulate actions to protect the public and environment.

Membership will depend upon the nature of the emergency and the scientific and technical advice required.

14.3.3 What further action(s) would you take?

- Attend multi-agency meetings as appropriate to your agency's involvement.
- Contribute to ongoing multi-agency communications addressing the concerns of the local community. Perceived fears arising from incidents such as a fire should not be underestimated and need a strong, proportionate, and appropriate response.
- Consider the potential impact of the plume (dispersion modelling predictions and visual observations from the scene are invaluable in supporting the risk assessment).
- Undertake ongoing risk assessment with available environmental monitoring data.

14.3.4 **Key scenario information**

Air quality monitoring undertaken at sensitive receptor locations during a fire can support the public health risk assessment, public health advice, and shelter/evacuation decisions. An indication of the level of pollutants at specific locations may be available from the local Automatic Urban and Rural Network (AURN), through an Air Quality Cell (AQC), or following the decision made by the local authority (LA) to provide reassurance to the local community.

14.3.4.1 Air Quality Cell (AQC)

An AQC (England and Wales) may be convened during the response phase for major chemical incidents, where there is the potential to affect the public's health. The AQC gives interpreted air quality information to a multi-agency group to assist with decisions regarding the impact of air pollution on health throughout the acute phase of the fire.

14.4 **Scenario update # 2**

- ◆ The LA has called regarding a nursing home located within the plume. Residents have been advised to shelter. However, there are concerns because it is a hot day and windows are usually open for ventilation. They are considering evacuation of the residents, as the elderly with underlying health conditions are particularly at risk of heart and respiratory problems in very hot conditions.

14.4.1 **What further action(s) would you take?**

- ◆ Consider the vulnerability of and risk to residents: some individuals may experience greater harm by being moved.
- ◆ Provide:
  - advice to keep residents cool (e.g. how to cool properties, drink plenty of cool fluids, wear loose clothing (PHE 2014)),
  - tailored sheltering messages for residents, and
  - health advice for symptomatic individuals.
- ◆ Interpret monitoring data to predict potential impact of the plume on residents' health—consider locating any air quality monitoring equipment at property.
- ◆ Consider the use of existing syndromic surveillance to identify unusual local health effects.

14.4.2 **Key scenario information**

Syndromic surveillance (SyS) is the (near) real-time collection, analysis, interpretation, and dissemination of health-related data to enable the early identification of the impact, or absence of impact, of potential threats. SyS systems can identify unusual patterns in healthcare presentation. SyS data from the affected areas can be compared with data from the same period in previous years, and unaffected areas, to identify statistically significant increases in relevant indicators. During a large fire, compare GP consultations for asthma and wheeze, and NHS 111 calls for difficulty in breathing with data from previous years. If levels observed are no different from those expected (using historical data for the time of year), reassurance can be provided to the public that there are no major local health impacts (see Chapter 21, section 21.5.3.6).

14.4.3 **Top tips**

- ◆ Tailor communications to the public as the incident progresses.
- ◆ Address local fears and concerns in all communications to the public.

- Give detailed protective actions to minimize exposure to smoke and in relation to when the property is no longer located in the plume (e.g. open windows and ventilate the property).
- Advise those suffering persistent health effects to seek medical attention.

14.5 **Scenario update # 3**

- The FRS has reported that the asbestos sheeting of the roof of the warehouse has broken up into fragments and been deposited downwind on the neighbouring housing estate and primary school. Locals are concerned regarding the risks to health. STAC has been asked for advice.

14.5.1 **Key scenario information**

Material which contains a proportion of asbestos (e.g. corrugated asbestos cement roofing panels, insulating board) is usually described as asbestos-containing material (ACM). Fires involving ACMs are relatively common and can cause significant public concern if debris is carried in the smoke plume and deposited in residential areas.

Unless ACM is weathered/friable, the majority of fibres in ACMs are held tightly within the material, even when an ACM is damaged. Respirable fibres are a small fraction of the total particles released. Atmospheric dispersion and dilution further reduce the concentration of airborne fibres. During an acute incident when sheltering advice is issued, the public exposure will be very low, minimizing the health risk. Available epidemiological evidence shows that long-term health effects from fires involving ACM are negligible (Smith and Saunders 2007). If appropriate clean-up procedures are followed, there is no significant public health risk.

14.5.2 **What further action(s) would you take?**

- Support the LA in producing a strategy to identify areas requiring decontamination.
- Maintain multi-agency communication with the local community throughout clean-up, providing clean-up advice, responding to queries to alleviate anxiety and input into press releases if required.
- Confirm with the LA that clean-up has been completed.

14.5.3 **Top tips**

- Appropriate clean-up of deposited ACM debris is paramount, as is prevention of further off-site recontamination (e.g. appropriate containment of incident site and off-site debris).
- Previous air sampling after fires involving ACM has not revealed significant levels of asbestos fibres. While it may be considered for public reassurance, in most cases air sampling for asbestos is not necessary.

14.6 **Scenario update # 4**

- **Recovery:** four days later the fire is out. In the transition from acute to recovery phase the incident has been handed over to the LA.

14.6.1 **What do you need to consider in terms of recovery?**

- whether an RCG has been established,
- site clean-up, including clean-up expectations and waste disposal (e.g. waste remaining on site, water run-off, waste materials involved in fire),

- off-site clean-up of contamination (e.g. residential properties, agricultural land, allotments) including ash and waste materials,
- ongoing multi-agency communication regarding recovery decisions and actions, residual waste on site, materials deposited off-site and clean-up advice,
- any further public health advice (e.g. regarding fears around residual waste), and
- ask if there is a need for a public health risk register of those exposed? Alternatively, consider with epidemiologists the need for a population cohort for further study.

14.6.2 **Key scenario information**

Public health issues can be associated with waste remaining on site following the fire, if clean-up is inadequate. During recovery, waste not dealt with promptly has the potential to decompose and become odorous, posing nuisance concerns (dust, pests). Migration of pests off site can be a potential public health risk (zoonotic infections). Ensure there is a strategy in place to address these issues, produced as part of the RCG.

14.7 **What if ... ?**

The fire continued for a number of weeks?

- What is the likely impact on the local community and how will you address the resulting concerns and fears?
- How is the incident response likely to change?
- What are the potential impacts on your organization?
- What is the likely media response to the ongoing incident?

14.7.1 **Key scenario information**

Certain fires, such as waste fires, have the potential to smoulder for weeks to months due to the volume and types of material involved. Long-burning fires can cause significant concern in the local community due to ongoing exposure to the plume, odour from smouldering waste, and the potential impact on local air quality. The response to long-running fires can be very resource-intensive for all agencies involved.

The incomplete combustion of waste materials at lower temperatures and poor oxygen availability can result in the production of complex molecules such as polycyclic aromatic hydrocarbons (PAHs) and dioxins, with production dependent on the materials involved and conditions of the fire. While the risk from a single acute exposure is considered likely to be very low, there can be significant concern in the local community. Continuing communication is key to address these concerns.

All public communication should be multi-agency, coordinated, and be consistent, timely, clear, and accurate to ensure community fears, which can be exacerbated during a protracted incident, are allayed. Perceived risk can affect the community as much as the actual risk (Stewart et al. 2010).

Public advice should continue to include protective actions for individuals to take throughout the incident and health advice for those suffering symptoms following exposure to smoke. Use of multiple communication channels ensures public health messages reach a wide population. The Internet and social media can be invaluable; however, they have potential to cause concern if multi-agency messages are not consistent and clear.

14.8 **Lessons learned**

◆ Fires, in particular long-burning fires, with the potential to smoulder for weeks to months, can cause significant health concerns within local communities.

◆ Any smoke can be an irritant. Smoke can cause symptoms including eye irritation, coughing and wheezing, and breathlessness, and can exacerbate existing conditions. Individuals with pre-existing underlying respiratory or heart conditions, children, and the elderly are particularly susceptible.

◆ A coordinated, multi-agency response is key to addressing the concerns of the local community. This ensures awareness of protective actions to minimize exposure to the smoke plume and actions to undertake if individuals experience health effects thought to be associated with the plume.

14.9 **Further thinking**

◆ What can be done to capture any potential health effects that may arise from fires (and other incidents) through routine data collection systems?

◆ What should be the response to media, public, and political pressure to assess perceived adverse health effects from low-level and short-term exposure (hours/day) to smoke or other pollutants?

◆ What further actions could be taken to improve the understanding of non-health protection professionals and the public around risks to health that may arise from fires?

◆ How can the challenges in multi-agency communications be identified better and addressed more effectively, given the variety, complexity, and paucity of significant incidents and responses?

References

Public Health England and NHS England. 2014. *Heatwave Plan for England 2014, Protecting Health and Reducing Harm from Severe Heat and Heatwaves*. http://www.nhs.uk/Livewell/Summerhealth/Documents/heatwave-plan-for-england-2013.pdf (accessed 8 March 2016).

Smith KR, PJ Saunders. 2007. *The Public Health Significance of Asbestos Exposures from Large Scale Fires*. HPA-CHaPD-003. Didcot: Health Protection Agency. www.brandweerkennisnet.nl/publish/pages/1092/thepublichealthsignificanceofasbestosexposuresfromlargescalefires.pdf (accessed 8 March 2016).

Stewart AG, P Luria, R Reid, et al. 2010. Real or illusory? Case studies on the public perception of environmental health risks in the North West of England. *International Journal of Environmental Research and Public Health*, 7(3): 1153–73.

Wakefied JC. 2010. *A Toxicological Review of Products of Combustion*. HPA-CHaPD-004. Chilton, Didcot: Health Protection Agency. cvoed.imss.gob.mx/COED/home/normativos/DPM/archivos/HDRM/health_topics/chemical_safety/a_toxicological_review.pdf (accessed 8 March 2016).

Further reading

Barker H. 2010. Air quality in major incidents, *Chemical Hazards and Poisons Report*, 18: 4–5. https://www.gov.uk/government/publications/chemical-hazards-and-poisons-report-issue-18 (accessed 8 March 2016).

Cabinet Office. 2007. *Guidance on the Establishment of a Science and Technical Advice Cell (STAC) within the Multiagency Strategic Co-ordination Centre (SCC)*. https://www.gov.uk/government/publications/

provision-of-scientific-and-technical-advice-in-the-strategic-co-ordination-centre-guidance-to-local-responders (accessed 8 March 2016).

Cabinet Office. 2013. *Emergency Response and Recovery.* https://www.gov.uk/emergency-response-and-recovery (accessed 8 March 2016).

Kibble A. 2010. Health Protection Agency experience on the public health aspects of fires involving waste materials. *Chemical Hazards and Poisons Report*, **18**: 6–8. https://www.gov.uk/government/publications/chemical-hazards-and-poisons-report-issue-18 (accessed 8 March 2016).

NHS England. 2014. *Emergency Preparedness, Resilience and Response (EPRR). Planning for the Shelter and Evacuation of People in Healthcare Settings.* http://www.england.nhs.uk/wp-content/uploads/2015/01/eprr-shelter-evacuation-guidance.pdf (accessed 8 March 2016).

Public Health England. 2013. *UK Recovery Handbook for Chemical Incidents.* https://www.gov.uk/government/publications/uk-recovery-handbook-for-chemical-incidents-and-associated-publications (accessed 28 April 2016).

Stewart-Evans J, N Brooke, J Isaac, et al. 2013. Conference Paper. *Protective Actions during Chemical Incidents and Fires: Evacuate or Shelter in Place?* Didcot: Public Health England. https://www.researchgate.net/publication/268503540_Protective_actions_in_acute_chemical_and_radiological_incidents_evacuate_or_shelter-in-place (accessed 28 April 2016).

Wakefield JC. 2010. *Combustion Products: A Toxicological Review.* HPA-CHaPD-004. https://www.gov.uk/government/publications/combustion-products-a-toxicological-review (accessed 8 March 2016).

Waste Industry Safety and Health Forum (WISH). 2014. *WASTE 28 Reducing Fire Risk at Waste Management Sites.* http://authority.manchesterfire.gov.uk/documents/s50003213/Appendix%20A%20Reducing%20fire%20at%20waste%20management%20sites.pdf (accessed 8 March 2016).

World Health Organization. 2013. *Health and Environment: Communicating the Risks.* http://www.euro.who.int/__data/assets/pdf_file/0011/233759/e96930.pdf?ua=1 (accessed 8 March 2016).

Chapter 15

Flooding and health: Immediate and long-term implications

Angie Bone, Alan Wilton, and Alex G. Stewart

OVERVIEW

After reading this chapter, the reader will be familiar with:

• the acute response: identification of immediate health hazards, risks and impacts, public health actions,
• the medium-/long-term response: multi-agency working and engagement, medium- and long-term health and social impacts, use of routine surveillance and health registers, and wider public health role including communication, and
• the clean-up and recovery: health and social impacts, community resilience.

Terms

Flood guidance statement (FGS) Issued by the Flood Forecasting Centre (FFC): provides a daily flood risk assessment up to five days in advance by county for responders in England and Wales.

Flood warnings Issued by the Environment Agency (EA) and available to the public. Three levels:

♦ **flood alert**: flooding possible; be prepared,
♦ **flood warning**: flooding expected; immediate action required, and
♦ **severe flood warning**: severe flooding; danger to life.

Health register A rapid way to collate basic details of individuals affected by an incident in the immediate aftermath of an event. Epidemiological rigour and ethical approval are applied later for follow up studies.

Multi-Agency Flood Plan (MAFP) developed by the Local Resilience Forum (LRF); complements existing major incident plans; recommended due to the complex and sustained response required for floods.

Secondary stressor An event/policy indirectly related to the primary event that results in psychosocial stress (e.g. loss of possessions, resources, infrastructure failure, interruption of daily life).

Responders Category 1 responders assess risks to communities and plan to deal with emergencies (e.g. emergency services, local authorities, public health); Category 2 responders (e.g. utilities) support Category 1 (Civil Contingencies Act 2004).

Science & Technical Advice Cell (STAC) Brings together experts from all relevant agencies to provide a single point of advice to the Strategic Coordinating Group, during a major incident.

> **Strategic Coordinating Group (SCG)** Composed of all relevant agencies to agree high-level objectives and guide response during a major incident; led by Strategic Coordinator (usually police, but may change as incident progresses).
>
> *(See further list of terms in the Glossary.)*

15.1 Background facts: flooding and health

Serious flooding can happen at any time of year in the UK; it can occur anywhere, not just to communities living near rivers or the coast. In England, 5.4 million properties (1/6) are at risk (Defra 2013). As our climate warms, flooding is expected to occur more frequently, through a combination of sea-level rise and increasingly severe and frequent rainfall.

There are different types of flooding; several may co-exist:

♦ **Coastal**: high physical impacts including erosion, destruction to property, and salt water contamination,

♦ **River** (fluvial): highly variable impacts depend on location,

♦ **Surface water** (pluvial): usually the result of intense rainfall; location and severity difficult to predict,

♦ **Rapid response catchments**: steep catchments where time between rain falling and river rising can be less than an hour; flooding difficult to predict, dangerous, highly destructive, and

♦ **Groundwater**: the water table rises, days or weeks after heavy rainfall; may persist for weeks.

Both coastal and inland flooding feature prominently on the UK's national risk register (Cabinet Office 2015), and are well-recognized within many community risk registers. However, there is generally poor public acceptance of the risk of flooding except in communities where flooding has already occurred.

15.1.1 Key scenario information

Flooding is an environmental emergency; health agencies take a largely supportive role (Defra 2013).

In England, responsibilities are:

♦ **Defra**: overarching, national policy on flood management,

♦ **Environment Agency**: managing risk from main rivers, reservoirs, estuaries and the sea, and

♦ **Lead local flood authorities**: managing risk from surface water, groundwater, and ordinary watercourses; lead on community recovery.

15.1.2 Effects of flooding on health and wellbeing

Flooding has extensive and significant impacts on health and wellbeing. However, these impacts are not well quantified because of challenges in linking health effects with flood exposures. Much of our knowledge comes from case studies and qualitative research from high-income countries such as the UK, summarized in systematic literature reviews (e.g. Menne and Murray 2013). Effects include:

♦ Immediate and early (warning and response phases):

  • drowning,

  • injuries (e.g. from hidden hazards, moving furniture, electrocution), and

  • distress;

◆ Medium to longer term (during recovery):
  • infectious disease outbreaks (water, rodent, or vector borne),
  • carbon monoxide (CO) poisoning (use of fuel-driven generators/heaters, etc. indoors),
  • common mental health disorders, and
  • post-traumatic stress;
◆ Secondary stressors:
  • loss of utilities (e.g. water, sewage, power, communication),
  • disrupted healthcare (e.g. access difficulties, loss of medicines/devices),
  • disrupted work or education,
  • loss of possessions and difficulties with recovery (repair, insurance), and
  • loss of amenity.

The risk of health effects depends on a complex interaction of factors including, the severity and rapidity of the flooding, the availability and accessibility of warning, and the rapidity of response.

Whilst anyone can be at risk of health effects, certain groups may be more vulnerable, including older people, pregnant women, children, individuals with poor health, those with physical, cognitive, or sensory impairments, people with language or cultural-based vulnerabilities, tourists. Some groups, who may not be thought of as vulnerable (e.g. young men) may put themselves at risk (e.g. driving through floodwater or by helping others).

15.1.3 **Components of the local response to flooding**

The LRF is composed of Category 1 and 2 responders, and other invitees. It aims to plan for localized incidents and emergencies to prevent and/or mitigate the impact on their local communities. In theory, efforts are focused on more vulnerable sections of society, although in practice such individuals can be difficult to identify, hence plans often focus on geographic and infrastructure risks. The detail of the approach may differ from area to area. Generic information on roles and responsibilities in emergency planning, response, and recovery is available (Cabinet Office 2013) (see Chapter 3).

As flood events are highly dependent on location and context, and the impacts are often complex, sustained and diverse, a well-coordinated multi-agency plan and response is required. Generic flood planning information is available (Defra 2013); the local plan will detail local decisions regarding roles, responsibilities and processes and expectations of public health.

Communities themselves have an important role in preparing and responding to incidents such as floods and are encouraged to be aware of their flood risk and warnings and develop individual and community flood plans.

15.1.4 **Health protection actions in response to flooding (with others through mechanisms such as SCG/STAC)**

◆ Scientific and technical advice regarding:
  • health effects,
  • vulnerable groups, and
  • interventions (e.g. safe disposal of sandbags);
◆ Public-facing health advice, accessible to a wide range of individuals, diverse in delivery, but consistent in content:
  • written (leaflets/booklets/posters, notice boards/bus shelters),
  • traditional (press releases/interviews),

- social media, and
- public meetings;
◆ Surveillance and evaluation of health impacts:
  - acute,
  - medium to long term, and
  - academic research to improve future response;
◆ Business continuity:
  - ensuring other health protection functions are maintained, and
  - considering need for mutual aid from teams in unaffected areas.

15.2 What's the story?

◆ An emergency planner informs you that a Flood Guidance Statement (FGS) has been issued for your area.

◆ The FGS states that, due to a forecast of exceptionally heavy rain, there is a **high likelihood of severe disruption** from river and surface water flooding to communities along the local river and three nearby towns in the next 48–72hrs. The risk may continue for several days.

◆ You are required to attend the SCG to provide advice about the likely health impacts.

15.2.1 Top tips

◆ The FGS is available to all Category 1 and 2 responders.
◆ Be aware that similar flooding events may be forecast beyond your geographical area which may have implications for the local response.

15.2.2 Tools of the trade

◆ local MAFP,
◆ knowledge about flooding and health (see section 15.1.2 and references), and
◆ sources of health surveillance (including syndromic) data, laboratory reports and outbreak investigations (PHE 2014).

15.2.3 What immediate action(s) would you take?

◆ Familiarize yourself with the FGS and MAFP, focusing particularly on local arrangements for protecting vulnerable sites (e.g. hospitals, care homes, Control of Major Accident Hazards (COMAH) sites) and individuals (e.g. on home oxygen/dialysis, requiring regular visits from services) (Cabinet Office 2008).

◆ Liaise with health emergency planners regarding alerting the health protection system, business continuity/mutual aid, and action to protect critical health infrastructure and/or divert demand.

◆ Familiarize yourself with rapidly available health surveillance data; agree plans for collection, analysis, and reporting.

◆ Start developing appropriate written information and a holding press statement with communications colleagues, in consultation with wider SCG communications.

◆ Liaise with neighbouring and national public health colleagues to ensure appropriate, joined-up, and consistent approaches.

(**Note:** this scenario concerns a situation with a high likelihood of severe disruption. Where there is less confidence about what will happen or the impact is expected to be less severe, actions will need to be adjusted in consultation with the SCG.)

15.2.4 **Key scenario information**

◆ Hospitals and care homes are required to have major incident plans; many have flood plans.

◆ Loss of critical infrastructure, such as utilities, may have significant health impacts, particularly for individuals who are highly dependent on these supplies and may have difficulties sourcing alternatives.

◆ Key health messages for the public during the warning phase may include:
  • stay informed (EA flood warnings, local radio, telephone helplines),
  • pack a flood kit; switch off gas/electric if flooded,
  • follow advice—evacuate if asked,
  • avoid contact with flood water; if unavoidable be aware of potential hazards and maintain hygiene, and
  • look out for the vulnerable in your community, but don't put yourself at unnecessary risk.

15.3 **Scenario update # 1**

◆ The SCG assesses the risks to the community and infrastructure. Plans are rehearsed and twice daily incident management meetings are agreed. A press release is issued, as part of the multi-agency communications strategy, alerting the community to recommended actions to protect health.

◆ Flooding starts earlier and more rapidly than expected and affects a wider area. Approximately 2000 homes have been flooded, and local authority rest centres have been set up. These are dealing mainly with the most vulnerable, as many residents have made their own provision through friends and relatives. Some rest centres are approaching maximum capacity and overnight accommodation at local hotels and guest houses is limited.

◆ A number of people have refused to leave their homes despite flooded ground floors. Seven people have had to be rescued from cars and one person has drowned after assisting a pet dog in fast-flowing water. The electricity substation has been flooded, with loss of power to over 10,000 homes and the water treatment facility, leading to a loss of mains water.

◆ STAC has been established to provide specialist health and other scientific advice to the local responders; you provide the public health input.

15.3.1 **What further action(s) would you take?**

◆ Update public health communications to reflect new risks associated with loss of power and water, as part of the wider SCG approach.

◆ Inform surveillance teams of areas affected by flooding, power, and water loss to ensure all flooding-related health impacts are captured as far as possible.

◆ Consider establishing a health register to support and follow up the population directly and indirectly affected (see 15.3.3) (PHE 2014).

15.3.2 **Key scenario information**

◆ Power loss may result in loss of light, control of temperature, water and sewage treatment, communications, storage of foods and medicines, use of mains-operated equipment, and medical devices.

◆ Loss of utilities may cause indirect health effects (e.g. CO poisoning through the inappropriate use of generators and barbecues indoors; burns from boiling non-potable water).

◆ Power and water companies are required to have plans to deal with unexpected loss of supply to:
  • restore services as quickly as possible, prioritizing vulnerable individuals (signed up to priority service registers) and institutions such as hospitals, care homes, and schools, and
  • lead public-facing communications on restoration of supply, 'boil water' notices, and access to alternative supplies.

◆ Health protection specialists provide:
  • specialist advice (e.g. on hygiene, food and water safety, and vulnerable groups),
  • public communications regarding health issues,
  • health impact surveillance, and
  • own business continuity.

◆ Key health messages for the public during flooding:
  • reinforce pre-flood messages,
  • do not use petrol or diesel generators indoors. The exhaust gases contain carbon monoxide, which can kill, and
  • distress is normal—friends and family can help.

15.3.3 **Top tips**

◆ Weather and flooding forecasts continue to improve, but flooding can be more severe and sudden than predicted.

◆ Consider ways to communicate that do not rely on power supplies (e.g. loud hailers, posters on telegraph poles) and avoid posting paper-based materials to flooded homes. Text messages can be useful, particularly for those displaced from home.

◆ People can be anxious about leaving their homes for fear of looting/uncertainty about the alternative.
  • There is no legal basis in the UK to force people to evacuate; however, those that stay in their homes may harm their health and put emergency personnel at greater risk.
  • Public Health has a role in encouraging people to leave homes when flooded, whilst recognizing personal autonomy, and reinforcing safety messages.

◆ Health registers offer the possibility to assure more complete and longer surveillance of health effects following flooding.
  • They are helpful in situations when people exposed are displaced; rapid registration enables collection of contact details.
  • They need quick implementation, are resource intensive, and should offer the population some direct benefit.
  • They should be implemented with full multi-agency agreement and support.
  • Resources and protocols should be agreed locally prior to any major flooding to facilitate rapid and effective deployment.

15.4 **Scenario update # 2**

◆ Eight days later the water is receding and people are assessing the damage. Power and mains water have been restored. Long-term temporary accommodation for displaced persons is being arranged by insurance firms, local authority and support organizations, and short-term arrangements in local hotels and rest centres are ceasing.

◆ Many residents are upset and angry. You are asked to address a public meeting about the health risks.

◆ An older gentleman in the community, who continued living alone in his flooded house, has just been admitted to hospital for an unknown reason; rumours are circulating. You call the A&E department. The gentleman has CO poisoning, the likely source being a disposable barbecue he had been using to keep warm.

◆ Chief among people's concerns are infection risk and why the flood waters haven't been tested, risk of leptospirosis, how to clean up safely, and disposal of sewage. Some worry about possible chemical contamination of the water.

15.4.1 **What further information do you need?**

◆ Others who will attend the meeting (e.g. colleagues from the local authority, NHS, EA).

◆ Up-to-date information on the extent of the flooding, any hazardous chemical sites affected and any health impacts identified from surveillance.

15.4.2 **Key scenario information**

◆ Whilst flood water in the UK is likely to be contaminated by disease producing micro-organisms from sewage, the risks of serious infection are low because:

  • high-risk enteric infectious diseases (e.g. cholera, typhoid) are not endemic, and leptospirosis is rare,

  • the diluting and dispersing of potential sources of infection further significantly reduces any risk,

  • basic hygiene measures (handwashing and rubber boots/gloves) are easily accessible, and

  • microbiological testing of the flood water is likely to find disease causing micro-organisms, but very unlikely to require a change in public health advice, so is not recommended.

◆ The dilution and dispersal of any chemical contamination is also likely to substantially reduce any risk to health, although specialist advice should always be sought.

◆ Risks such as CO poisoning can be overlooked and need emphasizing.

◆ While experiencing a flood is the primary cause of stress, the clean-up can also be very stressful, once the emergency services have moved on and secondary stressors become apparent.

◆ Distress is a normal reaction to a flood.

  • 'Psychological first aid' (practical supportive responses to meet basic needs that can be performed by anyone) rather than specialist counselling is recommended by the WHO following disasters.

  • Distress is usually temporary; but some people may go on to develop mental health problems.

- If a person's symptoms persist, they should visit their GP to identify further sources of support.
- Key public health messages should continue to reinforce basic hygiene messages, warn about the risks of CO poisoning, and acknowledge distress as being normal.

15.4.3 Top tips

- Before speaking at a public meeting check with your department; they may prefer a senior staff member to speak.
- If you do speak, make sure that you are prepared with key messages and have checked all the relevant information is correct and up to date. Guidance on recovery is available (PHE 2014).
- Stick to facts—not speculation. Be pragmatic (e.g. in relation to hand hygiene and toilets—no point in insisting on hot water and soap if no water/power).
- Respect confidentiality.

15.4.4 What further action(s) would you take?

- Usual actions in relation to CO poisoning (see Carbon Monoxide SIMCARD p. 386).
- Continue to reinforce public health messages during the recovery process.

15.5 Scenario update # 3

- It is six months later and most people have returned to their homes. Some remain displaced and many people are anxious about the impact on house insurance, house prices, and their livelihoods.
- An active community group has been established who are keen to develop a community flood plan. You are asked for advice about what to include from the health perspective.

15.5.1 What would you suggest?

- Get informed about flood risk, warning systems, household defences, and local and national support groups.
- Make a flood plan for your household and work with others in your community to develop a community flood plan.
- Think about how to help responders identify and support those most vulnerable in the community, remembering that not all who are vulnerable will be getting services and may be unrecognized.
- Build on existing mechanisms such as neighbourhood watch, parish council, faith groups, or other community sector organizations.
- Make contact with community flood groups in other regions to share information, ideas, and lessons learned.

15.5.2 Key scenario information

- Individuals and communities in flood risk zones are encouraged to prepare flood plans to help them take action before and during a flood.

- The EA has template plans available to help people prepare in advance of flooding; there are a number of case studies of communities working together to reduce their risk.
- The National Flood Forum is a charity dedicated to supporting and representing communities and individuals at risk of flooding. Several other national and local community sector groups work with statutory organizations to help prepare and respond to emergencies such as flooding.

15.6 **What if ... ?**

15.6.1 **It was a coastal flood?**

- Impacts may be faster and more extreme, but areas at risk of coastal flooding may be more prepared and better warned than others.
- People may put themselves in danger on harbour walls/promenades to watch the waves; SCG communications messages may need to advise against this.
- Coastal flooding can be particularly destructive and exacerbate existing problems with coastal erosion, loss of property, and livelihood. Large numbers of people may be asked to evacuate. The health effects of evacuation in the UK are not well understood.
- Coastal areas may have high proportions of older residents and temporary residents, low employment levels and high seasonality of work, physical isolation and poor transport links.

15.6.2 **It was ground water flooding?**

- Impacts may be more insidious and water may appear unexpectedly through the floorboards; traditional methods for flood protection (e.g. sandbags) may not be effective.
- Pumping is often used to prevent or reduce water inundation; if fuel-driven equipment is used inappropriately, there is a risk of CO poisoning.
- Septic tanks frequently have problems when ground water levels rise.

15.6.3 **There was an outbreak of gastrointestinal disease?**

- See Chapter 20 regarding management of an outbreak.

15.6.4 **A hospital/care home was flooded?**

- All hospitals should have assessed flood risks and addressed the issues either through their business continuity plans (see Chapter 13) or a specific flood plan for the premises.

15.7 **The unanswered question(s) around flooding and health and wellbeing**

- There is limited quantification of the health impacts of flooding (e.g. mortality, mental health effects, and health service use). Quantifying the health impacts is important so that the full costs of flooding can be incorporated into cost benefit analyses of interventions such as flood defences.
- There is even less evidence on the effectiveness of interventions that aim to protect health and wellbeing (e.g. warnings, evacuation, flood risk maps).

15.8 **Lessons learned**

◆ The effects of flooding on health and wellbeing can be underestimated and often relate to the indirect rather than the direct effects of the flood water. They are not well quantified, however, meaning that the health and wellbeing costs of flooding are not always fully included in cost–benefit analyses of interventions such as flood defences.

◆ The public is often most concerned about risks of serious infection, although these are rare in this country as long as basic hygiene measures are followed. Risks associated with CO poisoning and mental health impacts due to secondary stressors can be overlooked or underestimated.

◆ Climate change will increase the risk of flooding in the UK. This will have a negative impact on both communities and critical infrastructure and it is important that we continue to prepare for this.

15.9 **Further thinking**

◆ How can we encourage individuals and communities to be aware of current and future flood risk and the steps they can take to reduce the damage (without causing undue anxiety)?

◆ How can we improve our knowledge of the impacts of flooding on health and wellbeing?

◆ How can we use surveillance data to go beyond infectious disease risks?

◆ What is the role of health services in the preparation, response, and recovery from flooding?

◆ How can individual and community resilience be strengthened?

References

Cabinet Office. 2008. *Identifying People Who Are Vulnerable in a Crisis: Guidance for Emergency Planners and Responders*. https://www.gov.uk/government/publications/identifying-people-who-are-vulnerable-in-a-crisis-guidance-for-emergency-planners-and-responders (accessed 8 March 2016).

Cabinet Office. 2013. *Preparation and Planning for Emergencies: Responsibilities of Responder Agencies and Others*. https://www.gov.uk/preparation-and-planning-for-emergencies-responsibilities-of-responder-agencies-and-others (accessed 8 March 2016).

Cabinet Office. 2015. *National Risk Register of Civil Emergencies*. https://www.gov.uk/government/collections/national-risk-register-of-civil-emergencies (accessed 8 March 2016).

Department for Environment, Food & Rural Affairs (Defra). 2013 (updated Dec 2014). *National Flood Emergency Framework for England*. https://www.gov.uk/government/publications/the-national-flood-emergency-framework-for-england (accessed 8 March 2016).

Menne B, V Murray (eds). 2013. *Floods: Health Effects and Prevention in the WHO European Region*. Copenhagen: WHO. http://www.euro.who.int/__data/assets/pdf_file/0020/189020/e96853.pdf (accessed 8 March 2016).

Public Health England (PHE). 2014. *Flooding Health Guidance and Advice*. https://www.gov.uk/government/collections/flooding-health-guidance-and-advice (accessed 8 March 2016).

Further reading

Vardoulakis S, C Heaviside (eds). 2012. *Health Effects of Climate Change UK*. Didcot: Public Health England. https://www.gov.uk/government/publications/climate-change-health-effects-in-the-uk (accessed 8 March 2016).

Defra. 2013. *The National Adaptation Programme. Making the Country Resilient to a Changing Climate*. London: The Stationary Office. https://www.gov.uk/government/publications/adapting-to-climate-change-national-adaptation-programme (accessed 8 March 2016).

Section 4

Environmental Public Health practice case studies and scenarios

Chapter 16

Ambient air pollution and health

John Reid, Giovanni Leonardi, and Alex G. Stewart

OVERVIEW
....

After reading this chapter the reader will be familiar with:
- the common pollutants, sources, and scales of air pollution (local to global),
- the measures that could support pollution control and mitigate health effects,
- the available data on air pollution,
- the relative impacts of indoor and outdoor air pollution,
- the roles of public health and other agencies, and
- communicating risks and resolutions.

Terms

Ambient air Average outdoor air conditions (over a time period, e.g. 15 minutes, month, year) versus indoor air.

Air Quality Management Area (AQMA) Geographically and legally defined areas where local authorities estimate air pollution levels above regulatory standards. Part IV Environment Act 1995 requires UK local authorities to conduct Local Air Quality Reviews with Action Plans for each AQMA.

Particulate Matter (PM) Small respirable particles that may penetrate the lungs to alveolar levels. The diameter of the particle is described in the name and is measured in microns: $PM_{10} = <10$ microns; $PM_{2.5} = <2.5$ microns; $PM_{0.1} = <0.1$ microns (ultrafine particles).

(See further list of terms in the Glossary.)

16.1 Background facts: ambient air pollution and health

♦ Average levels of commonly measured air pollutants have decreased in the UK (and Europe) since the Clean Air Acts (1956, 1968, 1993) but the related health burden remains high.

♦ Current UK public health interest concentrates on small airborne particles and oxides of nitrogen (NOx), although there are other pollutants that are monitored under legislation (see Table 16.2).

♦ A key public health indicator of air quality is $PM_{2.5}$, but it is not measured as frequently as PM_{10}.

16.1.1 Key scenario information

♦ Requests for investigations of actual/suspected increased incidence of disease are made by a range of people, including health professionals, members of the public, Environmental Health Officers, and local elected members.

- Such requests can be made to any branch of Public Health.
- The requests may point to a suspected cause or a community concern that needs to be investigated.

16.1.2 Key points in an investigation

It is difficult to measure the health effects of chronic air pollution at a local population level. Evidence derived from large (often multi-centre) studies needs to be applied, via multidisciplinary specialist teams, possibly with modelling of pollution or health outcomes, to understand local impacts. A multi-agency Advisory Group on Health (Reid et al. 2005; Mahoney et al 2015) (see Table 20.3 for template agenda for an Advisory Group on Health) could be tasked to examine the problem and wider situation, including evidence from environmental and health sciences, relevant contexts and needs of different groups. The Director of Public Health (DPH) or Consultant in Public Health or Health Protection could chair the meeting.

Membership and terms of reference of the Advisory Group on Health should be agreed, based on the nature of the review and skills needed. The group may include a Health Protection Consultant, specialists in toxicology and environmental science, epidemiologist or analyst, Environmental Health Officer, and communications manager.

A structured and systematic process, including environmental monitoring or modelling, exposure estimation, and/or epidemiological risk assessment, underpinned by robust science, should highlight any potential legal or technical challenges. This process should share historic local authority Air Pollution Review and Assessment reports, including detailed assessments of AQMAs and previous assessments of pollution sources (source apportionment) and percentages of transport types used locally (modal share). Other useful information may include Met Office reports of Daily Air Quality Index (www.metoffice.gov.uk/guide/weather/air-quality).

16.2 What's the story?

- Local physicians are concerned that hospital admissions for asthma and chronic obstructive pulmonary disease (COPD) have increased 10% over five years, with associated deaths.
- They are concerned about three main roads into the town, each of which has an AQMA: two in residential areas and one near schools.
- The town (population 200,000) has a central regeneration zone around brownfield sites, plus residential and economic zones on the outskirts. There are static air quality monitoring stations (PM_{10}, NOx) at selected points (e.g. busy road junctions where air quality is considered to be poor).
- The local authority air quality officer read the major UK expert report (COMEAP 2010) on effects of $PM_{2.5}$ on health (Table 16.1). She is concerned that the council has no $PM_{2.5}$ monitors and wonders what the report means locally. Elected members ask how to reduce local ill health from air pollution and she turns to Public Health for advice.
- The DPH agrees to review the issues and evidence.

16.2.1 Key scenario information

- **Asthma** can be exacerbated by ambient air pollution but is not usually caused by it.
- **Air pollution** is a significant environmental trigger for exacerbations of COPD and cardiovascular problems, leading to increasing symptoms, emergency department visits, hospital admissions, and even death.

Table 16.1 Examples of air quality measures recommended for human health. Objectives and legal limits, derived from health-based guidance values (see Table 16.2)

Pollutant	Health effects	Public health significance	UK national air quality objectives	Guidance values
PM_{10}	Long-term exposure increases all-cause mortality, particularly lung cancer, cardiovascular disease	May contain harmful chemicals and other particles (e.g. dusts, pollens, moulds)	Annual mean 40µg/m^3 24-hour mean 50µg/m^3 Not to be exceeded more than 35 times per year	Annual mean 20 µg/m^3 24-hour mean 50 µg/m^3
$PM_{2.5}$	As above; penetrates deeper into the body than PM_{10}	Generated by human activity, may cause nearly 29,000 deaths in the UK and 340,000 life years lost (COMEAP 2010). Predicts mortality better than PM_{10}	Annual mean 25 µg/m^3	Annual mean 10 µg/m^3 24-hour mean 25 µg/m^3
SO_2	Irritant to airways causing breathing problems	Major decreases in UK ambient levels in last 30 years. Important in acute releases (e.g. large fires)	One hour mean of 350 µg/m^3 not to be exceeded more than 24 times a calendar year One day mean of 125 µg/m^3 not to be exceeded more than 3 times a calendar year	24-hour mean 20 µg/m^3 10-minute mean 500 µg/m^3
NO_2	Irritant to airways causing breathing problems	Contributes to photochemical smog and ground ozone levels	Annual mean 40 µg/m^3 1-hour mean 200 µg/m^3 not to be exceeded more than 18 times per year	Annual mean 40 µg/m^3 1-hour mean 200 µg/m^3
O_3	Ground-level ozone arises from photochemical smog; triggers asthma and exacerbates lung conditions	May increase daily mortality rate, especially cardiovascular	8-hour mean 100 µg/m^3 not to be exceeded more than 10 times per year	8-hour mean 100 µg/m^3

Source: data from World Health Organisation. WHO Air quality guidelines for particulate matter, ozone, nitrogen dioxide and sulphur dioxide – Global update 2005. Geneva: WHO, Copyright © 2006 WHO; Defra. The Air Quality Strategy for England, Scotland, Wales and Northern Ireland (Volume 1), (Department for Environment, Food and Rural Affairs in partnership with the Scottish Executive, Welsh Assembly Government and Department of the Environment Northern Ireland, 2007), © 2007 Crown Copyright, https://www.gov.uk/government/uploads/system/uploads/attachment_data/file/69336/pb12654-air-quality-strategy-vol1-070712.pdf, accessed 01 Oct. 2015.

16.2.2 Tools of the trade

♦ There is a range of relevant public health indicators available to local Public Health departments, including air quality indicators.

♦ The GP Quality and Outcomes Framework (QOF) requires practices to keep chronic disease registers and monitor patients with COPD and asthma.

16.2.3 What immediate action(s) would you take?

♦ Step back and look at the wider picture around the immediate question. Ask yourself and others what else needs to be understood to address the situation.

Table 16.2 The health background to statutory pollutant controls within the UK and Europe (For information on the UK national air quality objectives see https://uk-air.defra.gov.uk/air-pollution/uk-eu-limits and links therein)

Pollutant	Sources	Risks	WHO Guidelines
Benzene	Combustion: cigarettes, petrol; industry; petrol evaporation	Bone marrow depression; genotoxicity; carcinogenicity	No safe exposure; excess lifetime risk of leukaemia 6 x 10^{-6} for 1 $\mu g/m^3$
1,3-Butadiene	Incomplete combustion of fuel	Carcinogenicity, some CNS irritation	No definitive conclusions
Carbon monoxide	Incomplete combustion, tobacco smoking	Hypoxia, neurological damage, cardiovascular mortality and infarction; perinatal deaths, behavioural effects in infants & young children	90 ppm (100 mg/m^3) for 15 mins; 10 ppm (10 mg/m^3) for 8 hours
Lead	Water pipes, solder, paint, lead crystal & lead-glazed pottery, folk medicines, dust & soil, batteries, fishing weights, roof flashing	Neurological changes at low doses (cognition, hearing, peripheral nerves); anaemia, gastrointestinal symptoms, renal damage, death at higher doses	No safe level. No guidelines for ambient air.
Nitrogen dioxide and other oxides of Nitrogen.	Combustion: road transport (47%), power sources (22%), domestic (4%), natural sources (minor)	Decreased lung function	200 $\mu g/m^3$ for 1 hour; 40 $\mu g/m^3$ for annual mean
Ozone	Short-wave solar radiation effect, on anthropogenic pollutants like NO_2 & hydrocarbons. Long-term impact of climate change is expected to worsen Ozone levels in polluted areas	Particularly from increased short-term exposures, respiratory effects (including exacerbating asthma and COPD), also cardiovascular disease; current interest in further research to estimate effects of chronic exposure on atherosclerosis, asthma, reduced life expectancy	100 $\mu g/m^3$ daily maximum 8 hour mean
Particles (PM_{10})	Combustion: industry (38%), road transport (24%), power stations (16%), domestic power use (17%). Natural PM_{10} is much less toxic	Respiratory & cardiovascular disease, reduced survival, lowered life expectancy	20 $\mu g/m^3$ annual mean; 50 $\mu g/m^3$ 24 hour mean
Particles ($PM_{2.5}$)	As for PM_{10}; diesel > petrol > petrol with catalytic convertor	As for PM_{10} with greater emphasis on cardiovascular disease; also adverse birth outcomes and childhood respiratory disease	10 $\mu g/m^3$ annual mean; 25 $\mu g/m^3$ 24 hour mean
Sulphur dioxide	Power generation (esp. coal) (65%), industry (24%), commercial & domestic heating (6%), road transport (diesel) (2%)	Respiratory problems	20 $\mu g/m^3$ for 24 hours; 500 $\mu g/m^3$ for 10 minute mean

Source: data from World Health Organisation. WHO Air quality guidelines for particulate matter, ozone, nitrogen dioxide and sulphur dioxide – Global update 2005. Geneva: WHO, Copyright © 2006 World Health Organization, http://apps.who.int/iris/bitstream/10665/69477/1/WHO_SDE_PHE_OEH_06.02_eng.pdf; World Health Organization. Air Quality Guidelines for Europe. 2nd edition. Copenhagen: World Health Organization Regional Office for Europe Copenhagen, Copyright © 2000 World Health Organization, pp. 91, http://www.euro.who.int/__data/assets/pdf_file/0005/74732/E71922.pdf

♦ Decide if a Advisory Group on Health (see Chapter 20 and Table A20.1) should be established to support the review agreed by the DPH.

16.2.4 **Key scenario information**

♦ **The report on PM$_{2.5}$ particulate matter and deaths in local authority areas** (PHE 2014) gives data (number of deaths, life years lost before age 75) for this and neighbouring areas and those of similar socio-economic mix: the contribution to overall adult mortality varies (~2.5% in rural Scotland to 8% in some London boroughs).

♦ **National guidance physical activity and Active Travel** by the four UK Chief Medical Officers (CMOs 2011) expressed concerns, and supports safer walking and cycling to promote physical activity levels.

16.2.5 **Top tips**

♦ Use support from scientific staff in specialist health protection services (environmental/toxicology) and air quality specialists in local authorities.

♦ Academic colleagues may offer expertise or research support.

♦ Consider a structured analysis of key local issues and any sensitive or complex organizational dynamics (e.g. stakeholder map, a Force Field analysis of competing influences (http://www.institute.nhs.uk/quality_and_service_improvement_tools/quality_and_service_improvement_tools/force_field_analysis.html)), or a PESTEL issues analysis (Political, Economic, Social, Technical, Environmental and Legal).

16.3 **Scenario update # 1**

♦ The Advisory Group on Health reviewed local and wider evidence and requested further information.

♦ The Advisory Group on Health noted 4.8% of local adult deaths are due to PM$_{2.5}$ outdoor pollution.

♦ Another expert report (Straif et al. 2014) concluded air pollution is carcinogenic.

♦ The first Advisory Group on Health meeting recognizes increased evidence covering the significant burden of disease that air pollution contributes in UK and globally.

16.3.1 **Key scenario information**

♦ Ambient air pollution was globally estimated to cause 3.7 million deaths in 2012 with 4.3 million deaths due to indoor air pollution (WHO 2014).

♦ Removing all anthropogenic (man-made) PM$_{2.5}$ air pollution could save the UK population approximately 36.5 million life years over the next 100 years (COMEAP 2010).

♦ Particulate air pollution is estimated to reduce average life expectancy in the UK by ~6 months, worth £16 billion per year (DEFRA 2013).

16.3.2 **What further action(s) would you take?**

♦ Consider the underlying local social, political, and communication challenges. These will not be addressed without publicizing the local facts openly, engaging widely with policy-makers and communities, and a meaningful rethink on local transport policies.

♦ Advocate within the local authority for strong strategies (see Box 16.1).

Box 16.1 Ambient air pollution case studies

London, UK

- 60 years since the 1952 Great Smog, London has again become notable for excess air pollution deaths.
- PHE (2014) estimates 7.2% (3389) of all 47,998 deaths age ≥25 in London (2010), and 41,404 life years lost, were associated with higher levels of exposure to man-made $PM_{2.5}$ pollutants.
- Estimated deaths were highest in several internationally known, affluent boroughs (Westminster (8.3%), Kensington and Chelsea (8.3%)).
- Evidence is emerging that London may need to adopt stringent measures to meet air quality standards and reduce the large associated burden of disease.
- Failure to meet air quality standards threatens to undermine London's reputation as a world-leading city.
- London has been at the UK forefront of developing healthy environmental policies and Active Travel.
- Improving the Health of Londoners—Transport Action Plan 2014, recognizes needed integrated action; over £4 billion is promised over 10 years to achieve goals for physical activity, air pollution, road traffic collisions, noise and improving access and mental health.
- Key priorities include action for 'healthy streets', improved on-street air monitoring, better public transport, 'light segregation' of cyclist paths, and the 'Legible London' project to inform and promote safer pedestrian way-finding.

Aarhus, Denmark

- Aarhus is Denmark's second largest city (population 300,000). In 1994, the municipality adopted a plan to reduce the use of individual motor vehicles and increase the use of sustainable transportation.
- The cycling programme (1995–96) initially focused on the use of bicycles, and later public transport. Aarhus already had a well-developed network of bicycle paths and most residents lived within cycling distance of the city centre. Nevertheless, previous campaigns had been unsuccessful in convincing people to cycle to work, whereas this initiative achieved a sustained success by changing the general attractiveness of cycling (Surborg 2002).

16.4 **Scenario update # 2**

- The elected member with the environmental portfolio is sceptical of linking respiratory health effects to air pollution, suggesting high levels of smoking and deprivation are the main causes of poor local respiratory health.
- The DPH is concerned that focusing on air pollution alone could distract staff from the local efforts to reduce smoking and high levels of obesity, hypertension, and diabetes.

16.4.1 **What further action(s) would you take?**

♦ Include local smoking and physical activity levels in the Advisory Group on Health overview so their contribution to the local burden of respiratory and cardiovascular disease is understood. Smoking remains a critical factor for respiratory and coronary heart disease, while the effects of physical inactivity contribute significantly to risks for cardiovascular diseases, including coronary heart disease and stroke (CMOs 2011). Air pollution adds to those disease rates.

♦ Summarize key strengths and weaknesses of the local transport plan which should support healthier options to reduce coronary heart disease, diabetes and other diseases associated with low physical activity (WHO recommends 150 minutes moderate intensity exercise for adults weekly). Safer cycling and walking will also reduce injuries. Other health benefits of increased physical activity include reduction in osteoporosis, better mental health and reduced colon cancer and breast cancer rates (Pucher et al. 2010).

16.4.2 **What further information do you need?**

♦ Consider other relevant strategies such as changes in transport: demography, economics, public services.

♦ Useful regional and national health and environmental data can be accessed from the Public Health England or the Department for Environment, Food & Rural Affairs (Defra) websites: https://www.gov.uk/government/organisations/public-health-england and https://www.gov.uk/government/organisations/department-for-environment-food-rural-affairs.

16.4.3 **Tools of the trade**

♦ Geographical Information Systems can map air pollution levels and localities where Guideline Values are exceeded, show local baselines, and current street-level facilities (cycle paths and traffic free areas).

♦ There may be limited local modelling capacity for exposure of populations: look for expertise in nearby local authorities or academic departments.

♦ Health Impact Assessments can identify how to integrate plans to demonstrate public health outcomes such as healthy travel and environments. Tools and examples can be found via the HIA Gateway web portal (http://www.apho.org.uk/default.aspx?QN=P_HIA).

♦ The review should include all localities in the area.

16.5 **Scenario update # 3**

♦ The local community believes the industrial sites on the town outskirts are major contributors to local air pollution. These sites include a chemical works, which has had a number of leaks over the past few years, and an incinerator which has generated smoke complaints. A pressure group wants to close them both, as they are perceived to be bad for health. However, the council considers them an important source of local employment.

16.5.1 **Key scenario information**

New incinerators often arouse passionate opposition, which may be based on well-documented health issues arising from older, less clean and less well-regulated operations. Modern incinerators, like many other polluting commercial enterprises, are regulated under EU directives and UK environmental regulations.

16.5.2 **What further action(s) would you take?**

♦ Consider holding public meetings to capture local residents and user perspectives.

♦ Consider meeting pressure group leaders and discussing the wider issues. They may be willing to shift their focus, but gaining an insight into their perspective is even more important.

♦ Consider Equality Impact Assessment duties (Equality Act 2010) if a new policy is being developed and the views of protected groups are to be recognized fully.

♦ Study relevant parts of local air quality review and assessment documents. Seek air emissions data and other details from the pressure group and plant operators and liaise with local authority environmental health or the Environment Agency concerning their concerns and complaints database, including statutory nuisance reports.

16.6 **Scenario update # 4**

♦ The local radio station wants a panel discussion on air quality; you attend, along with the local air quality officer and pressure group members. During the discussion you are asked about the links between deaths and air pollution.

16.6.1 **How would you respond in the radio interview?**

♦ Ensure that communications officers in local authority, public health, and other organizations are aware of the investigation and support joint working.

♦ Agree key messages with the local DPH, other involved officers, and agencies.

♦ Provide full media technical press briefing notes to underpin their shorter coverage and headlines.

♦ Visit sites so you know the locality.

♦ Brief key leaders.

♦ Emphasize that public health actions related to air quality will improve health by supporting other essential healthy living priorities: cycling, walking, public transport, reducing car usage, reducing obesity.
  • Increasing physical activity from sedentary to moderate levels could reduce metabolic syndrome and diabetes by 30–40% (CMOs 2011).
  • 'Active and safe travel' is one of the nine key health-related priorities recommended for local authorities (Buck and Gregory 2013).

♦ Refer to the work of local stakeholders to reduce air pollution. Success of interventions rests on local support.

♦ Highlight win-win of alternative transport plans for local and global solutions (Woodcock et al. 2009).

16.7 **What if … ?**

♦ There is air pollution forecast for a local sporting event attracting large numbers of participants? (consider smog; see Giles and Koehle 2014).

♦ Indoor air pollution is raised as a key local concern? (see Box 16.2).

♦ There are sources outside the local community (e.g. long-range transport of pollutants from Europe)—what do you communicate and how do you reach the unreachable (e.g. elderly)? (see cf. Lamb 2014).

♦ The local authority air quality officer raised issues about the health effects of ozone? (see COMEAP 2015).

Box 16.2 Indoor air issues

Worldwide, indoor air pollution accounts for similar burden of disease to outdoor. Low- and middle-income countries are badly affected. The predominant effects are through exposure to particulates from indoor fuel combustion, causing death and morbidity in childhood (respiratory infections including pneumonia). Long-term adult exposure can cause COPD and exacerbation of chronic conditions. Replacement of traditional fuel burning devices with modern, affordable equipment is central to prevention.

Home environments are particularly important for the most vulnerable groups—ill or older people and pre-school children, who spend a higher proportion of their time indoors (see UK Parliament 2010).

Other indoor UK environments are regulated through occupational exposure limits (e.g. workplace and leisure setting smoking ban).

The European burden of disease from household environmental hazards has been calculated (Braubach et al. 2011). Air pollutants that increase the burden of disease are: carbon monoxide (CO), secondhand tobacco smoke, formaldehyde, radon, solid fuel indoor smoke, dampness, and moulds. Indoor air, including allergens, is important in asthma causation.

Current UK indoor air issues

Exposure at home and in private vehicles to environmental tobacco smoke is a major current priority for public health action. The significance of indoor emissions from electronic cigarettes remains uncertain.

CO, a byproduct of incomplete combustion of carbon-based fuels, kills through acute poisoning. Lower level exposure to CO is more important in terms of burden of disease, contributing to decline or exacerbations in pre-existing chronic conditions and elderly people. Annual campaigns raise awareness of dangers of CO, the importance of maintenance checks of heating and cooking systems, CO alarms, and signs of poisoning.

Radon (radioactive gas) causes ~1100 deaths in the UK each year, chiefly from lung cancer. Affected areas are determined by the underlying geology. Advice on monitoring and treatment of affected homes is available at: http://www.ukradon.org/

16.8 **Some unanswered questions**

+ What are the impacts of mixed indoor and outdoor exposures in causing ill health or effects of different mixes of pollutants?

+ Can new technologies make it easier to collect personal health and environmental exposure data, including personal sensors (Austen 2015)?

+ How will the interactions between air quality and health inequalities be studied and managed?

+ Will further research confirm the role of particulate pollution in an increasing number of common conditions (Brauer 2015), such as forms of stroke (Shah et al. 2015) or anxiety states (Power et al. 2015)?

+ Will future research confirm suspected adverse health impacts on neurodevelopment in young children or cognitive decline in older age (Guxens and Sunyer 2012)?

16.9 **Lessons learned**

♦ Local air pollution problems are difficult to link to routine health data.

♦ Fears and perceptions may arise by erroneously linking data from air pollution monitoring and crude health indicator data. Expert public health and environmental science analysis is usually required to inform public or professional understanding of risk.

♦ Public health specialists should take an active interest in the collection and analysis of routine scientific data, and advise on likely health issues. This also assists in leadership during air pollution crises and peaks.

♦ To assess risk, complex sources–pathways–receptors models may be needed, recognizing multiple pollution sources, geographical footprints, meteorology, and local population distribution and demographic mix.

♦ Regular communications and updates can be made via websites and social media.

♦ Identify lessons and discuss/share good practice by reviewing the situation as a 'public health case study' (see Box 16.1).

♦ The Local Transport Plan should be strong on Active Travel and health issues.

♦ Local authorities are required to promote public health.

16.10 **Further thinking**

♦ What can be done to embed consideration of air pollution interventions in the context of wider strategies and societal changes?

♦ What can be done to incorporate new technology such as Personal Exposure Monitoring Sensors (cheaper, lighter technology, transmitting data remotely) to improve data quality and support the evidence base?

♦ How can the public health community promote 'Citizens' Science': local, lay study of environmental or health problems?

♦ What can be done to facilitate sharing the learning, such as local experiences in sustainable transport, from other global towns of similar size (e.g. car-free centres do not detract from local business) (Fletcher and McMichael 1997)?

♦ What is the best way to encourage the public health community and wider multi-agency partners to consider and evaluate the wide range of interventions reported in the literature?

♦ What can be done locally to contribute to national and global issues: such as climate change, foreign travel and exposure, and long-distance air pollution movements?

References

Austen K. 2015. Pollution patrol. *Nature*, **517**: 136–38.

Brauer M. 2015. Air pollution, stroke and anxiety. *BJM*, **350**: 8.

Braubach M, DE Jacobs, D Ormandy. 2011. *Environmental Burden of Disease Associated with Inadequate Housing.* Copenhagen: WHO Regional Office for Europe.

Buck D, S Gregory. 2013. *Improving the Public's Health. A Resource for Local Authorities.* London: The King's Fund.

CMOs. 2011. *Start Active, Stay Active: A Report on Physical Activity for Health from the Four Home Countries.* Chief Medical Officers. UK Health Departments.

Committee on the Medical Effects of Air Pollution (COMEAP). 2010. *Long-term Exposure to Air Pollution: Effect on Mortality.* Didcot: Public Health England.

COMEAP 2015. *Quantification of Mortality and Hospital Admissions Associated with Ground-level Ozone.* Didcot: Public Health England.

Department for Environment, Food & Rural Affairs (Defra). 2007. *The Air Quality Strategy for England, Scotland, Wales and Northern Ireland (Volume 1).* (Department for Environment, Food and Rural Affairs in partnership with the Scottish Executive, Welsh Assembly Government and Department of the Environment Northern Ireland). https://www.gov.uk/government/uploads/system/uploads/attachment_data/file/69336/pb12654-air-quality-strategy-vol1-070712.pdf (accessed 8 March 2016).

Defra. 2013. *Abatement Cost Guidance for Valuing Changes in Air Quality (May 2013).* London: Defra. https://www.gov.uk/government/uploads/system/uploads/attachment_data/file/197898/pb13912-airquality-abatement-cost-guide.pdf (accessed 8 March 2016).

Fletcher T, AJ McMichael (eds). 1997. *Health at the Crossroads.* Chichester: John Wiley and Sons.

Giles LV, MS Koehle. 2014. The health effects of exercising in air pollution. *Sports Medicine,* **44**: 223–49.

Guxens M, J Sunyer. 2012. A review of epidemiological studies on neuropsychological effects of air pollution. *Swiss Medical Weekly,* **141**: w13322.

International Agency for Research on Cancer (IARC). 2014. *World Cancer Report 2014.* Lyon: IARC.

Lamb P. 2014. 'Le pong'—A Public Health Incident. *Chemical Hazards and Poisons Report,* Sept.(24): 10–14. https://www.gov.uk/government/publications/chemical-hazards-and-poisons-report-issue-24 (accessed 8 March 2016).

Mahoney G, AG Stewart, N Kennedy, et al. 2015. Achieving attainable outcomes from good science in an untidy world: case studies in land and air pollution. *Environmental Geochemistry & Health,* **37**: 689–706. doi:10.1007/s10653-015-9717-9

Power MC, M Kiomourtzglou, JE Hart, et al. 2015. The relation between past exposure to fine particulate air pollution and prevalent anxiety: observational cohort study. *BMJ,* **350**: h1111.

Public Health England (PHE). 2014. *Estimating Local Mortality Burdens Associated with Particulate Air Pollution.* Didcot: PHE.

Pucher J, R Buehler, DR Bassett, et al. 2010. Walking and cycling to health: a comparative analysis of city, state, and international data. *American Journal of Public Health,* **100**(10): 1986–92.

Reid JR, R Jarvis, J Richardson, et al. 2005. Responding to chronic environmental problems in Cheshire & Merseyside – Systems and Procedures. *Chemical Hazards and Poisons Report,* **4**: 33–35. https://www.gov.uk/government/publications/chemical-hazards-and-poisons-report-issue-4 (accessed 8 March 2016).

Shah ASV, KL Lee, DA McAllister DA, et al. 2015. Short term exposure to air pollution and stroke: systematic review and meta-analysis. *BMJ,* **350**: h1295.

Straif K, A Cohen, J Samet (eds). 2013. *Air Pollution and Cancer.* IARC Scientific Publication No. 161. Lyon: IARC.

Surborg B. 2002. *Århus Bike Bus'ters,* Tools of Change. http://www.toolsofchange.com/en/case-studies/detail/131 (accessed 8 March 2016).

UK Parliament. 2010. *UK Indoor Air Quality, November 2010: POST Note 366.* London: UK Parliament. http://www.parliament.uk/documents/post/postpn366_indoor_air_quality.pdf (accessed 8 March 2016).

Woodcock JP, C Edwards, BG Tonne, et al. 2009. Public health benefits of strategies to reduce greenhouse-gas emissions: urban land transport. *Lancet,* **374**(9705): 1930–43.

World Health Organization. 2000. *Air Quality Guidelines for Europe.* 2nd edition. Copenhagen: World Health Organization Regional Office for Europe Copenhagen.

World Health Organization. 2005. *WHO Air Quality Guidelines for Particulate Matter, Ozone, Nitrogen Dioxide and Sulphur Dioxide—Global Update 2005*. Geneva: WHO.

World Health Organization. 2014. *Ambient (Outdoor) Air Quality and Health: Fact Sheet N°313*. Geneva: WHO. http://www.who.int/mediacentre/factsheets/fs313/en/ (accessed 8 March 2016).

Further reading

Beatley T. 1999. *Green Urbanism: Learning from European Cities*. Washington, DC: Island Press.

Rayner G, T Lang. 2013. *Ecological Public Health: Reshaping the Conditions for Good Health*. Abingdon: Routledge.

Chapter 17

Cancer and chronic disease clusters

Alex G. Stewart, Sam Ghebrehewet, and Richard Jarvis

OVERVIEW

After reading this chapter the reader will be familiar with:
- the stepwise, structured approach to investigating clusters,
- the criteria for when to consider stopping investigating,
- the process of defining a realistic outcome(s) for an environmental investigation,
- the role of a multi-agency incident team, and
- the process of integrating health studies and environmental investigations.

Terms

Cancer registry Inventory of all malignant tumours in residents of an area.
Exposure Measure of the concentration of a chemical that affects someone.
Hazard Something that can threaten health.
Health criterion values Benchmark concentrations protective of human health.
Risk Probability that a substance will cause harm under specific conditions.
Source–pathway–receptor Source = environment; pathway = route of exposure (inhalation, ingestion, and contact); receptor = people or indicative animal; all three are necessary before a plausible public health problem needs investigating.
Toxicity Biological effect of a substance.
(See further list of terms in the Glossary.)

17.1 Background facts: cancer and chronic disease clusters

♦ A disease cluster is a grouping of cases that appear related in space (e.g. number of cancer cases in one street), time (e.g. suspected increase in incidence of congenital abnormalities in the past year), person (e.g. cancer cases in a family), or a mixture of these. Most reports of clusters indicate some worry that there is a preventable cause, often environmental.

♦ Not all reported clusters stand up to investigation, but all are worth some level of investigation because of the concerns they raise, whether to the lay public or professionals.

♦ Investigations of disease clusters can be time-consuming and resource-intensive and may not lead to the establishment of a clear aetiology.

♦ A cluster may be the result of chance or coincidence; it may be real or perceived (i.e. is there a definable cluster or is the cluster due to a mixed group of biologically unrelated diagnoses?);

it may arise from a bias introduced by a change in measurement, classification, or other factor (e.g. catchment area or target population).

♦ Clusters are often over-investigated, wasting resources. A structured, stepwise investigation alleviates this, proceeding to the next step only if positive findings have been found at the preceding one.

♦ Involvement of those concerned, at an early stage in the investigation, understanding their fears about the disease and possible determinants, as well as their hopes about the outcome of the investigation, is vital.

♦ Environmental investigations can be complex.

♦ Rare diseases are challenging in a different way from common diseases, as it is easier to rule out chance in common diseases than in rare diseases.

17.1.1 Key scenario information

♦ Requests for investigations of disease clusters come from a wide range of people, professionals and lay members of the public.

♦ While many requests are couched generally ('There are a lot of people dying from cancer in our street'), some are specific observations by professionals ('Five cases of testicular cancer in our general practice in the preceding two years').

♦ Requests can be made to general public health or specialist health protection practitioners, and to surveillance and epidemiology teams within public health/health protection/academic departments.

17.1.2 Stepped approach to cluster investigation

Aims and objectives of the whole investigation are:

♦ to examine whether there is an unexpected increase in the observed rate/numbers compared to the expected rate/numbers of the specific disease in question,

♦ to explore any increased disease rate or determine the necessary investigations, and

♦ to offer to those who raised the concern or enquired about the situation an appropriate and plausible explanation for the cluster.

Those concerned should be assured of a full investigation to the appropriate level, but not of any particular outcome.

♦ **Step 1**: define the case/disease or situation:
  - a single, recognized illness or event,
  - distinct basic characteristics (e.g. age, sex, occupation),
  - demarcated geographical boundary (critical, to reduce over- or under-investigation),
  - clear timespan (critical, to avoid over- or under-investigation), and
  - suitable, appropriate comparator.

If there is no relevant case definition, stop the investigation and discuss with those concerned, perhaps following with a written report.

♦ **Step 2**: accepting the need for further investigation, determine if the observed/expected ratio is greater than 1 and statistically significant:
  - search for other cases or events that meet the case definition (e.g. check registries, hospital episode data, routine surveillance, contact relevant health or other professionals serving the relevant catchment area),

- compare observed number of cases to the expected number (e.g. from routine surveillance or national rates applied to the local population). The Standardized Incident Ratio (SIR) (same calculation as Standardized Mortality Ratio (SMR)) is the easiest approach; other methods are complex and require specialist support,
- if there is an increase in numbers of observed cases, consider if they can be explained by:
  - chance—e.g. examine p values or confidence intervals to determine significance,
  - bias—examine the case ascertainment, time, and geographical boundaries to determine whether or not there is the possibility of distortion; correct and re-analyse,
  - confounding—examine any possible factor that may contribute to the disease causation to determine if it may influence the formation of the cluster (e.g. an unusually high number of at-risk people in the catchment area), or
  - if none of these explanations are likely, then the cluster may be real and the investigation should proceed to the next step.

If there is no clear or significant increase in the numbers of cases when compared to the expected numbers, stop the investigation and discuss with those concerned, perhaps following with a written report, if appropriate (Burls 1999). Note: this differs from step 1, since further investigation of a non-significant increase may be needed because of other factors outside the science of cluster investigation (note: the p value or confidence limits are not absolute limits and there is room for judgement, taking account of the wider context and interests of relevant individuals, exploring opportunities for positive health promotion).

- **Step 3**: assuming further investigation is warranted, check for a plausible explanation and consider possible hypotheses.
  - Through the literature and specialist colleagues, check the aetiology and biological plausibility of all possible explanations using the source–pathway–receptor concept:
    - genetics,
    - biological cause (e.g. predisposing condition or emerging infection),
    - environment (air, land, water):
      - radiological exposure,
      - chemical exposure, and
      - other change in environment (e.g. flood, heatwave);
    - lifestyle issues (e.g. alcohol, smoking, diet, physical activity), or
    - major event (e.g. predisposing major surgery, radiotherapy or prior exposure to a major incident such as war or fire);
  - Consider the possibility of a novel exposure or aetiology.

If there is no clear or plausible explanation, stop the investigation, discuss with those concerned, and prepare a written report. Explore opportunities for positive health promotion. This does not exclude unknown factors or the possibility that, with further understanding, an explanation may arise.

- **Step 4**: if continuing, check possible exposures:
  - Examine the source–pathway–receptor linkage for any alleged or suspected exposure.
  - Source—is there a known presence of a plausible explanatory factor (e.g. contaminated land/landfill site)?
  - Pathway—can this factor reach the patients through inhalation, ingestion, or skin contact?

- Receptor—who is exposed—a specific group or the whole population? Are (were) the cases living in the right place or did they have a behaviour that would place them at risk from the pathway?
- The source–pathway–receptor linkage needs all three components present before the possible exposure can be considered to be actual.

If there is no significant linkage, stop the investigation and discuss with those concerned; prepare a written report. Explore opportunities for positive health promotion. This does not exclude unknown factors or the possibility that, with further understanding, an explanation may arise.

♦ **Step 5**: any further investigation should examine possible exposure levels.

- A source–pathway–receptor linkage, if confirmed, needs exploring to determine if the link is association or causation.
- If the evidence indicates possible causal exposure, examine exposure levels in further detail:
  - explore the toxicology of the suspected causal factor,
  - consider modelling the exposure,
  - consider biological sampling for a bio-marker, and
  - explore other approaches with relevant experts.

If the exposure is too low to cause illness, it may not be possible to rule out association. Nevertheless, consider stopping the investigation through discussion with those concerned, and the preparation of a written report.

♦ In the real world it may not be possible to work through these steps in such a clear logical order; several steps may need to be considered at the same time. However, the stepped approach enables a confident and appropriate response to those concerned and to the initial enquiry, addressing perceptions that might appear unjustified to the professional. Furthermore, following the steps reassures those involved and keeps the investigation from escalating and consuming unnecessary resources, while offering an internationally recognized, scientific means to explain and justify the response to those concerned (Coory et al. 2012; Abrams et al. 2012; Goodman et al. 2012).

17.1.3 Risk factors for clusters of chronic disease or cancer

♦ land contamination,
♦ water contamination,
♦ air pollution,
♦ radiation leak,
♦ conflict (national, international), instruments of war (e.g. chemical, biological, gas), and terrorism,
♦ climate change (e.g. heatwave, flooding),
♦ poor industrial practice or regulation, or
♦ inappropriate use of harmful substances.

This list is not exhaustive but covers common or important risks.

17.1.4 Key points to note in the investigation

Case definition, time period and geography, local communications and links to local authority colleagues (including elected members) are critical to enable appropriate and proportionate investigation.

17.2 **What's the story?**

♦ A local oncologist reports that he has just seen a second child from the same town die from the same rare subtype of acute myeloid leukaemia within a year of the first.

♦ The father of this second case is concerned because their garden adjoins that of the first case. The father has asked if the cause of his daughter's illness is the same as that of his neighbour's child.

17.2.1 **Key scenario information**

Leukaemia is the commonest cancer in children (~30%) with ~160 cases per year in English children aged <15 years (2009–11), with 18 annual deaths (England: 2010–12) (http://www.cancerresearchuk.org/health-professional/cancer-statistics/childrens-cancers/incidence).

About 15% of childhood leukaemias are acute myeloid leukaemia, commonest in infants. Acute myeloid leukaemia is really an adult disease (http://www.cancerresearchuk.org/health-professional/cancer-statistics/statistics-by-cancer-type/leukaemia-aml#heading-Zero).

17.2.2 **Top tips**

Childhood deaths are emotive, as are cancer clusters, even in adults. Beyond the immediate family, local residents are likely to be concerned, and clusters may become known to the media.

17.2.3 **Tools of the trade**

♦ good medical history with laboratory data, clear case definition and descriptive epidemiology,

♦ surveillance of relevant indicators (e.g. mortality and morbidity), and

♦ a public health risk assessment (see figure 3.2) (Reid et al. 2005; Mahoney et al. 2015).

17.2.4 **What immediate action(s) would you take?**

♦ Step back and look at the wider picture around the immediate question, as per the public health risk assessment. Ask yourself and others what understanding is necessary to address the situation.

♦ Consider what epidemiological, chemical, toxicological, and environmental information may be needed to help public health management.

♦ Obtain as much information about the current case as possible:

  • patient and GP details,

  • admission details (place, time, attending physician),

  • basic clinical details including date of onset, and

  • relevant laboratory test results (e.g. pathology).

♦ Ask the cluster reporter to obtain as much information as possible about other cases and for any thoughts about the cause.

♦ Consider the early formation of a multi-agency incident management team to support an investigation and handle media relations. The team should:

  • understand the situation,

  • explore the causes and results by examining the risks, and

  • involve everyone who might have a part to play.

♦ Plan how to collect the information and analyse it.

17.2.5 **Key scenario information**

An **incident management team** (see Chapter 20) should be comprised of relevant professionals and representatives of relevant agencies; the Director of Public Health or Consultant in Public Health/Health Protection could chair the meeting.

Members of the incident management team may include a Health Protection Consultant, a representative from technical support within Public Health England, Health Protection Scotland or similar body (e.g. toxicologist, environmental scientist), an epidemiologist or analyst, an Environmental Health Officer from the local authority, and communications manager.

Note: membership should be reviewed according to the nature of the incident and may differ between incidents or change during the management of the incident. All investigations should be coordinated through the incident management team to ensure synergy, avoid duplication and improve efficiency.

17.2.6 **Key scenario information**

♦ **Epidemiological investigations** may cover mortality records, hospital and general practice records for the relevant time, persons, and place.

♦ **Environmental investigations** may include historical review of maps for land use, intrusive investigations of soils or sediments, air and water sampling covering appropriate geography and time.

♦ **Laboratory**—relevant investigations (e.g. biochemistry or pathology).

17.3 **Scenario update # 1**

♦ The incident management team comprises experts in haematology, cancer epidemiology, environmental health, toxicology, health protection, and communication, and is chaired by the Director of Public Health.

♦ Epidemiological, environmental, and laboratory investigations are undertaken. The children lived on a small social housing estate, whose residents ask 'Is it safe to live here?'

17.3.1 **Key scenario information**

The **aim of an incident team** is to:

♦ understand the extent of the problem,

♦ understand the public's concerns,

♦ explore the hazards, risks, causes, and outcomes,

♦ involve everyone who might have a part to play,

♦ act transparently, building trust,

♦ plan and communicate key messages, and

♦ determine if there are measures that might prevent or mitigate a similar situation.

Good communications with the local community are essential:

Simple: use words people understand,

Timely: give information as soon as possible,

Accurate: give up to date, correct information,

Relevant: give factual responses to questions, and

Credible: openness is key to credibility.

17.3.2 **What further action(s) would you take?**

For investigations which are expected to be prolonged or emotive, regular meetings of concerned parties are recommended, in a safe, neutral environment.

A local resident/elected member chairing the meeting, with advocacy and support, will build trust.

17.4 **Scenario update # 2**

- Three working groups are established within the incident management team to undertake epidemiological and environmental studies, and to ensure effective communications.
- Realizing that the houses were built on an old, unrecorded landfill, a year-long environmental investigation is begun, looking at the air, land, and water for pollutants (chemicals, radioactivity) that might move from the landfill into the houses, gardens, and surrounding areas at possibly harmful concentrations.
- Independent environmental consultants investigate environmental issues, funded by the local authority, but chosen by the residents.
- The results of all environmental investigations are fully shared with the residents in a timely manner.

17.4.1 **Key scenario information**

Sharing information with residents and professionals at the same time is not common. Usually professionals wish to see the raw data for analysis and interpretation. However, by sharing the raw (environmental) data, any suggestion of professional manipulation of the information was removed. Residents soon realized that they needed professional help to understand the data.

17.4.2 **What further action(s) would you take?**

Explain all data at residents meetings by the relevant professional in straightforward language. Take residents' questions seriously, regardless of their relevance, i.e., even if the questions seem irrelevant to professionals investigating the situation.

17.4.3 **What further information do you need?**

- validated laboratory data,
- toxicology of chemicals found,
- an understanding of any source–pathway–receptor links, and
- quantification of residents' exposures to chemicals found.

17.4.4 **Tools of the trade**

Expert toxicological interpretation of data, applied to the situation, contributes to the professional public health risk assessment.

17.4.5 **Top tips**

- Consult widely and think broadly.
- Never underestimate public concern. Treat seriously any issue relevant to, or raised by, members of the public.
- Communicate often and openly, in plain language.
- Report frequently to the incident management team.

17.5 **Scenario update # 3**

♦ The case definition is based on (1) the children's locality of residence, (2) a defined time frame, and (3) diseases related to their diagnosis. Further cases are sought through local general practice records, national and regional cancer registries, and coroner's records of unexplained childhood deaths.

♦ The local epidemiology of acute myeloid leukaemia and childhood cancers is examined (death certificates; cancer registries; hospital episode statistics; Congenital Abnormalities Register for relevant space-time clusters). The general health of the community is explored through comparison of local and regional calls to the national telephone health helpline and through analysis of routine data.

♦ GP and obstetric records are unremarkable. GP records of long-term residents of the estate show no unexpected conditions, indicating no unusual situation in the neighbourhood.

♦ No further cases of acute myeloid leukaemia in children are found. The number of local cases of all leukaemias and all cancers is not raised over the expected number.

♦ An assessment of life-long exposure to chemicals in the landfill is undertaken, for children and a 70-year-old adult. Benzo(a)pyrene, nickel, and mercury have elevated ratios in children, exceeding their respective health criterion values by factors of five or more. A toxicological review reveals no suggestion that these would be the cause of uncommon cancers in children.

♦ However, elevated levels of carbon monoxide, with a risk of asphyxiation, and landfill gas (methane), with a risk of explosion, are found. Neither gas causes cancer. The landfill was excavated and suitable gas-tight membranes fitted to the houses.

♦ The incident team finds it impossible to decide the cause of the children's leukaemia, but is able to reassure the families and community that it is safe to live in their houses.

♦ Local media asked several questions: 'Was the investigation a failure? Was the cost of the investigation justified? Would you undertake such an extensive investigation again in a similar situation?'

17.5.1 **Key scenario information**

Exposure calculations can be compared to health criterion values, which are calculated with large safety margins from known toxicology. Exceeding these values indicates further thought should be given to the situation, not that remediation or other response is necessary.

For example, a five-fold exceedance in a single year is a long way from a harmful exposure, since a harmful exposure level is usually calculated for a lifetime exposure. There would need to be continued exposure over several years or decades at the single-year exposure level before there were real possibilities of health effects.

The investigation costs approximated, per household, the cost of one month's in-patient treatment for acute myeloid leukaemia for an infant.

17.5.2 **How would you respond to the media enquiry?**

♦ Be prepared for unexpected questions (e.g. questions relating to emotional experiences and feelings, rather than the facts and science).

♦ Be clear about the message you want to communicate; take time to include it in your answers.

♦ Answer the question asked, before adding the message you want to deliver; this generates trust, making listeners more receptive to your message.

♦ Do not feel obliged to answer every question; be confident about saying, 'I don't know.' This will add to your credibility and trustworthiness, rather than undermine your position.

17.6 **What if … ?**

17.6.1 **The cases attended a school/college/university?**

♦ Collect as much information about these cases in the same way as for any other cases. It is important to investigate and understand the situation, explore the causes and risks, including the relevant school/college/university setting and involve all relevant parties.

♦ Although an open mind is important, given the nature and duration of exposure required for the development of cancer, unless there are more cases from the same setting, it is advisable and pragmatic to rule out any common exposure outside the educational setting before launching wider investigations into the educational establishments.

17.6.2 **The following year, after the investigation had closed, there was another, nearby, childhood case of acute myeloid leukaemia?**

♦ This will raise concerns again in the local area, regardless of any plausible link to the previous cases. Therefore, it is paramount that a multi-agency incident management team is convened promptly, not only to look into any possible link and support the wider investigation, but also to manage communications and to guide the handling of media and public relations.

17.6.3 **A family member who resides locally is reported to have developed a related illness?**

♦ In line with the principles of investigating clusters, there is a need to gather all relevant clinical information and check if the reported individual meets the original case definition.

♦ The investigation can only be initiated if the case definition is met. If not, the individual concerned, local professionals, and members of the public should be reassured, as appropriate. However, if the reported case meets the case definition, then a multi-agency incident management team should be convened and wider investigations initiated promptly.

17.7 **Some unanswered questions around cancer and chronic disease clusters**

♦ The pathogenesis of cancer and other chronic diseases is complex and unclear; the role of environmental chemicals and the contribution of the patient's genetic processes to carcinogenesis remains uncertain.

♦ Differentiating between causation, association, confounding, or proxy effects in epidemiological studies may be impossible, while experiments may be unethical. Genetic fingerprinting of tumours may help identify carcinogens; it is likely that many cancers have several different subtypes, each related to a different carcinogen and exposure pathway.

♦ The trans-generational effects of chemical exposure are unknown.

♦ Could unknown infections influence the aetiology of some cancers and chronic diseases?

♦ The lead time between exposure and disease (whether cancer or other) is usually unknown, making aetiological studies difficult.

17.8 **Lessons learned**

♦ Taking a stepwise approach conserves resources and builds trust.

♦ Engage the public from the outset.

♦ Be honest and open, making every effort to respond seriously to all public concerns.

♦ Do not promise anything that you are not certain about (e.g. finding the source, or even completing the investigation).

♦ Do not underestimate the value of clear risk communication, including unknown risk, with those concerned and relevant stakeholders.

♦ Do not communicate information with the media prior to informing relevant stakeholders.

♦ Remember, environmental investigations should be evidence based as much as possible, but should not be evidence bound, as alleviating local communities/populations concerns and anxiety is paramount.

17.9 **Further thinking**

♦ How can evidence-based environmental public health risk assessment be strengthened?

♦ What can be done to improve professionals' understanding of environmental public health risk assessment and risk communication?

♦ What can be done to develop environmental public health surveillance (tracking) to predict and identify cancer or chronic disease clusters?

♦ What can be done to build the capacity and capability of local public health professionals in order to undertake good standard environmental public health investigations?

♦ Given limited public health resources available to undertake environmental public health investigations, at what geographical footprint should such resources be available?

♦ How can the public be reassured if it becomes obvious that there is little value in undertaking an environmental public health investigation?

♦ What can be done when formal environmental public health investigations fail to reassure the public?

References

Abrams B, H Anderson, C Blackmore, et al. 2013. Investigating suspected cancer clusters and responding to community concerns: guidelines from CDC and the Council of state and territorial epidemiologists. Recommendations and reports. *Morbidity and Mortality Weekly Report*, 62(RR08): 1–14.

Burls AJE. 1999. Childhood leukaemia—communicating with a worried public. *International Statistical Institute*. 52nd Session. http://iase-web.org/documents/papers/isi52/burl1012.pdf (accessed 8 March 2016).

Coory MD, S Jordan. 2012. Assessment of chance should be removed from protocols for investigating cancer clusters. *International Journal of Epidemiology*, 42(2): 440–47.

Goodman M, JS Naiman, D Goodman, et al. 2012. Cancer clusters in the USA: what do the last twenty years of state and federal investigations tell us? *Critical Reviews in Toxicology*, **42**(6): 474–90.

Mahoney G, A Stewart, N Kennedy et al. 2015. Achieving attainable outcomes from good science in an untidy world: case studies in land and air pollution. *Environmental Geochemistry & Health*, **37**(4): 689–706.

Quinn E, T Merritt, ME Buckland, et al. 2014. An update on the epidemiology and key issues associated with the diagnosis and management of Creutzfeldt–Jakob disease cases in NSW. *Public Health Research and Practice*, **25**(1): e2511409.

Reid JR, R Jarvis, J Richardson, et al. 2005. Responding to chronic environmental problems in Cheshire & Merseyside—Systems and Procedures. *Chemical Hazards and Poisons Report*, **4**: 33–35.

Further reading

Bennett P, K Calman, S Curtis et al. 2010. *Risk Communication and Public Health*. 2nd edition. Oxford: Oxford University Press.

Health Protection Network. 2008. *Communicating with the Public About Health Risks. Health Protection Network Guidance 1*. Glasgow: Health Protection Scotland. http://www.documents.hps.scot.nhs.uk/about-hps/hpn/risk-communication.pdf (accessed 8 March 2016).

Scotland & Northern Ireland Forum for Environmental Research (SNIFFER). 2010. *Communicating understanding of contaminated land risks*. Edinburgh: SNIFFER. http://www.sniffer.org.uk/files/6313/8202/5406/SNIFFER_risk_communication_booklet.pdf (accessed 8 March 2016).

Section 5

Health protection tools

Chapter 18

Hospital and community infection prevention and control (IPC)

Paul Shears, Andrea Ledgerton, and Rita Huyton

OVERVIEW

After reading this chapter the reader will be familiar with:
- the key principles of infection prevention and control (IPC) in both hospital and community settings,
- the key issues and strategies of IPC in hospitals and in the community,
- the role of health protection teams in IPC, and the hospital and community infection control interface,
- the practical components of IPC including hand hygiene and surveillance of infections, and
- the relevant IPC policies and guidelines.

18.1 Introduction to hospital and community infection prevention and control (IPC)

Infections acquired in hospitals or in community-based health and social care settings are responsible for significant morbidity, resulting in extended hospital stays, increased pressure in residential and nursing homes, and increased costs to the health sector. Up to 10% of patients in hospital may acquire a healthcare-associated infection. The prevention and control of infection is the responsibility of the care provider, but health protection staff have a role in ensuring that adequate (and in some cases statutory) provisions are in place, and in managing infection incidents and outbreaks.

18.2 The key principles of IPC

Effective IPC programmes combine both the microbiological/epidemiological aspects of infection and the organizational and management structures and procedures necessary for implementation. These components are summarized in Table 18.1.

18.3 Organizational requirements

The IPC programme in both hospitals and community should be managed by an IPC team, comprised of an infection control doctor (ICD), usually a consultant microbiologist, and specialist infection prevention and control nurses (ICNs) with specific responsibilities, and supported by dedicated secretarial and information technology/data management support. The programme is coordinated by an infection prevention and control committee, which should include clinical and nursing members, estates and facilities departments, hospital or community management, and a health protection representative. Other sectors may be represented according to the issues to be

Table 18.1 The components of infection prevention and control programmes

Infection/epidemiology	Infection prevention and control practice	Organization/management
• Close liaison with microbiology laboratory • Surveillance of infections • Specific pathogens including MRSA, *C.difficile*, CPEs, VREs, norovirus • Hospital infections including bloodstream, respiratory, catheter-associated urinary tract, wound, skin, and soft tissue infections • Infections in special units including intensive care, burns, neonatal, surgery • Community infections including bloodborne viruses, infection clusters in schools, care homes	• Hand hygiene • Standard and transmission-based precautions • Isolation and cohorting • Personal protective equipment (PPE) • Environmental hygiene/cleaning/ • Waste/sharps disposal • Instrument decontamination • Wound management • Care bundles • Outbreak management	• IPC Team • Infection Prevention and Control Committee • Policies/guidelines • Training/education • Support from senior management • Secretarial and information technology support • Liaison with Health Protection Team • Liaison with local authority

considered. It is advisable that the IPCC has representation on the executive management committee or board. In England, the Director of Infection Prevention and Control fulfils this role.

18.4 **Infection prevention and control practice**

18.4.1 **Hand hygiene**

Appropriate hand hygiene, in both hospital and community settings, is the most important component of infection prevention and control that can be undertaken by staff. Staff must observe the principles of the Ayliffe technique for hand hygiene (Fraise and Bradley 2009), '*the five moments for hand hygiene*' (World Health Organization 2015), and bare below the elbows (NICE 2012) to enable hand hygiene to be performed effectively.

Settings where service users have dementia, mental health, or other complex needs present particular difficulties for the provision of point-of-care hand hygiene facilities and a risk assessment should be carried out. Where point-of-care hand hygiene facilities cannot be safely provided, alternative methods must be made available and these must be clearly documented.

The most commonly available *waterless hand hygiene products* are alcohol-based sanitizers and wet wipes. Alcohol-based sanitizers are not sporicidal (and therefore not active against *C. difficile*) and are not effective against non-enveloped viruses such as norovirus. Hands must be visibly clean for alcohol-based sanitizers to work.

18.4.2 **Infection prevention and control policies**

Policies must be available to ensure all staff are aware of their responsibilities in delivering preventative strategies. It is when these policies are not followed that lapses in care may happen, often resulting in hospital- or community-acquired infections or infection outbreaks.

It is essential that policies are regularly updated, and that all staff are aware of current procedures.

18.4.3 **Education and training**

Education and training are important aspects of any prevention and control strategy and staff should be updated regularly in relation to current IPC issues. The IPC team should be actively involved in providing education to all levels of staff from clinicians to ancillary workers.

18.4.4 **Surveillance of infections**

Surveillance of infections, through collecting, analysing, and reporting infection data, and with clear case definitions for infections, enables IPC teams continually to be aware of infection issues and to direct resources appropriately, and prompts the need for education and change through timely feedback.

18.4.5 **Infection prevention and control precautions and isolation guidelines**

Infection precautions are required to prevent staff acquiring infections from patients, and to prevent infections being transmitted between patients and service users. Most health and community facilities now follow guidelines based on the definitions from the Centers for Disease Control and Prevention (CDC Atlanta): Standard Infection Control Precautions (SICPs), and Transmission Based Precautions (TBPs). These have replaced earlier terms such as universal precautions, barrier nursing, and isolation precautions. SICPs include hand hygiene, gloves, aprons, other personal protective equipment (PPE) as required, and care of sharps. TBPs are additional to SICPs, and should be applied when caring for patients with symptoms of infection, asymptomatic patients who are suspected or incubating an infection, or patients colonized with an infectious agent (Siegel et al. 2007).

Under the Control of Substances Hazardous to Health (CoSHH) Regulations, blood and body fluids or excretions are classed as biological hazards and the employer is required to assess the risk of exposure to their employees and to manage those risks. The correct use of PPE is a critical factor in ensuring safe working procedures and good infection prevention and control. Guidance for the use of PPE is outlined in Table 18.2, based on the CDC defined Standard and Transmission Based Precautions (Siegel et al. 2007).

18.4.6 **Environmental hygiene**

Staff who undertake cleaning duties should be trained and provided with the necessary PPE and equipment required for the task. The segregation, disposal, and storage of waste (including sharp items) in accordance with current legislation is extremely important in ensuring a safe and hygienic environment (Department of Health 2013).

In community settings, cleaning with a general-purpose detergent is sufficient in most situations. Care should be taken to clean surfaces thoroughly, rinse, and allow to dry. Important considerations in the community are:

♦ the adequate cleaning of soft furnishings and fabric items,

♦ the correct use and dilution of detergents and disinfectants,

♦ the segregation (i.e. colour coding), storage, and decontamination of equipment used to clean the environment, and

♦ access to steam cleaning (e.g. following an outbreak).

A spillage is any uncontained release of blood, body fluids, or other excreted bodily substance. Key principles apply when dealing with spillages. There should be training for staff and readily available instructional aids. Appropriate PPE should be available. Spillages should be contained

Table 18.2 Use of personal protective equipment (PPE)

- PPE should be stored hygienically until it is required
- Staff must be trained in the correct donning, use, and removal of PPE including fit testing of appropriate mask/respirator where required
- Remove PPE as soon as task is complete
- Always change PPE between tasks and patients
- Dispose of PPE promptly and safely
- Always wash hands after removing PPE

Type of task	PPE required	Rationale	Comment
Contact transmission (direct and indirect)			
• Close personal care • High-dispersal activities With *no* anticipated exposure to blood, body fluids/excretions Examples: assisting a person bathing, changing beds	Disposable plastic apron	• Protect clothing from becoming wet • Protect clothing from picking up high numbers of bacteria that are commonly found on the skin, i.e. *Staphylococcus aureus* inc. MRSA	The front of clothing is the area where most contact occurs. Aprons protect this area; long-sleeved gowns are not required for routine tasks
• Any task where contact with blood, body fluids/excretions is anticipated With *no* anticipated splashing to the face Examples: assisting a person to use the toilet, changing nappies/continence aids, handling soiled laundry, handling soiled instruments	Disposable plastic apron Disposable medical gloves	• Blood and body fluids/excretions can carry high numbers of potentially pathogenic organisms i.e. blood—bloodborne viruses such as Hepatitis B and HIV; faeces—*C. difficile*, *E.coli*, norovirus, antibiotic-resistant organisms such as carbapenemase producing *Enterobacteriaceae* (CPE)	Suitable materials for disposable medical gloves are: latex, nitrile, or vinyl Consider the risk of latex allergy Consider the dexterity required. Vinyl provides the least grip and dexterity but is adequate for social care tasks and most healthcare tasks Polythene gloves are not suitable for use
Droplet transmission			
• Any task where contact with blood, body fluids/excretions is anticipated *With* anticipated splashing to the face Examples: dental procedures, oral suctioning, cleaning of spillages on carpets • Exposure to respiratory droplets where a risk of infection is suspected	Disposable plastic apron Disposable medical gloves Disposable surgical mask Face visor or eye protection	Droplets are large particles. For practical purposes they are assumed to travel in the air for up to 1 m. They are too large to be directly inhaled in to the lungs but can contaminate the nose, mouth, and eyes. Most bacteria and viruses can be transmitted this way; specific examples include *Bordetella pertussis* (whooping cough), influenza virus, *Neisseria meningitidis*	Visors and eye protectors must protect the eye from multiple angles Spectacles do not provide sufficient eye protection If re-usable, carefully follow the manufacturer's instructions on safe decontamination before re-use

Airborne transmission

◆ Aerosol Generating Procedures (AGPs). See Public Health England (2014) for details ◆ Infections such as measles and chickenpox are airborne	Fluid-repellent long-sleeved gown Disposable medical gloves Disposable facial respirator (FFP3) Face visor or eye protection There is no consensus on the use of the above PPE for control of these infections Local procedures often recommend PPE as per droplet transmission	During AGPs, small microorganisms can become suspended in aerosols and remain infectious. Aerosols remain in the air for some time and can travel >1 m from the source. Aerosols are smaller and lighter than droplets. They can be inhaled directly in to the lungs	AGPs are unlikely to occur in the community

Outbreaks

Outbreaks of viral gastroenteritis	Disposable plastic apron Disposable medical gloves Disposable surgical mask (if caring for a patient who is vomiting, < 1m distance)	Mainly contact transmission but vomiting releases droplets which travel for <1 m	Community providers should have plans in place to respond to an outbreak
Seasonal influenza outbreaks	Disposable plastic apron Disposable medical gloves Disposable surgical mask (<1 m distance of a symptomatic person)	Mainly contact transmission but coughs and sneezes release large droplets which travel for <1 m	Community providers should have plans in place to respond to an outbreak

Rare and emerging infections

Examples: avian influenza, viral haemorrhagic fever, Multi Drug Resistant Tuberculosis (MDR TB), Middle East Respiratory Syndrome Coronavirus (MERS-CoV)	*Refer to specific guidance for each infection.* PPE may include: Fluid-repellent long-sleeved gown Disposable medical gloves Disposable facial respirator (FFP3) (Public Health England 2014) Face visor or eye protection	Highly pathogenic organisms. Immunity in the local population is generally low	Community providers must be prepared to respond to new and rare threats as they emerge

Source: data from Siegel JD, Rhinehart E, Jackson M, Chiarello L, and the Healthcare Infection Control Practices Advisory Committee (2007) Guideline for Isolation Precautions: Preventing Transmission of Infectious Agents in Healthcare Settings. Atlanta, GA, USA: Centre for Disease Control and Prevention. Copyright © 2007 Centers for Disease Control and Prevention. Available from: http://www.cdc.gov/hicpac/pdf/isolation/Isolation2007.pdf

Table 18.3 Decontamination of equipment and instruments

Category	Examples	Decontamination	Comments
Low-risk items			
All devices that are intended to:	*Items such as:*		
Come in to contact with intact skin Or not come in to contact with the patient	Beds, wash bowls, furniture, sport equipment, toys	Cleaning	Clean with water and detergent, rinse, and dry When there is specific risk of infection the IPC team may advise that disinfection is also required
Medium-risk items			
All devices that are intended to:	*Items such as:*		
Come in to contact with intact mucous membranes (excluding those inserted in to body cavities, see high risk) Or Low risk items contaminated by blood/body fluid/excretions Or Low risk items contaminated with particularly virulent or readily transmissible organisms Or Low risk items to be used on immunocompromised patients	Commodes, potties, suction equipment	Cleaning followed by disinfection or disposable	Heat or chemical disinfection
High-risk items			
All devices that are intended to:	*Items such as:*		
have close contact with non intact skin or mucous membranes be used in body cavities be used in sterile body sites	podiatry equipment wound care equipment tattooing equipment dental equipment vaginal speculum minor surgery instruments urinary catheters (single use preferred)	Use disposable single use items wherever possible; if not possible: cleaning followed by sterilization	Sterilization using pressurized steam is optimal. Sterilization should be undertaken in specialized accredited units wherever possible. For items that will be damaged by sterilization, high-level disinfection may be required. Advice of the IPC team should be sought

Source: data from Medicines and Healthcare products Regulatory Agency (MHRA). (2010) Sterilization, disinfection and cleaning of medical equipment: guidance on decontamination from the Microbiology Advisory Committee (the MAC manual): Part 1 Principles, 3rd edition May 2010 (London: MHRA, 2010), © 2010 Crown Copyright, http://naep.org.uk/members/documents/MHRAMACPart1.pdf, accessed 22 Nov. 2015.

in an absorptive material and the area disinfected. A disinfectant equivalent to 10,000 parts per million (ppm) available chlorine is recommended for blood spillages. 'Off the shelf' kits should be checked for chlorine availability.

18.4.7 Decontamination of equipment and instruments

The key principles of decontamination are outlined in Table 18.3.

18.5 Prevention and control of infection in hospitals

With the occurrence of new pathogens, the increasing prevalence of multiply antibiotic-resistant infections, and increasing budgetary constraints, hospital infection prevention and control programmes will face increasing pressures and it is essential they maintain adequate staff levels and are supported by the hospital management board.

18.5.1 Organizational arrangements for infection prevention and control

The IPC team must be involved in all aspects of the hospital infrastructure to ensure that decisions are made with the associated IPC risks taken into account. These include patient pathways, bed management decisions, ward reconfiguration/refurbishments, purchasing of medical devices, education/training, communications, and priority setting, in addition to the daily role in IPC.

18.5.2 The epidemiology and surveillance of hospital infection

Most hospital-acquired infections are caused by bacteria that are relatively uncommon pathogens in the community (though many are part of the normal human microbial flora) or by a limited

Table 18.4 The important pathogens and infections in hospital settings

Sites of infection	Pathogens
Gastro-intestinal/diarrhoea	*C. difficile*, norovirus, rotavirus in children
Pneumonia (including ventilator-associated pneumonia (VAP) in ITU patients)	*E.coli, Klebsiella*, other Gram negatives including *Enterobacter, Acinetobacter*, and *Pseudomonas* *S. aureus*, MRSA. Rarely, fungal infections
Other respiratory infections	Influenza (seasonal), respiratory syncitial virus in children, Legionnaires' disease, tuberculosis
Blood stream infections (bacteraemia/septicaemia)	Gram negatives as pneumonia above (mostly endogenous). *S. aureus*, MRSA, vancomycin-resistant *enterococci* (VRE), *S. epidermidis* in compromised patients with invasive devices, rarely, fungal infections (in haematology/chemotherapy patients)
Catheter-related urinary tract infections (UTIs)	*E.coli, Klebsiella*, other *Enterobacteria, Pseudomonas, S.epidermidis* While catheter-related UTIs are a major problem, distinguishing true infection from bacterial colonization may be very difficult
Wound infections, ulcers, pressure sores	MSSA, MRSA, coliforms, VRE, Group A *streptococcus*

number of viruses and fungi (Table 18.4). Further details on microbiology of infection can be found in Chapter 4.

Many hospital bacterial pathogens are resistant to multiple antimicrobials. These include those with specific resistance properties (e.g. Methicillin-resistant *Staphylococcus aureus* (MRSA), Vancomycin-resistant *enterococci* (VRE), and multiple antibiotic resistance in Gram-negative bacteria such as *E.coli* and *Klebsiella* species.

A hospital-acquired infection (nosocomial infection) is defined as an infection that the patient was not incubating on admission, and where the causative organism was not isolated, or symptoms did not develop, until at least 48hrs after admission. An example demonstrating issues around the distinction between hospital and community acquisition of infection is shown in Box 18.1.

Surveillance of infections in hospitals should be an ongoing programme, and digital data collection, analysis, and reporting, integrated with the hospital patient management system and the laboratory system, is essential.

Box 18.1 Example illustrating issues regarding hospital or community acquisition

A 95-year-old lady with complex morbidity was admitted from a nursing home with vomiting, likely due to urinary tract sepsis. Following a seven-day course of antibiotics prescribed by her GP, symptoms had not resolved and she was prescribed a further course of treatment whilst in the Emergency Department. The transfer notes from the nursing home also indicated that she had also had a two-day history of diarrhoea.

Clostridium difficile (*C.difficile*) toxin was detected from a specimen collected on day four of admission.

Whilst by surveillance definition this is reported as a hospital-acquired infection, there is a reasonable possibility that the patient was already infected with *C. difficile* on admission.

Learning from incident: There was a delay in identifying the infection and therefore appropriate treatment of the patient and IPC measures were also delayed. A stool sample should have been obtained on admission as the patient was symptomatic.

Box 18.2 Example of an MRSA reduction strategy

Using MRSA as an example, auditing compliance with practices associated with MRSA is essential. In one example of a hospital programme, two Infection Prevention and Control Assistants (ICAs) were recruited to review all positive and all previously known MRSA patients on a daily basis to ensure that all screens had been performed appropriately in a timely manner, decolonization therapy had been prescribed and appropriately administered, and care pathways commenced with education and reinforcement of practices provided along the way. The ICAs would feedback antibiotic regimes to the IPC nurses for discussion, if required, with the Infection Control Doctor. This focused proactive strategy resulted in a significant reduction in hospital-acquired MRSA colonization and clinical infection, with zero MRSA bloodstream infections over a 15-month period.

18.5.3 **Prevention and control strategies**

The introduction of national targets for specific infections can contribute to more focused infection prevention and control programmes, and result in reductions in important pathogens such as MRSA and *C. difficile*, and in specific infections such as catheter-associated urinary tract infections and ventilator associated pneumonia. In many cases, specific healthcare bundles have been developed to ensure standardization of practice and auditing of outcomes. As an example, MRSA screening and early identification of colonized patients can result in prompt action to decolonize, isolate, and initiate heightened infection prevention and control measures, thereby avoiding clinical infection occurring and/or transmission to another patient. An example of a local MRSA-reduction strategy is given in Box 18.2.

Hospitals should have adequate isolation facilities, combined with standard or transmission-based precautions, for selected infected patients.

Isolation facilities may be individual rooms in a general ward, or a dedicated isolation unit comprising several en-suite rooms. Alternatives include cohorting, where all patients with the same infection (e.g. norovirus) are managed in a single ward with designated staff, or where patients with low transmission risk (e.g. carriers of multiply resistant bacteria) can be managed on an open ward, with appropriate standard- or transmission-based precautions.

Box 18.3 Investigation of a hospital infection cluster/outbreak

+ Case definition, usually with laboratory confirmation.
+ Convene outbreak control committee.
+ Decide action to be taken on symptomatic cases: isolation/cohorting.
+ Decide if screening contacts appropriate.
+ Consider decisions about closing units, patient admission, and discharge.
+ Consider communication to all hospital personnel, media.
+ Clear decision when outbreak is over.

Box 18.4 Examples of situations requiring health protection input to hospital infections

+ an outbreak of infection in the hospital that is not contained (e.g. *C.difficile* affecting several wards),
+ an infected healthcare worker where there are many susceptible contacts (e.g. a TB-infected nurse in a neonatal unit),
+ infections occurring concurrently in the community and the hospital (e.g. norovirus, PVL *S. aureus*),
+ new infections where preparatory planning is required, as demonstrated in the response to H1N1 ('swine flu'), and relevant for future possible infections such as MERS-CoV and avian influenza, and
+ clusters of infection affecting several local hospitals where transfers may occur, e.g. CPE, VRE.

18.5.4 **Infection clusters and outbreaks**

While the emphasis of IPC programmes is to prevent infection transmission, there must also be robust plans for controlling infection clusters and outbreaks. Control activities, which may include cohorting patients, closing wards to admissions, extensive patient screening, and restrictions on admissions and discharges, can have a major impact on the normal functioning of the hospital. If necessary, an outbreak control team (OCT) will be convened at an early stage, comprising relevant clinicians and nursing staff, hospital management, estates and hotel services, and health protection representation, where appropriate. A summary of the investigation process for managing hospital clusters/outbreaks is given in Box. 18.3, and examples of hospital situations that require local health protection team input in Box. 18.4. Further details of general incident/outbreak management can be found in Chapter 20.

18.5.5 **Major incident plan**

The IPC team plays an integral role in the hospital major incident plan and is responsible for ensuring that it is updated for changing major and potential infection issues (e.g. influenza, Ebola). Areas that must be covered include laboratory support for infection diagnosis, bed management and isolation facilities, staff training in personal protective equipment, out-of-hours IPC cover, liaison with health protection colleagues, and regular data collection and analysis. For information on business continuity see Chapter 13.

18.5.6 **Health protection inputs to hospital IPC**

Close collaboration between the hospital IPC team and the health protection department is required when infection incidents arise that have a linked community aspect, or are of sufficient impact within the hospital to require external advice or support.

Table 18.5 Community infection prevention and control services—service provision

Service provision *may* include:	
Health and social care providers	**Other**
◆ community hospitals	◆ schools
◆ community nursing services	◆ nurseries
◆ care homes	◆ other childcare facilities
◆ hospices	◆ tattoo parlours
◆ intermediate care units	◆ body piercers
◆ specialist rehabilitation centres	◆ cosmetic and beauty services
◆ private hospitals	◆ prisons
◆ general medical practices	◆ hostels
◆ domiciliary social care	◆ sheltered housing
◆ general dental practices	◆ sea and airports
◆ learning disability services	◆ ships
◆ mental health services	◆ hotels
◆ custodial health services	◆ sport clubs
◆ optometrists	◆ gymnasiums
◆ podiatrists	
◆ local authorities	

The above health and social care services may be delivered by the NHS,
independent contractors (contracted by the NHS),
the private sector or the voluntary sector.

18.6 **The prevention and control of infection in the community**

18.6.1 **Overview of community IPC services**

The aim of IPC in the community is to protect individuals and groups from avoidable infections that have the potential to cause significant harm. In England, Directors of Public Health (based in local authorities) are responsible for ensuring that local arrangements for the prevention and control of infection in the community are in place. Health Protection Specialists should familiarize themselves with the services in their area: in particular, where they are based, contact details, methods of referral, hours of operation, arrangements for out-of-hours cover, and the scope of provision. The responsibilities of community IPC services are varied and wide-ranging (Table 18.5).

While each of these settings has different functions and some have different regulatory frameworks, adequate arrangements for preventing and controlling infections must be in place and include the key principles described in this chapter.

18.7 **Infection prevention and control at the hospital–community interface**

Hospitals and the community are part of a health/infection continuum, and there are increasing situations where collaboration is necessary between hospital and community IPC teams. Examples include the occurrence of norovirus in a hospital and feeder care homes, the discharge of patients colonized with antimicrobial-resistant organisms to the community, and communicable diseases such as measles, where there will be issues regarding exposed staff and contacts in the hospital, and contacts of community cases presenting to hospital facilities.

Hospital and community infection control staff should be represented on the infection control committee of each for regular information flows, and should work closely together when there are infection episodes affecting the hospital and community.

18.8 **Conclusions**

IPC has a wide remit, including ensuring that a comprehensive and robust IPC policy is in place. It is important that in both the community and hospital settings, IPC teams liaise closely with local health protection teams. The link between hospital and community infection prevention and control is vital to ensure a seamless IPC service in a given geographical area, ensuring good information flow and that teams work closely together, especially when there are episodes affecting both community and hospitals.

References

Department of Health. 2013. *Environment and Sustainability. Health Technical Memorandum 07-01: Safe Management of Health Care Waste.* https://www.gov.uk/government/uploads/system/uploads/attachment_data/file/167976/HTM_07-01_Final.pdf (accessed 8 March 2016).

Fraise AP, C Bradley. 2009. *Ayliffe's Control of Healthcare-associated Infection. A Practical Handbook.* 5th edition. London: Hodder Arnold.

Medicines and Healthcare Regulatory Agency. 2010. *Sterilization, disinfection and cleaning of medical equipment: guidance on decontamination from the Microbiology Advisory Committee (the MAC manual) Part 1: Principles.* 3rd edition. http://naep.org.uk/members/documents/MHRAMACPart1.pdf (accessed 8 March 2016).

NICE. 2012. *NICE Guideline CG139. Infection: Prevention and Control of Healthcare-associated Infections in Primary and Community Care.* First published in 2003, partially updated March 2012. https://www.nice.org.uk/guidance/cg139 (accessed 8 March 2016).

Public Health England (PHE). 2014. *Infection Control Precautions to Minimise Transmission of Respiratory Tract Infections (RTIs) in the Healthcare Setting.* https://www.gov.uk/government/uploads/system/uploads/attachment_data/file/452928/RTI_infection_control_guidance_PHE_v3_FPF_CT_contents2.pdf (accessed March 2016).

Siegel JD, E Rhinehart, M Jackson et al. 2007. *Guideline for Isolation Precautions: Preventing Transmission of Infectious Agents in Healthcare Settings.* Atlanta, GA: Centers for Disease Control and Prevention. http://www.cdc.gov/hicpac/pdf/isolation/Isolation2007.pdf (accessed 8 March 2016).

World Health Organization. 2015. *Clean Care is Safer Care. Five Moments for Hand Hygiene. Tools and Resources.* http://www.who.int/gpsc/tools/Five_moments/en/ (accessed 8 March 2016).

Further reading

Damani NN 2003. *Manual of Infection Control Procedures.* 2nd edition. New York: Greenwich Medical Media.

Department of Health. 2010. *The Health and Social Care Act 2008. Code of Practice on the Prevention and Control of Infections and Related Guidance.* Published in 2008, revised December 2010. Gateway Ref: 14805 https://www.gov.uk/government/publications/the-health-and-social-care-act-2008-code-of-practice-on-the-prevention-and-control-of-infections-and-related-guidance (accessed 8 March 2016).

Lawrence J, D May. 2007. *Infection Control in the Community.* London: Churchill Livingstone.

Penny C. 2007. *Infection Prevention and Control.* Oxford: Blackwell

Wilson J. 2006. *Infection Control in Clinical Practice.* 3rd edition. Oxford: Elsevier.

Chapter 19

Immunization

David Baxter, Sam Ghebrehewet, and Gill Marsh

OVERVIEW

··

After reading this chapter the reader will be familiar with:

• the importance of continuing immunization in the context of declining vaccine preventable diseases incidence,
• the types of vaccine that are currently in use,
• the common components of vaccines and why they are needed,
• the UK immunization programme and its objectives, and
• vaccine side-effects, adverse events, and contraindications.

19.1 Introduction to immunization

Vaccines have had a huge impact on human health and may, justifiably, be regarded as the medical intervention that is second only to safe drinking water in reducing deaths and disease. Vaccines utilize the body's natural defence systems to protect against a number of specific pathogens that have the potential to cause serious disease. Using either attenuated or non-disease-causing components of microbes, they activate the immune system to provide protection before natural exposure to the pathogens can occur.

Vaccines have been used in various forms since around the tenth century AD, when Chinese and Indian physicians provided protection against smallpox using either dried crushed smallpox scabs, which people inhaled, or blister fluid inoculated intradermally (scarification, also known as variolation). Although not without risk (5–20% of recipients developed smallpox; 2–3% died), the benefits of such approaches were evident during smallpox epidemics when death rates were as high as 50% in the unprotected. In the late eighteenth century Edward Jenner introduced a safer approach to smallpox control by using a similar virus from cows ('cowpox'), with comparable protection but fewer side-effects.

Strictly speaking, the process of generating an immune response to any disease is termed immunization, whereas vaccination refers to the same process for protection against smallpox using cowpox vaccine (*vacca* means cow in Latin). However, the terms vaccination and immunization continue to be used interchangeably.

19.2 Why immunize?

It is important to consider the reasons for continuing with immunization programmes as the diseases and infections caused by vaccine-preventable diseases continue to decline.

Below is an outline of the main reasons for continuing with vaccination and immunization programmes in the face of declining rates of vaccine-preventable diseases/infections.

19.2.1 **Vaccines work**

Vaccines are very effective. They may be used to eradicate disease, as happened with smallpox in 1980 and may soon happen with polio. Alternatively, they may reduce disease occurrence as seen after the introduction of diphtheria vaccine. A similar situation is seen with invasive *Haemophilus influenza b* (Hib) disease, the commonest cause of bacterial meningitis prior to the introduction of Hib vaccine in 1992, with annually reported cases in the UK having dropped from 850 prior to the introduction of vaccine to 19 in 2013, the majority (17) of which were in those aged >15 years (Table 19.1).

19.2.2 **Improvements in sanitation don't eliminate infection risk**

The major public health successes of the eighteenth to twentieth centuries (clean drinking water, efficient sewage disposal, nutritional improvement, and reduced overcrowding) were the foundation of the improvement in health in the more affluent nations. However, these measures do not necessarily reduce either the frequency or impact of those infectious diseases where human behaviour, or a zoonotic/environmental reservoir, are key risk factors. Respiratory viruses like influenza are almost impossible to control by sanitation alone; sexually transmitted diseases,

Table 19.1 Vaccination impact on disease incidence in England & Wales (E&W) and the United States (US)

Disease	Cases per year before vaccination (pre-vaccine era)*	E&W (cases in 2010) USA (cases in 2005)	% Reduction
Diphtheria	E&W = 75,000	E&W = 1	E&W = 99.9%
	US = 175,885	US = 0	US = 100%
Measles	E&W = 763,531	E&W = 380	E&W = 99.9%
	US = 503,282	US = 66	US >99.9%
Pertussis (whooping cough)	E&W = 170,000	E&W = 1519 (2008 data)	E&W = 99.1%
	US = 147,271	US = 25,616	US = 82.6%
Polio (wild)	E&W = 7,760	E&W = 0	E&W = 100%
	US = 16,316	US = 0	US = 100%
Rubella	E&W = Not Known	E&W = 12	E&W >99.9%**
	US = 47,745	US = 11	US >99.9%
Tetanus	E&W = Not Known	E&W = 4 (2008 data)	E&W >99.7%**
	US = 1,314	US = 27	US = 97.9%
Invasive Hib disease	E&W = 850	E&W = 37 (2009 data)	E&W = 95.6%
	US = 20,000	US = 9	US >99.9

* Maximum cases reported or estimated annually in pre-vaccine era.

** Based on US data.

Source: data from Centers for Diseases Control and Prevention (CDC). Summary of Notifiable Diseases—United States, 2005. Morbidity and Mortality Weekly Report (MMWR), Volume 54, Issue, 53: pp. 2–92, Copyright © 2007 CDC, http://www.cdc.gov/mmwr/preview/mmwrhtml/mm5453a1.htm; Yeh S and Lieberman J, Update on adolescent immunization: Pertussis, meningococcus, HPV, and the future. Cleveland Clinic Journal of Medicine, Volume 74, Issue 10, pp. 715, Copyright © 2007 Cleveland Clinic; Public Health England. Notification of Infectious Diseases (NOIDS): Notifiable diseases: annual totals from 1982 to 2014, © 2012 Crown Copyright, https://www.gov.uk/government/publications/notifiable-diseases-historic-annual-totals; Public Health England. Notifiable diseases: annual totals from 1912 to 1981, © 2012 Crown Copyright, https://www.gov.uk/government/publications/notifiable-diseases-historic-annual-totals

including human papilloma virus (HPV), are spread by human behaviour; and tetanus spores are widely distributed in the natural environment. Influenza, HPV, and Tetanus Toxoid vaccination can control but not eliminate these different infections.

19.2.3 **The body's defences do not always protect against disease**

A baby's defences against infection can remain immature for weeks or months after birth. Vaccination is a key protective measure during this potentially dangerous period. The immune system of a baby exposed to a pathogen may not protect it, but maternally derived antibodies, passively transferred before birth, i.e. specific antibodies, will provide enough protection until its immune system has matured sufficiently to protect it.

A similar situation, although due to different mechanisms, is found in older people who have an increased risk of infection and although they may not mount a particularly effective immunological response when vaccinated, nevertheless even suboptimal protection is useful.

Hepatitis B is an example of an infection against which the immune system at birth is less able to provide protection. As many as 90% of babies born to a mother who is a carrier of the virus will themselves become carriers because of exposure to infected maternal blood at or around the time of birth (PHE 2013a). However, hepatitis B vaccine and hepatitis B immunoglobulin are highly effective at preventing an exposed baby from becoming infected.

Polio is an example of a viral illness against which most peoples' immune systems are generally highly effective at providing protection. When large outbreaks of polio occurred in England and Wales from the 1940s to the early 1960s, most people who had polio virus infection either recovered without developing any obvious clinical signs and symptoms or had a influenza-like illness with fever and diarrhoea, which got better on its own. However, a few developed viral meningitis, and a small number (perhaps 1 in a 1000) developed paralytic disease, many of whom died (Christie 1948).

If newborns were exposed to polio, their immune system would be unlikely to protect them (as with hepatitis B) but maternally derived passively transferred antibodies would generally protect them until the immune system had matured sufficiently to provide protection.

19.2.4 **Changing lifestyles increase our infection risk**

International travel has increased, including travel to exotic areas with exposure to unfamiliar bacteria and viruses. Yellow fever, rabies, tick-borne encephalitis, and Typhoid are several examples of travel-associated vaccine-preventable infections. Hepatitis A might also be included, because more recent improvements in sanitation in high-income countries in the past 50 years have substantially reduced the numbers of childhood infections, resulting in fewer immune adults and so a greater infection risk to travelling adults.

Furthermore, for some vaccine-preventable diseases, the destination country may require proof of certain vaccinations before allowing entry. Travel to a yellow fever area will require prior vaccination if the individual has previously been in an endemic area. Travel by pilgrims to the Hajj and Umra requires meningococcal ACWY vaccination before the Kingdom of Saudi Arabia will issue an entry visa.

19.2.5 **Pathogen mutation**

Bacterial and viral mutations continue to challenge and reduce the effectiveness of available drugs and vaccines. For example, influenza viruses evade immune responses by changing the antigenic structure of two key surface molecules: Haemagglutinin, which attaches to cell surfaces and initiates infection, and Neuraminidase, which enables newly formed viral particles to exit an infected cell and spread infection. Consequently, some components of the Influenza vaccine are changed annually, resulting in the need to administer the vaccine each year. The development of penicillin resistance by up to 7% of *Streptococcus pneumoniae* species of the reported invasive isolates in England and Wales (George and Melegaro 2001, 2003) provides further justification for the routine use of conjugate pneumococcal vaccine in infancy.

19.2.6 Reducing occupational risk

Particular occupations can increase the risk of infection. For healthcare workers that risk involves bloodborne viruses like hepatitis B, and the potential to both acquire the infection from and spread it to patients.

As the workforce ages, more people are being employed who have an impaired immune system, resulting in the challenge of how to protect them and enable them to continue working. Although vaccines do not necessarily work particularly well in all individuals with an impaired immune response, nevertheless they provide good protection for a significant proportion (including the older population) from vaccine-preventable disease such as influenza and pneumococcal pneumonia.

Many people will become carers at some point. Vaccination may help carers remain well. A good example of this would be the UK recommendation that registered carers receive an influenza vaccine annually (Public Health England 2013b).

19.3 Different types of vaccine

In the UK, there are four types of commercially available vaccines classified by their immunogen as:

♦ toxoid,

♦ killed/inactivated,

♦ subunit, and

♦ live attenuated.

19.3.1 Toxoid vaccines

Tetanus and diphtheria are bacterial infections in which disease is caused by a bacterial-secreted toxin that either impairs cell function (tetanus) or kills cells (diphtheria). Some infections, for example, whooping cough, appear to be partly toxin-mediated.

Tetanus Toxoid (TT) vaccine is manufactured by growing a *Clostridium tetani* (*C. tetani*) strain that produces large amounts of toxin. The toxin is separated off and treated with formaldehyde to convert it into a toxoid, which is structurally similar to the wild toxin, but can induce cross-reacting antibodies. The changes produced by formaldehyde render it non-toxic. The rationale for tetanus vaccination is based on generating antibodies against the toxoid, which binds the wild toxin and prevents disease development in the event of exposure to *C. tetani*.

Because the incubation period for tetanus can be as short as 24hrs, it is important that tetanus antibodies constantly circulate throughout the bloodstream: hence the need to ensure completion of the five-dose programme for life-long immunity. Diphtheria toxoid vaccine works in the same way, by inducing cross-reacting antibodies that act to neutralize the wild *Corynebacterium diphtheriae* toxin, as in the case of tetanus vaccine.

Pure toxoid vaccines are weakly immunogenic, i.e. the immune response to them is limited. This has the obvious advantage that they rarely cause any serious side-effects or adverse events following vaccination, but it also means that the levels of antibody generated are low. In order to achieve an effective and long-lasting immune response, an adjuvant (see section 19.4.2) is added, which results in high and protective antibody levels.

There are two principal advantages of toxoid vaccines:

♦ As the vaccine antigens are not actively multiplying they cannot cause the disease they prevent and they cannot spread to unimmunised individuals.

♦ When stored, they are usually stable, long-lasting, and less susceptible to changes in temperature, humidity, and light.

19.3.2 **Killed/inactivated vaccines**

The term 'killed' generally refers to bacterial vaccines, whereas 'inactivated' is used to describe non-replicating viral vaccines. Typhoid was one of the first killed vaccines to be produced and was used in the British army at the end of the nineteenth century. Polio and hepatitis A are currently the most commonly used inactivated vaccines in the UK. In many countries whole cell whooping cough vaccine, used in the UK until 2004, continues to be the most widely used killed bacterial vaccine.

Killed/inactivated vaccines share the same advantages as toxoid vaccines and, in addition, as they contain the whole virus/bacteria, all the antigens associated with infection are present and will result in antibodies being produced against each of them. Killed/inactivated vaccines usually require several doses, as one dose does not give a strong signal to the immune system because the microbes are unable to multiply in the host.

A local inflammatory reaction at the vaccine site and a fever are quite common side-effects.

19.3.3 **Subunit vaccines**

Subunit vaccines are a more recent development of the killed vaccine approach. However, instead of generating antibodies against all the components of the pathogen, a particular component (or combination) is used and the antibody produced neutralizes or kills the micro-organism to prevent infection. The key requirement is to identify that particular immunogen (see section 19.4.1), or combination of immunogens, which generate antibodies to prevent infection.

Haemophilus influenza b (Hib) is an example of a bacterial subunit vaccine that uses only one immunogen (the polysaccharide capsule). The hepatitis B vaccine also uses only one protein from the viral surface produced using recombinant DNA technology. Influenza vaccine has two immunogens (both viral surface proteins).

Subunit vaccines are very safe, with the most common side-effects being a local reaction at the vaccine site and a fever, and by and large most subunit vaccines produce long-term protection.

19.3.4 **Live attenuated vaccines**

The vaccines described above only generate antibodies. However, antibodies do not usually cross cell membranes and so provide little or no protection against those micro-organisms that live and replicate inside cells, including all viruses. A complementary approach to immunization is required in this situation and this is provided by the use of live attenuated vaccines, which generate special cells (T lymphocytes) that are able to kill virus infected cells.

Variolation against smallpox, described earlier, worked because the micro-organism used was naturally weakened, a process termed 'attenuation'.

Measles, mumps, and rubella, as MMR, are live attenuated viral vaccines used in the UK children's immunization programme. BCG is a live attenuated bacterial vaccine, providing some immunity against disease progression and the extra-pulmonary forms of tuberculosis.

The administration of live attenuated measles vaccine imitates the natural infective process with both antibody and cytotoxic T-cells being generated. Serious illness very rarely results, because attenuation has made the measles virus multiply so slowly that these protective mechanisms eliminate the virus before it can cause typical disease. Features of clinical illness may develop but they are usually very mild and require no treatment.

An individual adequately immunized against measles will have both specific antibodies and cytotoxic T-cells in their body so that when wild measles virus is inhaled, cells infected by virus at the site of infection are killed by cytotoxic T-cells: measles viruses that evade these and spread through the bloodstream are then eliminated because antibodies bind to the virus particles and neutralize them.

One disadvantage of live attenuated vaccines is the possibility that they may cause serious features of the illness they are designed to prevent, either because they revert to a more virulent form, or because, for some individuals (e.g. the immunosuppressed), they are insufficiently attenuated. This is, however, an extremely rare occurrence (Mäkelaä et al. 2002; Demicheli et al. 2012).

Until recently it was advised that live attenuated vaccines should normally be given on the same day or four weeks apart, because of concerns that interferon (a cytokine produced in response to exposure from a wild or vaccine virus), may prevent the replication of the second vaccine virus (PHE 2013c). However due to the different immune mechanisms of the various live vaccines used currently this is no longer generalizable. Current advice is that intervals between vaccines should be based on specific evidence for any interference of those vaccines (PHE 2015a). All vaccines with the exception of MMR, yellow fever and chickenpox vaccines, can be given at any time before or after each other—however, yellow fever and MMR vaccines must not be administered on the same day, and chickenpox and MMR vaccines should be given on the same day or if administered separately, a gap of four weeks between them should be observed. When live vaccines are given simultaneously, an appropriate immune response will be mounted to each vaccine immunogen.

In addition, live vaccine should *not* normally be given in pregnancy or to the immunocompromised, due to the potential but rare risk of vaccine-induced infection. As a precaution, non-live vaccines (excluding influenza, diphtheria, tetanus, whooping cough and inactivated polio) should also be avoided in pregnancy. However, if the risk of infection is considered high further expert advice about their suitability should be sought.

A summary table of some currently available vaccines in the UK, by type of vaccines, is presented in Table 19.2.

19.4 **Vaccine components**

Vaccines may contain up to three separate groups of components:

+ the immunogen,
+ active components/ingredients, and
+ residuals from the manufacturing process.

19.4.1 **Immunogen**

An immunogen is the vaccine ingredient that gives rise to the adaptive immune response. It is so called because it *GEN*erates an adaptive *IMMUN*e system response, which has both antibody- and T-cell components. It is sometimes called an antigen, which is slightly different. An antigen *GEN*erates an *ANTI*body response only. Strictly speaking, in the context of live attenuated vaccines, immunogen is the more appropriate term.

Immunogens are derived from the appropriate disease-causing bacteria or viruses.

Table 19.2 Summary of vaccine types with examples of currently available vaccines in the UK

Vaccine type	Immunogen	Vaccine name example
Toxoid	Diphtheria	Pediacel; Repevax; Infanrix-IPV; Revaxis
	Tetanus	Pediacel; Repevax; Infanrix-IPV; Revaxis
	Cholera	Dukoral
Killed/Inactivated	Poliomyelitis	Pediacel; Repevax; Infanrix-IPV; Revaxis
	Hepatitis A	Avaxim; Epaxal; Havrix monodose; Havrix monodose; Vaqta Paediatrics; Vaqta Adult
	Rabies	Rabies Vaccine BP; Rabipur
	Japanese encephalitis	Ixiaro
	Tick-borne encephalitis	TicoVac
	Typhoid	Vivotif
Subunit	Hepatitis B	Engerix B; Fendrix; HBvaxPRO; HBvaxPRO Paediatrics; HBvaxPRO 40; Twinrix Adult (HepA&B); Twinrix Paediatrics (HepA&B)
	Pneumococcal conjugate	Prevenar13, Synflorix
	Pneumococcal polyvalent polysaccharide	Pneumovax Polysaccharide Vaccine
	Meningococcal Group C conjugate	NeisVac-C; Menjugate Kit; Menitorix
	Meningococcal Group B	Bexsero
	Meningococcal ACWY polysaccharide	ACWY Vax
	Meningococcal ACWY conjugate	Menveo, Nimenrix
	Human Papilloma Virus	Gardasil; Cervarix
	Haemophilus influenza type B	Pediacel
	Pertussis	Pediacel
	Influenza	Influvac
	Typhoid	Typhim Vi (polysaccharide vaccine); Hepatyrix (HepA&Typhoid) ViATIM (HepA&Typhoid) Typherix (Typhoid)
Live Attenuated	Rotavirus	Rotarix
	Tuberculosis	BCG
	Measles; Mumps; and Rubella	MMRvaxPro; Priorix
	Influenza	Fluenz Tetra
	Varicella (Chickenpox)	Varilrix; Varivax;
	Shingles	Zostavax
	Typhoid	Vivotif
	Yellow Fever	Stamaril

19.4.2 **Active components**

These are ingredients that have a defined use(s) within the vaccine and comprise:

- adjuvants,
- carrier proteins,
- stabilizers,
- preservatives,
- buffers, and
- solvents (or diluents).

19.4.2.1 Adjuvants

In order to ensure that they are safe and cannot cause serious adverse effects, most vaccine antigens/immunogens are weakened and do not give rise to strong protective immune responses. Therefore, vaccine manufacturers may add an adjuvant: an ingredient that helps the immunogen generate an adequate and protective response. The most commonly used adjuvants are aluminium hydroxide or aluminium phosphate, and these have been used in vaccines for more than 70 years (Centers for Disease Prevention and Control 2015).

19.4.2.2 Carrier proteins

A number of 'pure' bacterial or viral components are composed of carbohydrate molecules which are not recognized by T-cells and are thus in some ways immunologically inert. However, they can be modified by linking or conjugating them to a large-molecular-weight carrier protein, which makes them very effective vaccine immunogens because they can now activate T-cells. Typical carrier proteins are Tetanus Toxoid or the mutant diphtheria toxin, CRM_{197}. Vaccines with carrier proteins are known as conjugate vaccines (e.g. Hib, Men C, and Pneumococcal Conjugate Vaccine (PCV)).

19.4.2.3 Stabilizers

These enable the vaccine to remain unchanged in the presence of factors (e.g., heat, light, humidity, acidity) that could cause deterioration in the vaccine's efficacy. Lactose is a common stabilizer.

19.4.2.4 Preservatives

These are compounds that kill or prevent the growth of micro-organisms, particularly bacteria and fungi. They are used in vaccines to prevent microbial growth in case the vaccine is accidentally contaminated. A common preservative is 2-phenoxyethanol. Thiomersal, which contains small amounts of mercury, can be used; however, there have been theoretical concerns regarding toxicity related to the use of Thiomersal. Following a comprehensive review of the evidence. the WHO has published a statement confirming the safety of Thiomersal in vaccines (WHO 2006). Currently, no vaccines in the UK childhood programme contain Thiomersal.

19.4.2.5 Buffers

These are added to resist changes in pH, adjust tonicity, and maintain osmolarity that might affect the effectiveness of vaccines when they are injected into subcutaneous or muscle tissue (intramuscular). A common buffer used in vaccines is sodium chloride.

19.4.2.6 Solvents

These are needed to ensure that all the vaccine ingredients are at the correct concentration in the final product. The commonly used solvents are saline or sterile water.

19.4.3 **Residuals from the manufacturing process**

Residuals include antibiotics, emulsifiers, and vaccine production media in extremely low concentrations, usually parts per million or billion.

◆ **Antibiotics** are added to cell cultures to prevent extraneous bacteria damaging the vaccine during its manufacture. Common ones are neomycin, polymyxin, and streptomycin.

◆ **Emulsifiers** are needed for vaccines with an oil-in-water adjuvant because the oil will not mix with the water in its absence. Polysorbate 80 (Tween), which is made from sorbitol and oleic acid, is commonly used.

◆ **Vaccine production media**: vaccine immunogens are made in a variety of production media, and residuals of the growth media may be present. Polio can be grown in cultures of kidney cells, some proteins which may be present in the vaccine following production.

19.5 **Side-effects, adverse events, and unrelated events post immunization**

Side-effects are known and expected outcomes that occur after vaccine administration. In contrast an adverse event is a response that is both harmful and unintended and which occurs at the normal dose. Unrelated events comprise any outcomes, which are not a direct or indirect effect of the vaccine.

◆ **Side-effects**: these are commonly seen after vaccination and result from a direct effect of the vaccine immunogen or any of the vaccine components. For example, local redness and swelling at the injection site, or fever, due to an acute but expected inflammatory response.

◆ **Adverse events**: these are rare and unusual occurrences after vaccination, resulting from an immune mediated hypersensitivity reaction (e.g. anaphylaxis).

◆ **Unrelated events**: these events would have occurred whether the person would have been vaccinated or not – they are not caused by the administered vaccine.

Detailed information on individual vaccine side-effects and adverse events are documented in the Summary of Product Characteristics supplied with the vaccine or on the Electronic Medicines Compendium website (http://www.medicines.org.uk/emc/).

19.6 **Vaccine contraindications**

The (very few) contraindications to any vaccination are:

◆ previous anaphylactic reaction to the vaccine antigen or any other vaccine component,

◆ acute and systemic illness (acute febrile illness) on the intended day of vaccination, postpone until they have recovered, or

◆ an evolving neurological disorder or current neurological deterioration, including poorly controlled epilepsy, immunization should be deferred until the condition stabilizes—seek advice.

For live attenuated vaccines, extra contraindications are:

◆ immunosuppression or pregnancy (individual risk assessment is needed).

19.7 **Vaccination programme objectives**

The objectives of a vaccination programme are disease eradication, elimination, local control, or protection of special groups.

+ **Eradication** describes the permanent removal of the causal organism from the world. This happened with smallpox in the 1970s and should happen with polio in the next few years. Disease eradication requires a human-only pathogen, a vaccine with a high protective efficacy, global vaccine uptake rates resulting in both high individual coverage and herd protection (vaccination of a significant portion of a population providing protection for non-immune individuals), and a readily recognizable early disease state so that affected individuals can be isolated to prevent further disease transmission.

+ **Elimination** refers to complete disease removal at a country level. The requirements are the same as for eradication with the exception that once a disease has been eliminated vaccination is still required at levels that prevent disease spread because of the potential for reintroduction from endemic countries. The UK was declared polio free by the WHO in 2002 (WHO 2002).

+ **Local control** describes the reduction of disease frequency to acceptable lower levels. Tetanus is an example because the organism is ubiquitous in the environment, so cannot be eradicated.

+ **Protection of special groups** is similar to local control and is the objective of the influenza vaccination programme. Influenza virus constantly mutates, there is an animal source of infection, and the available amounts of vaccine considerably limit the numbers of people who can be immunized.

19.8 **The developing UK immunization programme**

The introduction of new vaccines in the UK has usually been in response to an identified epidemiological need, such as epidemics causing extensive morbidity and mortality. It is also influenced by the technological expertise in developing vaccines. An understanding that a toxin caused diphtheria led to the development of the toxoid vaccine in the early twentieth century. The ability to predict and subsequently identify bacterial proteins involved in disease pathogenesis led to the development of the new meningococcal B vaccine licensed in 2014.

Adults vaccinated as babies between the 1960s and 1980s generally received diphtheria, tetanus, whooping cough, and polio vaccines: protection was against eight diseases (including three whooping cough and three polio types) but used about 3,600 immunogens, because of whole cell whooping cough and polio vaccines, which contained all their pathogens' components. A baby born in 2011 will have received diphtheria, tetanus, whooping cough, polio, meningitis type C, Hib, and pneumococcal vaccines: protection was against 23 infections (including 13 pneumococcal types) but fewer than 100 immunogens, and better protection was associated with significantly fewer vaccine components, due to the development of subunit vaccines. The immune system can theoretically deal with tens of thousands of immunogens, but this complex discussion is rarely needed if it is understood that it is the immunogen content rather than the number of vaccines that matters in generating an immune response. This addresses the misconception around 'overloading the immune system with multiple vaccines'.

From the mid twentieth century, the UK national immunization programme (https://www.gov.uk/government/collections/immunisation) was initially focused on infants and young children with the aim of eliminating diseases like diphtheria, tetanus, whooping cough, polio, and tuberculosis. As these became better controlled, programmes to eliminate measles, rubella, certain forms of meningitis, pneumonia, and influenza were introduced, with considerable expansion of the programme into adolescence, young adulthood, and the elderly. More recently, targeted programmes to address occupational, travel, and patients at risk because of underlying diseases have been introduced, and vaccination is now considered to be a life-long activity. Table 19.4 shows the current England and Wales adolescent and adult immunization programme.

Table 19.3 Baby/child/adolescent vaccine schedule, UK (from September 2015)

Age	Vaccine	Route of administration	Comments
Birth	♦ Hepatitis B (HBV) ♦ Tuberculosis (BCG)	Intramascular (IM) Intradermal (ID)	Risk groups only
2 months	♦ Diphtheria, tetanus, acellular pertussis (whooping cough), Haemophilus influenza type b, inactivated poliomyelitis (polio) (DTaP-Hib-IPV)	IM	IM vaccine administered antero-lateral aspect of thigh
	♦ Pneumococcal conjugate (PCV)	IM	IM vaccine administered antero-lateral aspect of thigh
	♦ Meningococcal B (Men B)	IM	Introduced in 2015
	♦ Rotavirus (Rotarix)	Oral	–
3 months	♦ Diphtheria, tetanus, acellular pertussis (whooping cough), Haemophilus influenza type b, inactivated poliomyelitis (polio) (DTaP-Hib-IPV)	IM	IM vaccine administered antero-lateral aspect of thigh
	♦ Meningococcal C (Menjugate Kit or NeisVac—to be removed in 2016	IM	IM vaccine administered antero-lateral aspect of thigh
	♦ Rotavirus (Rotarix)	Oral	–
4 months	♦ Diphtheria, tetanus, acellular pertussis (whooping cough), Haemophilus influenza type b, inactivated poliomyelitis (polio) (DTaP-Hib-IPV)	IM	IM vaccines administered antero-lateral aspect of thigh.
	♦ Pneumococcal conjugate (PCV)	IM	IM vaccines administered antero-lateral aspect of thigh
	♦ Meningococcal B (Men B)	IM	Introduced in 2015
One year old	♦ Haemophilus influenza type b/ Meningococcal C (Menitorix)	IM	IM vaccines administered antero-lateral aspect of thigh
	♦ Pneumococcal conjugate (PCV)	IM	IM vaccines administered antero-lateral aspect of thigh
	♦ Meningococcal B (Men B)	IM	IM vaccines administered antero-lateral aspect of thigh
	♦ Measles, Mumps, Rubella (M-M-RVAXPRO)	IM or SC (Subcutaneous)	IM vaccines administered antero-lateral aspect of thigh

(continued)

Table 19.3 Continued

Age	Vaccine	Route of administration	Comments
2 years	♦ Influenza vaccine (reassortant, live attenuated) (Fluenz tetra)	Nasal spray	–
3 years	♦ Influenza vaccine (reassortant, live attenuated) (Fluenz tetra)	Nasal spray	–
4 years	♦ Influenza vaccine (reassortant, live attenuated) (Fluenz tetra)	Nasal spray	–
3 years 4 months or soon thereafter	♦ Diphtheria, tetanus, acellular pertussis (whooping cough), inactivated poliomyelitis (polio) (dTaP-IPV)	IM	Vaccine administered in deltoid
	♦ Measles, Mumps, Rubella (M-M-RVAXPRO)	IM or SC (Subcutaneous)	Vaccine administered in deltoid
5 years	♦ Influenza vaccine (reassortant, live attenuated) (Fluenz tetra)	Nasal spray	School Year 1
6 years	♦ Influenza vaccine (reassortant, live attenuated) (Fluenz tetra)	Nasal spray	School Year 2
12–13 years	♦ Human Papilloma Virus Vaccine (Gardasil). A two-dose schedule is recommended in girls under 15 years—second dose at least 6 months after the first dose. If course commenced late, girls aged 15 years and over should receive a three-dose schedule	IM	Female only programme Vaccine administered in deltoid
14 years (around)	♦ Meningococcal C (replaced by quadrivalent conjugate ACWY vaccine in August, 2015)	IM	Vaccine administered in deltoid
14 years (around)	♦ Diphtheria, tetanus, inactivated poliomyelitis (polio) (dT-IPV)	IM	Vaccine administered in deltoid
14 years (around)	♦ Measles, Mumps, Rubella (M-M-RVAXPRO) (Catch-up if not received two doses previously)	IM or SC	Vaccine administered in deltoid

Source: data from Public Health England. The complete routine immunisation schedule from summer 2014 (London: Public Health England, 2014), © 2014 Crown Copyright, https://www.gov.uk/government/publications/the-complete-routine-immunisation-schedule, accessed 2 Jun. 2015.

In 2015, a baby born in the UK, by 13 months of age, will have been offered a number of highly effective and very safe vaccines that provide protection against 31 different bacteria and viruses, including MenB and rotavirus, again using only about 100 immunogens (Table 19.3).

Diphtheria, tetanus, whooping cough, polio, and measles vaccines are core vaccines offered in all WHO countries. Other vaccines are added to this, partly as determined by the disease's epidemiology and the status of other preventable disease programmes, partly by the strength of the current immunization programme and health system, including availability, performance, and funding, and partly by vaccine availability. For example, in Nigeria yellow fever vaccine is offered to infants because the disease is endemic; in Japan the Japanese encephalitis vaccine is offered universally beginning at 3 years of age for the same reason (http://apps.who.int/immunization_monitoring/globalsummary).

Table 19.4 UK adolescent and adult vaccination programme, from September 2015

UK adolescent and adult vaccination programme 2015

Programme and vaccine	Age					Comments
	16–24	**25–64**	**65–69**	**70–79**	**≥80**	
Universal						
TdIPV	5 doses for lifetime protection					
MMR	2 doses for lifetime protection					Not likely to be required for those born before 1970, as they are less likely to be susceptible
Shingles	Not recommended		70-, 78-, and 79- year-olds on September 1st			1 dose Zostavax for 70 (routine) and 78/79 (catchup) year olds from September 2014
Targeted						
Men B	Give one dose to splenectomized individuals					Currently is Bexsero
Men C	1 dose if not previously given. If a dose is received <10 years of age, booster dose between 13–18 years or before starting higher education.	Not recommended				Meningococcal C was replaced by quadrivalent conjugate ACWY vaccine from August, 2015, i.e. due to increases in MenW cases in the UK
Pneumococcal	For at-risk groups 1 dose or 5 yearly*	Universal 1 dose				*5 yearly if in a group whose antibodies would be expected to drop more quickly
Influenza	1 dose annually for at risk groups	Universal annually				Children aged 6 months to < 9 years who are in clinical risk groups and not received influenza vaccine previously should be offered a second dose
HPV	3 doses*	Not recommended				*Females up to 18 years
BCG	1 dose*—up to 35 years (DH), or 65 years (NICE)					*If in at risk group
Varicella	adolescents (≥13 years) and adults 2 doses*					*If in at risk group—no data on use in elderly
Pertussis	1 dose*	Not recommended				*All pregnant women ≥ 20 weeks
Occupational/travel						
Hepatitis A	2 doses for long-term protection					The second between six and twelve months after the first dose
Hepatitis B	3 doses with post serology if Chronic Renal Failure (CRF)					Post serology if CRF or occupational

In addition, the public and private sector have come together internationally in the GAVI alliance with the aim of 'Saving children's lives and protecting people's health by increasing access to immunisation in developing countries' (GAVI the Vaccine Alliance 2015). They have made great progress with introducing some of the more costly vaccines into poor countries with high disease burden, most recently HPV vaccine (GAVI the Vaccine Alliance 2014).

19.9 **Vaccine efficacy and effectiveness**

One way of quantifying how well a vaccine prevents disease is to calculate its protective efficacy (PE). In a randomized controlled trial, where equal numbers receive vaccine and placebo, all subjects are followed for the same length of time, and none are lost to follow-up, PE (as a %) is calculated as:

$$\frac{(\text{Disease incidence in unvaccinated} - \text{Disease incidence in unvaccinated})}{\text{Disease incidence in unvaccinated}} * 100$$

The above formula measures the proportionate reduction in disease incidence following the introduction of a vaccine. Vaccine effectiveness is a similar measure but estimates how good a vaccine is under the real conditions of everyday use.

19.10 **Conclusions**

Immunization is a highly successful public health programme that protects infants, children, adolescents, adults, and the elderly against a range of common, and not so common, infections.

The success is such that health workers in the UK no longer see the infections that caused hundreds of thousands of deaths and sickness among the population in the mid-twentieth century.

With the knowledge acquired from vaccination against infections about how the immune system functions, it is very likely that the role of immunisation will expand in the near future to treat other diseases, including chronic diseases and cancers.

References

Centers for Diseases Control and Prevention (CDC). 2005. Summary of notifiable diseases—United States, 2005. *Morbidity and Mortality Weekly Report (MMWR)*, **54**(53): 2–92. http://www.cdc.gov/mmwr/preview/mmwrhtml/mm5453a1.htm (accessed 8 March 2016).

CDC. 2015. *Frequently Asked Questions about Adjuvants*. http://www.cdc.gov/vaccinesafety/Concerns/adjuvants.html (accessed 8 March 2016).

Christie AB. 1948. Poliomyelitis: clinical features. *Public Health*, **61**: 62–64. http://dx.doi.org/10.1016/S0033-3506(47)80090-3 (accessed 8 March 2016).

Demicheli V, A Rivetti, MG Debalini et al. 2012. Vaccines for measles, mumps and rubella in children. *Cochrane Database System Review*, **15**(2): CD004407. doi:10.1002/14651858.CD004407.pub3.

GAVI, the Vaccine Alliance. 2014. *206,000 More Girls to Benefit from HPV Vaccine with GAVI Alliance Support*. http://www.gavi.org/library/news/press-releases/2014/206-000-more-girls-to-benefit-from-hpv-vaccine-with-gavi-alliance-support/#sthash.DjfCcySW.dpuf (accessed 8 March 2016).

GAVI, the Vaccine Alliance. 2015. http://www.gavi.org/index.aspx (accessed 8 March 2016).

George AC, A Melegaro. 2001. Invasive pneumococcal infection, England and Wales 1999. *CDR Weekly*, **11**(21).

George AC, A Melegaro. 2003. Invasive pneumococcal infection, England and Wales 2000. *CDR Weekly*, 3–9.

Mäkelä A, JP Nuorti, H Peltola. 2002. Neurologic disorders after measles-mumps-rubella vaccination. *Pediatrics*, **110**(5): 957–63.

Public Health England (PHE). 2013a. *Hepatitis B: Immunisation against infectious disease - The Green Book, Chapter 18.* https://www.gov.uk/government/publications/hepatitis-b-the-green-book-chapter-18 (accessed 8 March 2016).

PHE. 2013b. *Influenza: Immunisation against infectious disease - The Green Book, Chapter 19.* https://www.gov.uk/government/publications/influenza-the-green-book-chapter-19 (accessed 8 March 2016).

PHE. 2013c. *Measles: Immunisation against infectious disease - The Green Book, Chapter 21.* https://www.gov.uk/government/publications/measles-the-green-book-chapter-21 (accessed 8 March 2016).

PHE. 2014. *The Complete Routine Immunisation Schedule from Summer 2015.* https://www.gov.uk/government/publications/the-complete-routine-immunisation-schedule (accessed 8 March 2016).

PHE. 2015. *Notification of Infectious Diseases (NOIDS): Notifiable Diseases: Annual Totals from 1982 to 2014. Notifiable diseases: Annual Totals from 1912 to 1981.* Didcot: PHE. https://www.gov.uk/government/publications/notifiable-diseases-historic-annual-totals (accessed 8 March 2016).

World Health Organization (WHO). 2002. *Certification of the Region's Polio-free Status in 2002.* http://www.euro.who.int/en/health-topics/communicable-diseases/poliomyelitis/activities/certification-and-maintenance-of-polio-free-status-in-the-european-region/european-regional-commission-for-the-certification-of-poliomyelitis-eradication/certification-of-the-regions-polio-free-status-in-2002 (accessed 8 March 2016).

WHO. 2006. *Global Vaccine Safety: Statement on Thiomersal.* http://www.who.int/vaccine_safety/committee/topics/thiomersal/statement_jul2006/en/ (accessed 8 March 2016).

Yeh S, J Lieberman. 2007. Update on adolescent immunization: Pertussis, meningococcus, HPV, and the future. *Cleveland Clinic Journal of Medicine,* **74**(10): 715.

Further reading

Plotkin SA, A Walter, WA Orenstein, PA Offit. 2013. *Vaccines,* 6th edition. Philadelphia: Elsevier Saunders.

Chapter 20

Incidents and outbreak management

Sam Ghebrehewet and Alex G. Stewart

OVERVIEW

....

After reading this chapter the reader will be familiar with:
- key definitions and steps in the investigation and control of incidents and outbreaks,
- practical approaches to managing incidents and outbreaks,
- steps and processes followed in providing an emergency response and managing environmental public health situations, and
- the overall approach to public health risk assessment in all three domains of health protection (communicable disease, emergency response, environmental public health).

20.1 Introduction to the public health management of incidents and outbreaks

This chapter covers the general principles and practice of incident and outbreak investigation and management in all three domains of health protection (communicable disease, emergency response, and environmental public health).

In the UK, the process of investigating and managing incidents and outbreaks in communicable diseases is well established. In England, local health protection teams follow the PHE outbreak control plan (PHE 2014), with similar approaches in the devolved administrations. The outbreak control plan describes the overall approach and responsibilities of different parties in responding to infectious disease outbreaks. However, every incident or outbreak has its own unique features, characteristics and complexities, even if the causative organism(s) and/or source are the same. The outcome depends on how well those specific characteristics are identified and managed.

20.1.1 Terms

Outbreak observed number of cases greater than expected for a defined place and time period, or two or more cases with a common source.

Cluster two or more probable/confirmed case with an epidemiological link (place, person and time) to warrant further investigation.

Incident one case of serious disease (e.g. Ebola/plague/anthrax).

Index case the first case to come to the attention of the investigator; not always the primary case.

Primary case the case that introduced the disease into the group or population.

Secondary case the case that contracted the infection from the primary case.

20.1.2 **Communicable disease incident/outbreak management**

Communicable disease transmission is underpinned by the agent–host–environment concept. In addition, for an outbreak to occur there needs to be a chain of transmission.

The key features of the agent are: infectivity (the capacity of the agent to cause infection in a susceptible host); pathogenicity (the capacity to cause disease in a host); and virulence (the severity of disease that the agent causes in the host).

The status of the host (susceptible or immune) determines the response to the agent (e.g., no illness, typical illness, atypical (modified) illness).

Environmental characteristics play a crucial role in the chain of transmission by influencing the interaction of the agent and host. They include socio-economic conditions (e.g. tuberculosis (TB) association with overcrowding and poor housing), climate (influences or controls malaria-carrying mosquito life cycles), and ecology (human–animal interaction).

20.1.3 **How do outbreaks come to light?**

Outbreaks that are caused by common organisms are usually identified by:

♦ routine surveillance data showing an increase over the normal background level for the particular place and time,

♦ GPs/hospital physicians reporting cases either formally or informally,

♦ laboratory reports or calls from microbiology laboratory staff, or

♦ environmental health officers.

Outbreaks that are acute or unusual are usually identified by:

♦ calls to health protection team from members of the public, NHS or local authority professionals, schools, hotel staff, media, etc.

20.1.4 **Why investigate outbreaks?**

Outbreak investigation is important to:

♦ take action to control further spread, and

♦ identify and control the source of the outbreak.

In addition, systematic investigation of an outbreak enables professionals and organizations to prioritize and release resources to:

♦ determine the nature and extent of the outbreak,

♦ manage internal and external communications effectively,

♦ identify lessons in order to prevent similar outbreaks in the future,

♦ obtain new or up-to-date evidence about the optimal way to manage similar outbreaks,

♦ understand better the behaviour of novel organisms, and

♦ provide assurance (organisational/societal/political), gather evidence for legitimate legal reasons, or alleviate public concerns.

20.1.5 **How to investigate an outbreak?**

It is important to investigate outbreaks promptly and convene an Outbreak Control Team (OCT) within three days of such a decision (PHE 2014) in order to implement timely controls that prevent further spread. The OCT leads the systematic collation of accurate, contemporaneous, and comprehensive information.

It is better to convene an OCT and stand down if it is unnecessary, rather than attempting to manage without one. A template agenda for an OCT meeting can be found in Table 20.1. If an OCT is not convened, the justification for the decision should be recorded along with a clear management plan that needs to be reviewed within 24–48hrs. However, it is our experience that most care-home-related diarrhoea and vomiting outbreaks continue to be controlled and managed safely and effectively without convening an OCT, i.e. following a thorough risk assessment and ruling out foodborne illness.

Table 20.1 Template agenda for OCT, STAC, and Incident Management Team (IMT) and/or Advisory Group on Health for managing health protection incidents and outbreaks

	Communicable Disease Control (OCT)	Emergency Response (STAC)	Environmental Public Health (Advisory Group on Health/IMT)
1	Introductions; check membership	Introductions; check membership	Introductions; check membership
2	Apologies	Apologies	Apologies
3	Review minutes and actions of previous meeting	Review minutes and actions of previous meeting	Review minutes and actions of previous meeting
4	Purpose of Meeting ♦ First meeting: agree ground rules and terms of reference	Purpose of Meeting ♦ First meeting: agree ground rules and main tasks	Purpose of Meeting ♦ First meeting: agree chair, ground rules, and main tasks
5	Review of Evidence ♦ Epidemiological ♦ Microbiological ♦ Environmental	Review of evidence ♦ Site: emergency services', and site owner's reports ♦ Risk: known and potential health or environmental impacts ♦ Actions: current response and context ♦ Other relevant reports	Review of evidence ♦ Epidemiology ♦ Toxicology, pathology, other health sciences ♦ Environmental sciences ♦ Other sources of evidence
6	Current Risk Assessment (severity, uncertainty, spread, intervention, context)	Review health risk analysis and agree updated advice ♦ Risk assessment ♦ Risk management options ♦ Risk communication messages	Review health risk analysis and agree updated advice ♦ Risk assessment (source, pathway, receptor) ♦ Risk management options ♦ Risk communication messages
7	Control Measures	Review immediate control measures	Review preliminary and long-term control measures
8	Further investigations ♦ Epidemiological ♦ Microbiological ♦ Environmental	Further investigations ♦ Consider need of risk register	Further investigations ♦ Epidemiology ♦ Toxicology, pathology, other health sciences ♦ Environmental sciences ♦ Other sources of evidence

Table 20.1 Continued

	Communicable Disease Control (OCT)	Emergency Response (STAC)	Environmental Public Health (Advisory Group on Health/IMT)
9	Communications ♦ Public ♦ Media ♦ Healthcare providers ♦ Other stakeholders	Communications ♦ Public ♦ Media ♦ Healthcare providers ♦ Other stakeholders	Communications ♦ Public ♦ Media ♦ Healthcare providers ♦ Other stakeholders
10	Agreed Actions Allocated tasks	Agreed Actions Allocated tasks	Agreed Actions Allocated tasks
11	Any other business ♦ Escalation needed?	Any other business ♦ Shift, handover, and timescales	Any other business ♦ Timescales
12	Next Meeting	Next Meeting	Next Meeting

IMT = Incident Management Team, OCT = Outbreak Control Team, STAC = Scientific and Technical Advice Cell

Source: data from Public Health England. Communicable Disease Outbreak Management: Operational Guidance. London: Public Health England, © 2014 Crown Copyright.

20.1.6 Who makes the decision to convene an outbreak control team (OCT)?

An outbreak is usually declared by the consultant in communicable disease control (CCDC) or consultant in health protection (CHP), following a thorough joint risk assessment with the local consultant microbiologist, and relevant professionals such as a senior environmental health officer (EHO) for foodborne outbreaks, and a chest physician for a respiratory illness, e.g., TB.

Communicable disease outbreaks identified and declared in hospitals or similar healthcare premises are managed by hospital infection control teams usually led by the Director of Infection Prevention Control/Hospital Infection Control Doctor. The local CCDC/CHP is a core member of the hospital OCT.

20.1.7 Who are members of an Outbreak Control Team?

OCTs convened to manage community outbreaks are usually chaired by the Consultant in Communicable Disease Control or senior health protection staff (Table 20.2).

Table 20.2 Members of an Outbreak Control Team

Usual members	Additional members to be invited depending on the nature of the outbreak (not exhaustive)
CCDC/CHP (Chair)	Community Infection Control Nurse
Consultant Epidemiologist	Consultant Physician/General Practitioner
Consultant Microbiologist	NHS Representative
Director of Public Health/Deputy	Local authority education department
EHO	Water company
Communications Officer	Veterinary scientists (Animal Health)
Administrative support	Food Standard Agency

20.1.8 What are the key steps in the investigation of an outbreak?

The key steps in the investigation of incidents or outbreaks of communicable diseases are: case ascertainment, confirmation of outbreak, case identification, conducting descriptive epidemiology, generating a hypothesis, considering further investigation including testing hypothesis using analytical studies (if appropriate), interpretation of results, writing an outbreak report, and communication (Table 20.3). Communication of findings and implementation of control measure should be considered at all stages, and reviewed regularly at each stage of investigation.

Table 20.3 Key steps in the investigation of health protection incidents and outbreaks, arising from a communicable disease, an emergency response, or an environmental situation

		Communicable disease	Emergency response	Environmental situation
1	Health Leadership	Outbreak Control Team (OCT)	Scientific and Technical Advice Cell (STAC)	Incident Management Team (IMT) and/or Advisory Group on Health
2	Process			
2.1	Case ascertainment	Check reports and notifications against the standard/agreed case definition of the particular disease	Check with ambulance service and local hospitals for patients possibly affected by situation; case definition may be needed	May not be possible if the focus is on risk and not outcomes. Check any relevant registries and GP records against agreed case definition where possible
2.2	Confirmation of outbreak or situation	Confirm epidemiological links (place, person, and time) that meet the outbreak definition for the particular infectious outbreak	Confirm details of the incident, including details of source and possible chemicals, pathways, and receptors (affected population)	As for emergency response, plus epidemiological links that meet definition for situation
2.3	Case identification	Identify unreported cases through communication with local GPs, hospital staff, and other relevant health and non-healthcare settings	Identify affected individuals and unreported cases through emergency services, including A&E departments, walk-in centres	Identify potential cases who may meet case definition, but are not reported, through relevant departments (e.g. specific disease registry, GP)
2.4	Conduct descriptive epidemiology	Place, person, and time. Analyse and interpret, including drawing an epidemic curve (see Chapter 22) showing disease propagation, to enable a point source (in time) to be distinguished from an ongoing source, and the efficacy of control measures to be checked	Often point source, but good descriptive epidemiology will help define the situation more effectively	Point source common, but diffuse sources or putative clusters need careful interpretation of descriptive epidemiology to understand the situation and check the efficacy of control measures

Table 20.3 Continued

		Communicable disease	Emergency response	Environmental situation
2.5	Generate hypothesis	Often possible following comprehensive descriptive epidemiology, but may involve implementation of a questionnaire to gather relevant information from those exposed and affected (e.g. foods eaten, places eaten at, travel history etc.)	Often possible following description of incident, but may need interrogation of emergency services or exposed people. Best done within a multi-agency setting	Often possible following comprehensive descriptive epidemiology; a good hypothesis will focus thinking around the situation. Likely to need multi-agency input
2.6	Consider further investigations	Further investigations such as microbiological, epidemiological, and environmental investigations may be needed if the descriptive epidemiology does not provide enough information to implement control measures	Undertake what is necessary for public health advice. Ensure information from other agencies is integrated before decision about further investigation is made	Likely to involve health sciences (e.g. toxicology, pathology), appropriate environmental sciences, and expert opinion. May be complex and need academic or multi-agency approach
2.7	Test the hypothesis	Usually through analytical studies (case-control, cohort)	Not usually undertaken. However, a Risk Register of exposed people can provide relevant cohort, if considered appropriate	Case-control and cohort studies useful; perhaps modelling of local situation in light of wider scientific understanding rather than direct analytical study. May also involve a qualitative approach, including stakeholder and case interviews, mapping of cases or complex statistical methods (seek advice)
2.8	Interpret results	Make sense of all the data, and produce intelligence that informs public health control measures. Note: If already implemented, control measures may need to be reviewed in light of analytical study results plus microbiological, environmental, and epidemiological investigations	Consider dose, signs and symptoms, site and situation, toxicology on short timescale (immediate response) and longer (Risk Register)	Full results might take extended time to obtain, but preliminary results may need to be interpreted to aid public health actions

(continued)

Table 20.3 Continued

	Communicable disease	**Emergency response**	**Environmental situation**
2.9 Consider wider public health issues	Consider the technical interpretation of results within the wider structure of a full public health risk assessment, taking context and stakeholder accounts (see Chapter 3 Section 3.3.4)	A full public health risk assessment (see Chapter 3 Section 3.3.4) will help with fear and perception issues, which play major roles in emergencies	Wider public health risk assessment (see Chapter 3 Section 3.3.4) is vital to ensure community engagement, informed decisions, and sensible public health advice and control measures
2.10 Write report	Final summation of the outbreak, investigation, and control measures, identifying any lessons that can reduce the likelihood of such outbreaks occurring in the future and improve the response and control	Contribute to hot and cold multi-agency debriefs to identify what went well and what did not in immediate response. Reports considering management processes and lessons are not common; an area ripe for development	Health reports considering management issues and peer-reviewed publications not written enough, particularly in complex situations run by non-health organizations where different agencies contribute at different times and health is not responsible for the overall management
2.11 Communicate results	During and after the outbreak, to relevant parties, including partners and the public (press statements, letters, etc.) and professionals (peer-reviewed publications, e.g. Eurosurveillance for preliminary reports)	Regular communication with professionals, those at risk, and the public, is crucial. This includes recovery phase, particularly if prolonged	Engagement with those affected, at risk, and the local community, through regular communications, including meetings if appropriate, cannot be emphasized enough, due to longer timescales

Source: data from Hawker J, Begg N, Blair I, Reintjes R, Weinberg J, and Ekdahl K. Communicable Disease Control and Health Protection Handbook, 3e. Chichester, UK: John Wiley & Sons, Ltd., Copyright © 2012 John Wiley and Sons, Ltd.

20.1.9 **When to declare an outbreak is over?**

The conventional view is that once a period of twice the incubation period of the causative agent has elapsed without identification of any new case, subject to reliable surveillance, then a communicable disease outbreak can be declared over. However, for outbreaks caused by organisms with a short incubation period (e.g. fewer than ten days) it may be pragmatic to observe a period three times the incubation period to allow adequate time for delay in notification or reporting, diagnostics, and other surveillance-related delays.

Once the outbreak is declared over, a final written report, ideally agreed by all members of the OCT, should be prepared within 12 weeks (PHE 2014).

20.2 **Investigation and control of emergency responses**

The investigation and control of acute incidents follow the same principles as for communicable disease outbreaks. However, emergency response is provided under the Civil Contingencies Act (2004). Responders (Category 1 and 2) are subject to civil protection duties. Category 1 responders are subject to the full set of civil protection duties, which include: assessing the risk of emergencies, and putting in place emergency and business continuity management plans. Category 2 responders are described as 'coordinating bodies' and their primary duty is to cooperate and share information with other Category 1 and 2 responders.

Under Civil Contingency a major incident is defined as a situation that seriously threatens human health or disrupts services. It gives rise to an agreed multi-agency response as already defined in the local Major Incident Plan. A variety of emergency situations are possible (e.g. fire in a COMAH (Containment of Major Accident Hazard) site, chemical leak in an occupational setting, fire on a waste site, or a weather-related event). Notification of a major incident mainly comes to the attention of health protection via the emergency services (ambulance, fire, and police).

The reasons for investigation are similar to communicable disease control—to control the source and mitigate further harm—but includes addressing anxiety and fear arising from perceptions of the incident.

If a major incident is declared, then a Strategic Coordinating Group (SCG) is convened by the police, and, if appropriate, a Scientific and Technical Advice Cell (STAC) is established to advise the SCG (see Table 20.1 for a template agenda for a STAC meeting) primarily on health matters in the initial phases, including public health communications. Members of STAC reflect those of an OCT, with relevant environmental, chemical, or toxicological scientists replacing microbiologists. However, any company involved in the incident provides a representative to STAC to give site-specific information, including chemical details.

Key steps in the investigation and management (Table 20.3) also mirror those for communicable disease: confirmation of what has happened, size of incident, chemicals or other hazards involved, nature and route of exposure, numbers affected, any resulting health issues, conducting a full public health risk assessment (Table 20.3), and reviewing management procedures and communication messages.

Decisions to close incidents are made by fire and police for the acute phase, and local authority for the recovery phase; health contributes appropriately to both phases and decisions.

20.3 **Investigation and control of environmental public health incidents**

The process of investigating and managing environmental incidents is less well established than the approach to communicable disease outbreaks or emergency incidents. However, although environmental incidents are often complex, long-lasting, and require judgements and health advice in the face of uncertainty, the approach remains similar.

A chronic environmental incident is often defined less by the disease than by the environmental situation, such as flood, fire, or chemical spill, although investigations into disease clusters putatively caused by environmental factors can be just as challenging (see Chapter 17).

Environmental public health is underpinned by the source–pathway–receptor framework. Sources are as diverse as a land previously contaminated by lead and arsenic on which houses and gardens have been standing for 50 years, a factory emitting odours or leaking toxins into the sewers or watercourses. There must be a full linkage of the environmental source through to the receptors, which in public health terms are people, with a plausible pathway (inhalation, ingestion, skin or eye contact). If any one of the three factors is missing, breaking the linkage, then there is no further need to investigate. Structured approaches to cluster investigations exists, but are not as well rehearsed as communicable disease management, due to their complexity and uncertainty.

Environmental situations can be reported by the public, the emergency services or other professionals (e.g. the public or Environmental Health Officers concerned about air pollution, ambulance requesting help around flooding, or GPs noting a disease cluster and wondering about local industry as a source). Investigations are important to determine any plausible linkage that can be controlled to reduce further exposure and possible ill health. Lessons can be learned and used to develop local and national responses to similar situations.

The structure and approach to environmental situations (Table 20.3) is parallel to communicable disease control in outbreaks, with the replacement of microbiological investigations and science with environmental investigations and science. The multi-agency meetings of an Incident Management Team (IMT), usually led by partners other than Public Health, may not be as frequent as those in an outbreak but are as important in identifying and investigating possible hypotheses, supporting control measures, and learning lessons.

Environmental issues may last months or years, unlike most outbreaks. In some chronic situations, as a subgroup of the IMT, an Advisory Group on Health may need to be established (for an example see Mahoney 2015). This group operates in a manner similar to the OCT, with parallel membership to STAC, offering a focused approach to the lead agency around public health risk assessment (see Chapter 3, section 3.3.4), advice about environmental investigations and remediation, public health messages, and assurance. This can be a vital contribution, without taking up time at the incident management meetings, and can direct an incident response in appropriate ways with relatively little resource. (See Table 20.1 for template agenda for an IMT or an Advisory Group on Health.)

Requests to establish an Advisory Group on Health can come from other agencies such as the local authority or the Director of Public Health, who may be responding to questions or complaints under their public protection role.

Decisions about closing the situation are usually taken by the multi-agency management team or the responsible Public Health bodies. Health protection involvement in environmental situations may last for the whole of the response or only contribute at specific times for focused questions, particularly in situations that last for years.

20.4 **Practical issues for communicable diseases**

20.4.1 **Leadership**

♦ The leadership of the management of any incident and outbreaks requires experience, understanding of local epidemiology, and situational analysis. These build into a personal, professional, and agency knowledge base that is critical for safe and effective management. Currently in the UK, this is provided by organizations such as Public Health England and Health Protection Scotland. Cross-border incidents require all this and more, including diplomacy and a clear agreement as to the lead agency and the level of leadership within each organization (PHE 2013).

♦ In managing outbreaks that require resources over and above the local capacity, the OCT needs to assess whether or not overall leadership should be escalated to a Strategic Coordinating Group (led by health) to ensure appropriate level of priority and commitment is given.

20.4.2 **The process**

♦ In complex incidents and outbreaks, it is best practice for the OCT to establish subgroups, such as epidemiological, microbiological, and environmental cells, that report to the OCT.

♦ Similarly, it may be more appropriate for multiple but common outbreaks to be managed by one OCT with contribution and representation from the professionals responding to the affected communities or settings.

20.4.3 **Evidence for public health action**

♦ Often, it is not possible to prove causation, or even association, beyond reasonable doubt. Therefore, a clear conclusion, agreed with relevant partners, matters; narrative is as useful an explanation to support and prioritize needed public health action as a statistical estimate linking cause and effect.

♦ As long as a comprehensive risk assessment is undertaken and due consideration is given to the benefits of public health action versus the costs of that action (including financial, reputational, and professional), then a robust defence can be made against criticism of action being too early (not enough statistical evidence) or too late (taking time to gather statistical evidence).

♦ Caution should be exercised in interpreting statistical significance, as it does not always prove association or causation and its absence does not rule either out. Results, even from analytical studies, are subjective and need to be interpreted in the context of findings from other investigations.

♦ Overall, any OCT/IMT needs to keep an open mind when synthesizing the evidence and concluding association or causation, especially if the cost of resulting public health action is going to be high. Identifying indistinguishable strains of organisms, both from those affected and a potential source, does not necessarily mean that a particular source is the cause, as it is possible that both have been exposed to and affected by a common source.

20.4.4 **Debrief**

♦ It is good practice for all relevant organizations to run internal debriefs as soon as the incident/outbreak is declared over (within four weeks).

♦ As a minimum, internal debriefs should provide information on: what went well; what did not go so well; and what can be improved upon, in relation to the following three areas: (1) internal organizational response; (2) multi-agency engagement; (3) overall management and leadership of the incident/outbreak.

♦ An overall multi-agency debrief should be undertaken within eight to ten weeks of the incident being declared over, in order to allow time for internal debriefs. The overall debrief should be structured in the same way as internal debriefs, with the aim of producing a plan that contains agreed action(s), identified responsible bodies, and a timeline. The lessons learnt reviewed within 12 months after formal closure of the outbreak.

20.4.6 **Communications**

♦ Subject to adhering to relevant confidentiality issues, proactive communication is preferred to reactive, and every opportunity needs to be used to engage the media, professionals, and the general public to enhance their contribution.

♦ It is good practice to establish regular communication with both professionals and the general public, as it would help the OCT to control the timing of communication, reduce incoming enquiries, and provide reassurance.

20.4.7 **Outbreak report ownership**

♦ The copyright will belong to the organization(s) which employ(s) the author(s); if a multi-agency sign-off procedure is in place, ownership of copyright and responsibility for formal disclosures needs to be agreed by the OCT (PHE 2014).

- It is crucial that OCT members understand that the responsibility for the report contents and conclusions lie with all OCT members and the organizations they represent.

20.4.8 Outbreak Control Plan

- Incidents/outbreaks can be related to unusual and rare diseases or situations; therefore, any learning in their management should contribute and inform the local Outbreak Control Plan, which should be reviewed regularly.
- For the same reason, caution needs to be exercised in modifying the day-to-day response to common sporadic cases or situations based on experience of managing unusual situations; change to day-to-day practice should be based on surveillance and the epidemiology of a disease or situation.

20.5 Practical issues for EPRR

In EPRR the practical issues are the same as for communicable disease, except that the OCT is replaced by STAC and the multi-agency SCG. Stand-down arrangements are more challenging than escalation and immediate response, as it is often difficult to find clear evidence of no or reduced risk of exposure on which to base decisions. Therefore, soft intelligence from emergency services is the usual basis for such decisions, which needs to be recorded accordingly. Good relationships and mutual support are vital for ease of making these difficult decisions.

Debrief reports are internal to each organization, with multi-agency debrief reports usually compiled by the police and owned by the local resilience forum. Similarly, the control plans, covering a variety of situations, are owned by all contributing agencies under the local resilience forum.

20.6 Practical issues for environmental public health

The practical issues related to environmental public health are the same as for communicable disease, except that there may not be a formal IMT. Decisions on evacuation or execution of public health actions are often not easy, especially when costs and consequences—financial, social, personal, environmental—may be high or unclear. Public health actions should probably be more pragmatic than solely precautionary, taking the wider context and interests of stakeholders into account.

Reports are often internal to each organization. Multi-agency reports are seldom written, and very little is published in peer-reviewed journals. There is little formal multi-agency planning and agreement on how to investigate and control environmental situations, leaving this as an area ripe for development.

20.7 Conclusions

Communicable disease outbreak investigation is one of the key health protection functions, and requires competent specialists in health protection to apply knowledge (science), skills (art), experience, and leadership to protect the public. The investigation of environmental situations and incidents is a developing area for competent professionals, where the same skills and leadership, but different competency and knowledge, are applied in more challenging and long-lasting situations, with the same end of protecting the public's health.

Once an outbreak of communicable disease or an environmental public health situation is declared, thorough technical and public health risk assessments should be undertaken, and the appropriate team (OCT, STAC, IMT, and/or Advisory Group on Health) convened promptly (if appropriate) in order to:

- ensure appropriate and effective control of infection or environmental health risks,
- get new evidence about:
  - optimal outbreak and incident management,
  - prevention of future outbreaks or incidents,
  - behaviour of novel organisms or toxins, or environmental issues; and
- address organizational, political, legal, or public concerns.

Outbreak investigation and OCT activities, as well as responses to emergency environmental situations (with or without STAC), must take priority over other work, and include the relevant expertise and adequate representation of relevant stakeholders. While chronic environmental situations are not so time-bound, their investigation should be given time and resources in a similar fashion.

An outbreak report that covers the nature and extent/size of the outbreak, the results of the investigation, and the outcome of the control measures taken must be produced within 12 weeks of an outbreak being declared over. Reports on chronic situations and environmental emergencies are likely to be compiled by other agencies. Thought should be given as to whether a separate health report, which enlarges on the contribution to the main report, would be beneficial.

In every outbreak investigation and management situation, it is of paramount importance to review the experience of all involved, to identify shortfalls and particular difficulties encountered, and to revise the Outbreak Control Plan in order to improve future response. Health protection contribution to a multi-agency debrief following emergency environmental situations is vital to ensure emergency preparedness, planning, and response continues to improve. The identification and dissemination of lessons from chronic environmental situations is less well structured or developed at this point, but no less important.

References

Hawker J, N Begg, I Blair, et al. 2012. *Communicable Disease Control and Health Protection Handbook*. 3rd edition. London: John Wiley & Sons.

Mahoney G, AG Stewart, N Kennedy, et al. 2015. Achieving attainable outcomes from good science in an untidy world: case studies in land and air pollution. *Environmental Geochemistry & Health*, 37: 689–706. doi:10.1007/s10653-015-9717-9

Public Health England (PHE). 2013. *Emergency Preparedness, Resilience and Response (EPRR) Concept of Operations (CONOPS)*. http://phenet.phe.gov.uk/Resources/emergencyresponse/Documents/EPRS%20 Concept%20of%20operations.pdf

PHE. 2014. *Communicable Disease Outbreak Management: Operational Guidance*. https://www.gov.uk/ government/uploads/system/uploads/attachment_data/file/343723/12_8_2014_CD_Outbreak_ Guidance_REandCT_2__2_.pdf (accessed 8 March 2015).

Further reading

Centers for Disease Control and Prevention (CDC). Atlanta: CDC. Emerging Infectious Diseases: Outbreak Investigations – A Perspective. Atlanta: http://wwwnc.cdc.gov/eid/article/4/1/98-0104_article (accessed 28 April 2016).

Food Standard Agency (FSA). 2008. *Management of Outbreaks of Foodborne Illness in England and Wales*. https://www.food.gov.uk/business-industry/guidancenotes/hygguid/outbreakmanagement (accessed 8 March 2015).

Heymann LD (ed.). 2014. *Control of Communicable Diseases Manual*. 20th edition. Washington, DC: American Public Health Association.

Chapter 21

Health protection surveillance

Roberto Vivancos, Giovanni Leonardi, and Alex J. Elliott

OVERVIEW

After reading this chapter the reader will be familiar with:
- the definition of surveillance, and how and when it is used in health protection,
- the different types of surveillance,
- the framework for assessing quality and the steps to follow when evaluating surveillance systems, and
- the different surveillance systems and tools including syndromic and environmental monitoring, and their application in health protection.

21.1 Introduction to surveillance

The most commonly cited definition of surveillance is 'the ongoing systematic collection, analysis, and interpretation of health data, essential to the planning, implementation, and evaluation of public health practice, closely integrated with the timely dissemination of these data to those who need to know' (Langmuir 1963). Surveillance is an integral part of epidemiology, but in the last few decades it has increasingly developed to become a field on its own.

Within this definition we can extract a series of steps that are involved in any surveillance system:

- Reporting: a system of detection of health events or disease and notification (e.g. reporting of clinical diagnosis of a specific disease).
- Data accumulation: collection and collation of data, including systems for quality assurance.
- Data analysis: this requires the skills to be able to manipulate and query the data collected so that it can be appropriately queried for the purpose for which the surveillance system has been set up. Descriptive epidemiology is used to describe health events and diseases in terms of who, when, and where. Continuous analysis over time allows for detection of unusual occurrences and exceedances over baseline levels.
- Judgement: interpretation of the analysis, which may also take into account additional information about the disease or health event (e.g. information about local epidemiology or known factors from the scientific literature).
- Action: the system should help inform what actions need to be taken in response to the health event.

Surveillance information can be used to:

- follow trends in the health status of a population over time,
- establish health care and public health priorities,

- ensure those with greatest need are prioritized,
- detect and respond to epidemics,
- evaluate the effectiveness of programmes and services, and
- develop hypotheses for research about risk factors for disease causation, propagation, or progression.

21.2 **Types of surveillance**

There are broadly four types of surveillance systems: passive, active, sentinel, and negative (Table 21.1).

Table 21.1 Types of surveillance systems

Surveillance system	Description	Example
Passive	<ul><li>Rely on the routine reporting of event or disease data by those individuals or organizations involved in the diagnosis or detection</li><li>Relies on the cooperation of these individuals and organizations</li><li>Provides basic information about a disease, mainly about incidence</li><li>Less expensive and in many countries participation is regulated in legislation</li><li>As the collector of data does not actively seek out information, these systems may suffer from underreporting</li></ul>	Scarlet fever, chickenpox
Active	<ul><li>Required for some diseases of importance or on occasions when more accurate information is needed</li><li>Public health professionals actively contact all individuals and institutions to ensure that they are collecting information on cases and that the information collected is as complete as possible</li><li>Results in a higher level of interaction between those reporting and the collector of data</li><li>These systems are more labour intensive to maintain, and may require incentives, and therefore tend to be more expensive to coordinate</li></ul>	Invasive group A streptococcal disease; measles; rabies
Sentinel	<ul><li>Required where it may not be practical to actively collect information from all providers</li><li>A representative subset of the providers is chosen to provide the desired information</li></ul>	Influenza
Negative	<ul><li>Required for rare or emerging diseases or events</li><li>Rely on reports of the absence to reassure those making decisions on control</li><li>Reporters are asked for a 'nil report' as well as reporting incidences</li></ul>	Ebola, MERS-CoV

21.3 **Assessing the quality of surveillance data**

To understand the strengths and limitations and to be able to assess the quality of a surveillance system, it is important to understand the attributes that constitute it. The following are attributes of quality of surveillance systems:

- Accuracy: the ability of a system to measure what it aims to measure. This is normally reported as sensitivity and specificity.
- Representativeness: the measure taken must come from the population of concern.
- Timeliness: a system may score high in accuracy and representativeness, but it has to provide the information in a timeframe that allows timely action to be taken.
- Simplicity: a complex system is more difficult to implement and maintain, which will impact on the reliability of the system, the quality of the data that it provides, and the resources required to maintain it.
- Flexibility: capacity to adapt to changing environment.
- Acceptability: what is asked of those reporting must be reasonable and achievable to allow concordance.

21.4 **Evaluation of surveillance systems**

The purpose of evaluating surveillance systems is to ensure that problems of public health importance are being monitored efficiently and effectively (German et al. 2001). The evaluation of a surveillance system is a consultative process where stakeholders (e.g. the secondary users of the outputs from the system) are engaged in defining what is being assessed about the systems, and in constructing any recommendations about the system, and includes the following steps:

- engagement of stakeholders in order to ensure that the evaluation addresses appropriate questions and that the evaluation assesses the relevant attributes of the systems,
- description of the surveillance system, which includes a description of the importance of the event under surveillance, the purpose and operation of the system, and the resources required to maintain it,
- the direction and process of the evaluation must be focused to ensure efficient use of resources,
- gathering of evidence to measure the performance of the surveillance system against the appropriate system attributes,
- when recommendations are made from the evaluation, these must be justified and take into account the attributes as well as the overall purpose of the system and opinion from stakeholders, and
- findings of the evaluation must be communicated and any lessons learnt implemented.

21.5 **Surveillance tools**

This section presents examples of surveillance tools used to monitor either infections and diseases, symptoms and events, or risk factors and precursors of disease.

21.5.1 **Infection and disease**

21.5.1.1 Notification of diseases

In order for public health authorities to monitor disease trends and to set up early warning systems for the detection of outbreaks, certain diseases are required by law to be reported to government authorities. These are called notifiable diseases (see Appendix 4). The list of notifiable diseases varies by country, although it usually includes diseases and syndromes of potential public health significance, such as anthrax or cholera, or more common ones, such as food poisoning. There is normally a statutory duty on agencies or practitioners to notify. Most countries also have lists of notifiable diseases in animals. Notification in animals may include diseases of importance to livestock (e.g. foot and mouth), but also significant threats to human health (e.g. avian influenza or rabies).

One of the limitations of notification of diseases is that under-reporting can be significant, and particularly more prominent in common diseases (e.g. food poisoning).

The World Health Organization (WHO) uses the International Health Regulations (IHR), a binding document of international law, agreed by 196 countries around the globe, to prevent and control the international spread of disease (e.g. diseases of extreme virulence such as viral haemorrhagic fevers, or diseases targeted for eradication such as polio). The original IHR of 1969 listed diseases of international concern; however, the updated revision of 2005 focused loosely on international disease threats and health risks, which allows for a more dynamic surveillance tool adaptable to emergent threats (e.g. severe acute respiratory syndrome (SARS) or Middle East respiratory syndrome (MERS)).

21.5.1.2 Laboratory reporting

Another way of counting cases of infection to monitor incidence and prevalence is to collect information from diagnostic laboratories directly. The way in which this is done varies considerably between countries and even within countries depending on the disease. Systems can be voluntary or statutory, or even sentinel, where only a selected number of laboratories report.

21.5.1.3 Prevalence surveys

This is the monitoring of disease or infection trends through surveys carried out at regular intervals. These surveys can give information about trends in prevalence of disease, and are a useful tool to assess quality of care through the measure of key performance indicators (e.g. measuring post-operative infections in different hospitals to be able to compare rates). Prevalence surveys are commonly used in the monitoring of healthcare-acquired infections or in measuring anti-microbial resistance to antibiotics, where ongoing routine collection of information may be more onerous.

21.5.2 Symptoms and event surveillance

21.5.2.1 Syndromic surveillance

Syndromic surveillance (SyS) is the (near) real-time collection, analysis, interpretation, and dissemination of health-related data to enable the early identification of the impact, or absence of impact, of potential threats (Triple S. 2011).

Originating in the US, some of the earliest examples of SyS systems were developed in direct response to '9/11' to monitor potential bioterrorist attacks. Subsequently, these systems were increasingly used to monitor the epidemiology of infectious diseases (e.g. using emergency department attendances and ambulance dispatch data to monitor 'chief complaints'), and the use of SyS is now spreading.

21.5.2.2 How does SyS work?

SyS differs from traditional surveillance in that it is not based on laboratory-confirmed diagnoses, but on non-specific clinical signs, symptoms, and proxy measures for health; these constitute a provisional diagnosis or syndrome. Data are usually collected for purposes other than surveillance and, where possible, are automatically generated to avoid imposing an additional burden on data providers. The general principle of SyS is to monitor health data to detect unusual increases in signal activity (e.g. a rise in the number of people attending emergency departments with respiratory symptoms) in near real-time.

The main aims of SyS are to:

♦ detect an unknown, novel, or emerging threat,

♦ provide reassurance by demonstrating a lack of public health impact of a known threat,

♦ provide 'situational awareness' to quantify and monitor the impact of an identified public health threat, and

♦ provide early warning of the start of an expected seasonal event (e.g. influenza season).

21.5.2.3 Limitations of SyS

SyS is not a case-based reporting system. Data are anonymized and are analysed and reported at population rather than individual level. SyS is therefore not suitable for detecting or monitoring small outbreaks. SyS also does not report on pathogen-specific data; therefore, increases in syndromic indicators cannot be linked directly to specific diseases.

21.5.2.4 Examples of SyS systems

Table 21.2 provides examples of SyS systems and the health data sources that they utilize.

SyS systems are flexible in their nature, enabling them to respond to a wide range of public health incidents. Table 21.3 illustrates a number of different public health scenarios that SyS can support.

21.5.2.5 Event-based surveillance (EBS)

Event-based surveillance (EBS) is the organized and rapid capture of information on infectious disease events of potential public health risk that may have significant impact or be the result of a major incident or event (e.g. mass gatherings or national floods). Unlike traditional surveillance, EBS is based on the capture of unstructured reports rather than the routine capture of data (WHO 2008).

21.5.2.6 How does EBS work?

The range of data sources that can be captured for EBS broadly fall into the following categories:

♦ medical setting: including healthcare service data (e.g. outbreaks, notifications) and public health intelligence from specialist public health services (e.g. laboratory reports), and

♦ community setting: including media and published sources, schools, pharmacies.

EBS is used particularly during specific incidents of public health significance. In these instances, the findings from EBS would be communicated by both national and local public health teams and the relevant information fed into a national incident response report, thereby incorporating a range of surveillance sources to monitor the progress of the incident.

Data collected by EBS is usually structured according to a minimum dataset including such information as:

♦ when/where the event happened,

♦ what has been reported,

♦ how many people have been affected,

♦ severity of the public health impact, e.g. deaths, and

♦ contact details of the reporting team to enable further dialogue/investigation.

Table 21.2 Examples of syndromic surveillance systems

Health data source	Data fields used for surveillance	Example systems	Established or developmental systems
Emergency department (ED)	ED attendances; triage; discharge; diagnosis code	(Elliot et al. 2012)	Established
General practitioner (GP)	Clinical codes recorded during GP consultation	(Harcourt et al. 2012)	Established
Ambulance dispatch (AmD)	Dispatch events including those taken to hospital; presenting complaint code	(Coory et al. 2009)	Established
Web queries	Search engine queries for particular health problems	(Ginsberg et al. 2009)	Established
Social Media (Twitter)	Number of tweets; tweets specific for certain search criteria	(Gesualdo et al. 2013)	Developmental
Telephone health services	Calls; symptoms presented; advice given to caller	(Anderson et al. 2014)	Established

Source: data from Coory MD, Kelly H, and Tippett V. Assessment of ambulance dispatch data for surveillance of influenza-like illness in Melbourne, Australia. *Public Health,* Volume 123, Issue 2, pp. 163–8, Copyright © 2009 Elsevier, Inc.; Ginsberg J, Mohebbi MH, Patel RS, Brammer L, Smolinski MS, and Brilliant L. Detecting influenza epidemics using search engine query data. *Nature,* Volume 457, Issue 7232, pp.1012–4, Copyright © 2009 Macmillan Publishers Limited; Elliot AJ, Hughes HE, Hughes TC, Locker TE, Shannon T, Heyworth J, et al. Establishing an emergency department syndromic surveillance system to support the London 2012 Olympic and Paralympic Games. *Emergency Medicine Journal,* Volume 29, Issue 12, pp. 954–60, Copyright © 2012 BMJ Publishing Group Ltd and the College of Emergency Medicine; Harcourt SE, Smith GE, Elliot AJ, Pebody R, Charlett A, Ibbotson S, et al. Use of a large general practice syndromic surveillance system to monitor the progress of the influenza A(H1N1) pandemic 2009 in the UK. *Epidemiology and Infection,* Volume 140, Issue 1, pp.100–5, Copyright © 2012 Cambridge University Press; Gesualdo F, Stilo G, Agricola E, Gonfiantini MV, Pandolfi E, Velardi P, et al. Influenza-like illness surveillance on twitter through automated learning of naïve language. *PLoS ONE,* Volume 8, Issue 12: e82489, Copyright © 2013 Gesualdo et al.; Andersson T, Bjelkmar P, Hulth A, Lindh J, Stenmark S, and Widerström M. Syndromic surveillance for local outbreak detection and awareness: evaluating outbreak signals of acute gastroenteritis in telephone triage, web-based queries and over-the-counter pharmacy sales. *Epidemiology and Infection,* Volume 142, Issue 2, pp. 303–13, Copyright © 2014 Cambridge University Press.

21.5.2.7 Limitations of EBS

EBS is based on extracting information from existing case management systems and reporting from local and national health protection teams. It can therefore only report on significant cases and incidents being managed by those teams. In addition, delays in notification of events may affect the completeness of EBS.

21.5.2.8 Examples of EBS

Table 21.4 provides a number of examples where EBS can be used to support the Public Health response to a particular event or incident.

21.5.2.9 Behavioural and lifestyle risk surveillance

Behavioural surveillance refers to the monitoring of changes in knowledge, attitudes, and behaviours associated with an outcome. Behaviour surveys are conducted at regular intervals (e.g. every five or ten years) to provide a cross-sectional overview and trend in risk factors for an illness or problem. It is most often used with the monitoring of behaviours associated with sexually transmitted infections (STIs), although it may refer to other lifestyles leading to important public

Table 21.3 Examples of public health scenarios that SyS can support

Health protection scenario	Potential health threat	SyS systems of particular value	SyS indicators used in response
Pandemic influenza	Respiratory illness; severe illness (depending on strain); secondary bacterial infections	General practitioner (GP); Emergency department (ED)	Respiratory indicators including influenza-like illness, acute respiratory infection, pneumonia
Industrial fire	Respiratory irritation from particulates/toxic fumes; exacerbation of asthma and cardiovascular problems	ED; GP	Asthma, wheeze, difficulty breathing; cardiac, myocardial ischaemia
Heatwave	Exposure to high day and night temperatures, particularly elderly and vulnerable population	Ambulance dispatch (AmD); ED; telehealth calls	Heat/sun stroke; cerebrovascular; cardiac
Flooding	Gastroenteritis from contaminated flood water; respiratory problems during post-flood drying out period (mould); psychological/ anxiety problems; CO poisoning from use of generators during power-outs	GP; telehealth calls; AmD	Gastroenteritis, diarrhoea, vomiting; asthma, wheeze, difficulty breathing; anxiety, stress, psychological problems, prescription of anti-depressants

health problems (e.g. diet and exercise habits and obesity). Most developed countries have HIV and AIDS behavioural risk surveys.

21.5.3 Environmental surveillance

21.5.3.1 Framework for environmental public health surveillance

A general framework for conducting environmental public health surveillance involves data from three points in the process by which an agent in the environment produces an adverse outcome in a host: hazards, exposures, and outcomes (Hertz-Picciotto 1996). This approach can be applied to public health information concerning any preventable adverse effect on health, whether infectious or not-infectious.

Table 21.4 Examples of EBS

Public health scenario	Potential health threat	EBS indicator
Norovirus outbreaks in hospital wards	At risk patients with comorbidities; closure of wards/institutions	Numbers of wards/hospitals affected; laboratory reports of norovirus
Returning healthcare workers from Ebola endemic countries	Symptomatic returnees transmitting virus to close contacts	Airport screening; contact tracing; local public health team reporting of suspect cases
Olympic Games	Outbreaks of disease	Local public health incident reporting; environmental health reporting of food poisoning; laboratory exceedence reporting.

21.5.3.2 Environmental precursors of infection

Monitoring of environmental circumstances, or hazards, associated with the incidence of air-, water-, and foodborne infections can provide opportunities for earlier interventions compared to outbreak monitoring. Environmental drivers are often epidemic precursors of disease such as malaria, dengue, chikungunya, hantavirus infections, Rift Valley fever, Lyme disease, plague, tularemia, and schistosomiasis, meaning that monitoring changes in environmental conditions can help predict upsurges in infectious disease (Semenza et al. 2013).

21.5.3.3 Occupational disease

In occupational health, monitoring of hazards in the workplace is an effective tool for prevention. Physician reports on diseases attributed to occupational exposures, including asthma, contact dermatitis, noise-induced hearing loss, carpal tunnel syndrome, and musculoskeletal disorders, have been monitored in several countries, providing crucial information to guide interventions and compensation (Stocks et al. 2015). Occupational disease surveillance can also detect emerging diseases in the population.

21.5.3.4 Definition and principles of environmental public health surveillance

Environmental health surveillance is used both to track changes in exposures that are known to have adverse health effects (such as lead or carbon monoxide) and to identify previously unrecognized hazards (such as potential impacts of persistent organic pollutants).

The term 'environmental public health tracking' (EPHT) has been used to describe the integration of environmental surveillance within a public health service (McGeehin et al. 2004). The interpretation of results within a surveillance system monitoring environmental hazards or exposures requires a conceptual framework that accounts for the several ongoing transitions that affect health and wellbeing (demographic, epidemiological, economic, energy, and others) (Rayner et al. 2012). In addition, the practical implementation of an environmental public health surveillance system requires a systematic framework and a concrete set of criteria to guide development, selection, and evaluation of environmental public health indicators (Malecki et al. 2008), as well as application of several analytical tools and data standards.

21.5.3.5 Food and water surveillance

Foodborne diseases represent a considerable public health burden and pose a major challenge to the public health system. Salmonellosis and campylobacteriosis are the most commonly reported foodborne diseases in Europe. Foodborne illnesses can also result from pesticides or medicines in food, and from naturally toxic substances. Given the decline in funding for sampling of food by public health authorities, food surveillance systems might be able to provide intelligence leading to targeted sampling. With the globalization of food markets, climate change, and increasing international travel, there are risks of new outbreaks of foodborne diseases globally. In addition, there is a challenge of anti-microbial resistance, partly related to use of anti-microbial agents in the food production sector (European Observatory on Health Systems 2013).

Because of the importance of waterborne diseases, provision of drinking water is strictly regulated in most countries, where resources are sufficient. Supplementation of water supplies, such as fluoridation aimed at reducing incidence of dental cavities, requires public health monitoring and communication with the local community. Public health agencies should devote special attention to potential exposures from private drinking water supplies and recreational use of water, and also consider factors such as interactions with activities in the agricultural sector, algal blooms, local geology, and incidents, including radiation releases, to be potential reasons for specific surveillance programmes.

Table 21.5 Examples of integrated health protection surveillance systems

Public health scenario	Risk factor/precursor	Outcome	Strategy for control/ prevention
Sexual health	*Sexual risk behaviour—* behaviour surveys conducted at regular intervals	*Sexually transmitted infections—*diagnosis at genitourinary medicine clinics or laboratory detections	*Health promotion—*advice on risk factors
	Contraception— long-acting reversible contraception prescription	*Teenage pregnancies—* maternity records	Targeting of health advice/ campaign
		Termination of pregnancy— hospital episodes data	Detection and investigation of clusters
		Emergency Contraception— prescriptions of 'morning after pill'	
Influenza	*Immunization—*uptake rates	*Advice seeking—*calls to remote help lines or web searches	Inform media campaigns
	Laboratory detections— information on prevalent strains and whether they are covered by vaccine	*Consultations—*consultation rates in primary care providers	Decision on use of antivirals for prophylaxis and treatment
		Laboratory detections— number of detections and type of influenza detected	Alert health services
		*Intensive Care Unit admission—*reports of cases admitted to ICUs	Evaluate impact of vaccination
		*Outbreaks—*reports of outbreaks in care homes or schools	Detect clusters
Air pollution	Environmental monitoring of air quality	General practitioner (GP) consultations for respiratory problems	Health promotion—advice on risk factors
	National pollution forecasts		Targeting of health advice/ campaign
Carbon monoxide (CO) poisonings	CO in indoor air	Deaths	Health promotion—advice on best practice to avoid hazards in relation to fuel combustion
		Hospital admissions	
		Emergency department attendances	Targeting of health advice/ campaign (beginning of heating season)
		GP and other primary care visits	
		Symptoms in the community	Guidance to health care workers

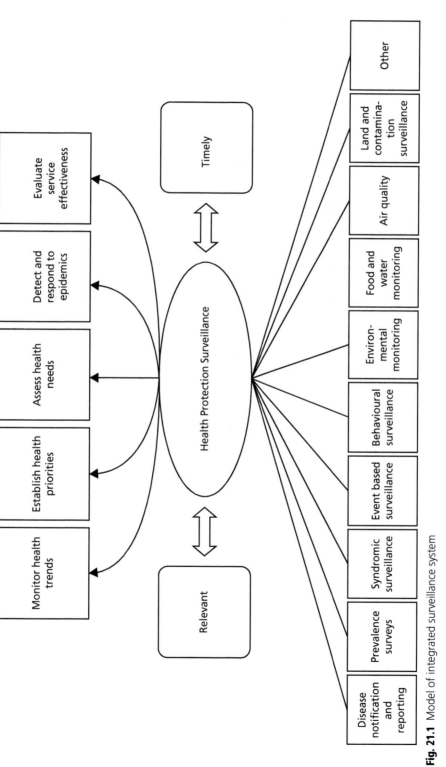

Fig. 21.1 Model of integrated surveillance system

21.5.3.6 Air quality surveillance

Air quality monitoring can be considered part of a health protection surveillance system in relation to interventions such as those discussed in Chapter 14. Indoor air quality includes several hazards that are potentially preventable, including volatile organic compounds and carbon monoxide (CO). Surveillance of CO may focus primarily on reports of incidents, as in France (Verrier et al. 2010) or attempt an integration of several sources of information to monitor overall preventable burden, as in the US (see Table 21.5) (Iqbal et al. 2012).

21.5.3.7 Land and contamination surveillance

The evidence base for health impacts from soil exposure includes hazards from helminths and chemicals such as metals and asbestos (Hough 2007). Contaminated sites are areas hosting (or having hosted) production and processing plants and facilities for chemicals, petrochemicals, manufacturing, waste disposal and/or treatment, cement, power generation, and mining and metals. In Europe, earlier industrialization and poor environmental management practices have left a legacy of thousands of contaminated sites. Past and current activities can cause local and diffuse contaminations to such an extent that they might threaten human health and the environment. In specific circumstances, surveillance may be of support to the monitoring and management of such legacy sites, as part of a risk assessment leading to remediation.

21.6 **Integrated surveillance**

The surveillance systems previously described in this chapter are rarely used in isolation to assess a public health situation or issue. It is more commonly the case that public health officials use information from various sources or systems in an integrated manner, to allow triangulation of information. An integrated system may look at the precursors, hazards, or risk factors of a public health problem, as well as measuring disease and other outcomes that are relevant, in order to support decisions on actions that may be required to prevent or control such as problem (Figure 21.1).

In these instances, interpretation relies on the understanding of the quality of each of the component surveillance systems. Table 21.5 gives a number of examples of integrated surveillance systems.

21.7 **Conclusions**

Surveillance is a core function of health protection, providing, through various approaches, essential information and intelligence on the robust prevention, control, and response programmes that can be established. A good understanding of surveillance is essential for all public health/health protection professionals who practise in any of the three domains of health protection (communicable disease control, emergency preparedness, resilience and response (EPPR) and environmental public health). The importance of surveillance in informing strategy and policy should not be underestimated. In addition, the all-hazards approach to health protection requires health protection professionals to be conversant with the common principles that underpin all surveillance systems.

References

Andersson T, P Bjelkmar, A Hulth, et al. 2014. Syndromic surveillance for local outbreak detection and awareness: evaluating outbreak signals of acute gastroenteritis in telephone triage, web-based queries and over-the-counter pharmacy sales. *Epidemiology & Infection*, **142**(2): 303–13.

Coory MD, H Kelly, V Tippett. 2009. Assessment of ambulance dispatch data for surveillance of influenza-like illness in Melbourne, Australia. *Public Health*, **123**(2): 163–68.

Elliot AJ, HE Hughes, TC Hughes, et al. 2012. Establishing an emergency department syndromic surveillance system to support the London 2012 Olympic and Paralympic Games. *Emergency Medicine Journal*, **29**(12): 954–60.

European Observatory on Health Systems and Policies. 2013. *Facets of Public Health in Europe*. http://www.euro.who.int/en/about-us/partners/observatory/publications/studies/facets-of-public-health-in-europe (accessed 8 March 2016).

German RR, LM Lee, JM Horan, et al. 2001. Updated guidelines for evaluating public health surveillance systems: recommendations from the Guidelines Working Group. *Morbidity and Mortality Weekly Report*, **50**(RR-13): 1–35; quiz CE1–7.

Gesualdo F, G Stilo, E Agricola, et al. 2013. Influenza-like illness surveillance on twitter through automated learning of naïve language. *PLoS ONE* **8**(12). http://www.ncbi.nlm.nih.gov/pmc/articles/PMC3853203/ (accessed 8 March 2016).

Ginsberg J, MH Mohebbi, RS Patel, et al. 2009. Detecting influenza epidemics using search engine query data. *Nature*, **457**(7232): 1012–14.

Harcourt SE, GE Smith, AJ Elliot, et al. 2012. Use of a large general practice syndromic surveillance system to monitor the progress of the influenza A(H1N1) pandemic 2009 in the UK. *Epidemiology & Infection*, **140**(1): 100–105.

Hertz-Picciotto I. 1996. Comment: toward a coordinated system for the surveillance of environmental health hazards. *American Journal of Public Health*, **86**(5): 638–41.

Hough RL. 2007. Soil and human health: an epidemiological review. *European Journal of Soil Science*, **58**(5):1200–12.

Iqbal S, JH Clower, M King, et al. 2012. National carbon monoxide poisoning surveillance framework and recent estimates. *Public Health Reports*, **127**(5): 486–96.

Langmuir AD. 1963. The surveillance of communicable diseases of national importance. *New England Journal of Medicine*, **268**(4): 182–92.

McGeehin MA, JR Qualters, AS Niskar. 2004. National environmental public health tracking program: bridging the information gap. *Environmental Health Perspectives*, **112**(14): 1409–13.

Malecki KC, B Resnick, TA Burke. 2008. Effective environmental public health surveillance programs: a framework for identifying and evaluating data resources and indicators. *Journal of Public Health Management Practice*, **14**(6): 543–51.

Rayner G, T Lang. 2012. *Ecological Public Health: Reshaping the Conditions for Good Health*. Abingdon: Routledge.

Semenza JC, B Sudre, T Oni, et al. 2013. Linking environmental drivers to infectious diseases: the European environment and epidemiology network. *PLoS Neglected Tropical Diseases*, **7**(7): e2323.

Stocks SJ, R McNamee, HF Molen, et al. 2015. Trends in incidence of occupational asthma, contact dermatitis, noise-induced hearing loss, carpal tunnel syndrome and upper limb musculoskeletal disorders in European countries from 2000 to 2012. *Occupational Environmental Medicine*, **72**(4): 294–303.

Triple S. 2011. Assessment of syndromic surveillance in Europe. *Lancet*, **378**: 1833–4.

Verrier A, C Delaunay, S Coquet, et al. 2010. Carbon monoxide poisoning episodes in metropolitan France in 2007 (French) *BEH Bull Épidémiologique*, **1**: 1–5. http://www.invs.sante.fr/beh/2010/01/ (accessed 8 March 2016).

World Health Organization. 2008. *A guide to developing event-based surveillance*. http://www.wpro.who.int/emerging_diseases/documents/docs/eventbasedsurv.pdf (accessed 8 March 2016).

Chapter 22

Essential statistics and epidemiology

Paul Cleary, Sam Ghebrehewet, and David Baxter

OVERVIEW

After reading this chapter the reader will be familiar with:
- the role and components of descriptive and analytical epidemiology,
- methods for summarizing categorical and quantitative variables,
- different patterns of epidemic curves and their interpretation,
- using analytical epidemiology to determine odds and risks ratios and understand issues of confounding, and
- using statistical tests in hypothesis testing.

22.1 Introduction to statistics and epidemiology

Health protection practitioners require an understanding of basic principles of statistics and epidemiology for several common scenarios:

- investigation of an outbreak of an infectious disease,

- monitoring infectious disease surveillance data,

- conducting surveys or other cross-sectional studies,

- contributing to research studies, evaluations or audits, and

- reading, reviewing, or writing scientific publications.

Most analyses in typical health protection scenarios use only a basic repertoire of statistical and epidemiological methods, which are outlined in this chapter; however, a wide and rapidly developing range of more advanced statistical and epidemiological methods are available, and there is growing interest in the use of relatively new data sources, such as genomic or network data.

In the investigation of an outbreak, the aims of data analysis typically include summarizing currently available information on the course, extent and impact of the outbreak (**descriptive epidemiology**); inferring the possible agent, source or mode of transmission from information on cases (**hypothesis generation**); or testing these hypotheses using **analytical epidemiology**.

The broad aims of analysis of infectious disease surveillance data include describing whether the occurrence of a disease or condition is changing over time (overall or for specific groups of people or disease subtypes), early detection of outbreaks, describing geographical variations in the occurrence of disease, and identification of populations at particular risk.

Surveys or other cross-sectional studies are commonly used to assess the proportion of a population having certain characteristics of interest at a given point in time, often based on information from a subset (or **sample**) of that population which can be selected in a number of ways.

22.2 **Summarizing different types of data**

The first step in data analysis is to recognize which types of data have been collected, as different types of data are summarized and analysed differently. In a typical epidemiological dataset we have a number of items of information (often referred to as **variables**) about each of a group of individuals. It is good practice to begin analysis by examining each variable individually using the following summary measures and visualizations.

22.2.1 **Categorical data: frequency distributions, bar charts**

Data representing categories are often called **categorical data**. Examples in health protection practice include:

♦ gender (male or female),

♦ clinical status (e.g. ill or not ill, whether a case had particular symptoms or not),

♦ age group (e.g. <1yr, 1–4 years, 6–9 years, 10–14 years, 15+ years),

♦ ethnic group, and

♦ region of residence.

Categorical variables may have an inherent order (as in the example of age group), in which case they are sometimes called **ordinal** variables; categorical variables without inherent ordering are sometimes called **nominal** variables. Categorical variables with only two categories are sometimes called **binary** or **dichotomous** variables.

Categorical variables can be summarized in a type of table called a **frequency distribution**, including percentages of the total number to show the **relative frequency** of each category, as in the simple example in Table 22.1.

Categorical variables can also be summarized visually using plots such as **bar charts or dot charts**, where the relative frequency of each category is indicated by the length of a bar or by the position of a dot, as shown in Figure 22.1. A **population pyramid** is a development of the bar chart to display population demographic structure; counts or percentages in each age group are typically shown as horizontal bars, to the left for one gender and to the right for the other.

22.2.2 **Quantitative data: measures of central tendency and spread; histograms and box-and-whisker plots**

Variables representing counts or measurements as numbers may be called **quantitative** variables. Examples in health protection practice include age in years, durations of incubation periods, or the number of cases of a given disease in a particular area at a particular time.

Summaries of quantitative variables need to convey at least three things: an indication of the 'middle' of the data (more formally called a **measure of central tendency**), an indication of the spread of the observations around this point (**measure of spread**), and the general shape of the distribution on a histogram.

Table 22.1 Example of a frequency distribution of gender

Gender	Frequency	Percentage
Male	95	47.5
Female	105	52.5
Total	200	100.0

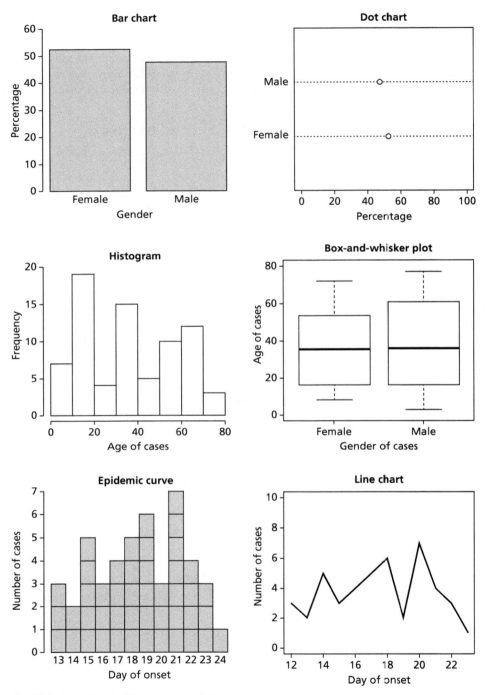

Fig. 22.1 Examples of different types of charts

Histograms, or box-and-whisker plots, as shown in Figure 22.1, may be used to summarize quantitative variables visually and to guide the method of summary. A **histogram** groups the values of a quantitative variable into several mutually exclusive **bins** and shows the relative frequency of each, as shown in Figure 22.1. It shows whether the distribution of a variable is symmetrical or **skewed**. Symmetrical, bell-shaped distributions are often described as **normally distributed**; this is a key prerequisite for certain statistical tests. A skewed distribution is a distribution with a 'long tail' on one side; distributions with a long tail to the right are most commonly seen and are described as **skewed to the right**. Sometimes a distribution has more than one peak, in which case it is described as **multimodal**.

The **mean** (sometimes called the **arithmetic mean**) is often the appropriate measure of central tendency and the **standard deviation** the appropriate measure of spread for a symmetrically distributed variable in which case approximately 95% of observations will fall within two standard deviations of the mean. Skewed variables (or variables with any unusually extreme values, known as **outliers**) are more appropriately summarized with the **median** as the measure of central tendency and the **interquartile range (IQR)** as the measure of spread.

The mean is obtained by dividing the sum of the values of the observations by the number of observations.

The **median** is found by rearranging the observations in order of size. If there are an odd number of observations, the median is the middle value, i.e. where approximately half of the observations are above and half are below. If there is an even number of observations, then the median is the mean of the middle two observations.

The interquartile range is the difference between the upper and lower quartiles. The **upper quartile** (or **75th centile**) is the point below which lie 75% of the observations; the **lower quartile** (or **25th centile**) is the point below which lie 25% of the observations. There are a number of different methods of calculating quartiles and the interquartile range, and it is usually simpler to use computer software to obtain this. A **box-and-whisker plot** may be useful to display the median and interquartile range visually (see Figure 22.1): the thicker central line shows the median, the height of the 'box' shows the interquartile range and any points beyond the 'whiskers' are outliers. Outliers may be defined as values lying more than 1.5 times the interquartile range from the 'box'. Outliers may arise due to mistakes in data collection but may represent unusual observations of particular interest and should be investigated.

22.2.3 Outbreak investigations: epidemic curves

A number of other figures can be useful for presenting descriptive epidemiology. Data grouped (or **aggregated**) by date or period are typically displayed in either of two ways: as epidemic curves or as line charts. In outbreak investigations, the number of cases over time is conventionally displayed by an **epidemic curve**, as in Figure 22.1. The course of the outbreak can provide useful clues.

♦ A single sharp peak with a subsequent fall to the baseline suggests a **point source outbreak**; that is, where the majority of outbreak cases resulted from a single brief exposure event.

♦ A sustained rise in the case count suggests a **continuous source outbreak**; that is, ongoing exposure to infection over a period.

♦ Multiple small peaks suggest transmission of infection by **person-to-person spread**.

♦ Where the incubation period (or the range of possible incubation periods) is known, it may be possible to infer the likely timing and duration of exposure to infection.

♦ Where the incubation period is unknown, it may be possible to infer this (and thereby the identity of the pathogen) from known dates of exposure and onset.

+ It may be possible to infer that an outbreak has ended if the latest case occurred a number of incubation periods ago (Note: a fall-off in case counts at the leading edge of the epidemic curve is commonly seen because of reporting delay and should not be interpreted as indicating resolution of the outbreak; methods sometimes described as **nowcasting** exist for predicting the likely number of cases not yet reported).

+ It is also possible to monitor the impact of intervention or control measures.

22.2.4 Line charts: trends, seasonality, and outliers

Line charts (see example in Figure 22.1) are useful for displaying important measures of disease occurrence commonly estimated from surveillance data, particularly incidence and prevalence. Line charts should be examined for the following informative features.

+ **Trend**: the general level and direction of change in the occurrence of disease. A number of **smoothing** methods exist for revealing trends. The most straightforward smoothing method is the **moving average** where we plot the mean of each value and one or more values to each side of it. Trends may differ during different periods; a change in trend (which may represent the effect of an intervention or other factors of interest) is sometimes called a **changepoint**.

+ **Seasonality**: a trend with a repeating cyclical pattern. Many gastrointestinal infections occur predictably more commonly during summer than during winter, while in temperate northern hemisphere climates influenza incidence rises during autumn or early winter and falls thereafter. Infections with seasonality are often plotted by **epidemiological year**, where the time axis begins at the time of lowest incidence and ends at the corresponding point in the next year.

+ **Outliers**: values which fall outside the expected range of variation in the occurrence of disease. Outliers may represent data errors but may also signal events of particular interest, such as outbreaks, and so require further investigation. A wide range of statistical methods is available to define the expected range of variation using historical data, for example **statistical process control** (SPC) methods.

Line charts may be made more informative by adding comparison data from previous years or data from a wider enclosing area (e.g. at region or country level). Data plotted by week may use one of a number of different definitions of week. In the UK the International Organization for Standardization (ISO) week date system is commonly used, where weeks begin on Monday and week 1 is defined as the week containing the first Thursday of the year, which results in years comprising 52 or 53 weeks.

Maps can concisely display geographical patterns in disease or other factors of interest. Systems for the storage and/or analysis of geographically referenced data are sometimes called geographical information systems (**GIS**). A **spot map** shows the locations of cases of disease or other events of interest as points on a map, which demonstrates the extent of the affected area and possible **clusters** (areas with unexpectedly high occurrence of disease), which may provide clues to causality. **Choropleth maps** typically show areas (often based on administrative boundaries such as regions) coloured according to intervals of a measure calculated for each area, such as incidence or prevalence (e.g. low incidence could be represented on a map as white areas, medium incidence as pink areas, and high incidence as red areas).

22.3 Surveillance data analysis: incidence and prevalence

Estimates of the occurrence of disease are often calculated from surveillance data. **Incidence** is an estimate of the probability (or **risk**) of new cases of disease occurring in a given population during a given period of time. In the simplest case it is calculated by dividing the number of reported cases in one year by the number in the **population at risk** of the disease at the midpoint of the year. For easier presentation, incidence may be presented as number of cases per X thousand population. For infectious diseases, the population at risk comprises persons without immunity who may conceivably be exposed to infection; often this is not known and the total population is used instead. (Point) **prevalence** is an estimate of the probability that an individual in a population at risk has a particular disease (or condition, such as immunity to a disease) at a given point in time. It is calculated by dividing the number of known cases by the total population at risk at a given point in time. It is often informative to calculate incidence or prevalence for specific subgroups (e.g. age groups).

Incidence, prevalence, and duration of disease are interrelated. A disease of short duration (days or weeks), such as influenza, may have low prevalence despite high incidence; in this case incidence would be a better representation of the impact of disease than prevalence. A disease of long duration (months or years), such as *Chlamydia*, may have low incidence despite high prevalence; in this case prevalence would be the preferred measure.

Two measures of **cumulative incidence** (the number of outcomes which have occurred up to a particular point in time in a defined group, divided the total number in that group) are in common use. An **attack rate** is the proportion in a group who have developed an outcome of interest by a particular point in time. For example, in an outbreak investigation we might be interested in the proportion of persons who went swimming who became ill. A **case fatality ratio** is the proportion of those with a particular disease who have died by a given point in time.

22.4 Analytical epidemiology: exposures, outcomes, measures of association

In analytical epidemiology we wish to determine if a particular **exposure** causes a particular **outcome** (**causal inference**). An 'exposure' is a term used in epidemiology to mean any characteristic, state, or external factor which may or may not cause or influence the development of a disease event or other condition of interest (an 'outcome'). For example, in an outbreak investigation we often wish to infer whether consumption of a particular food (exposure) which could have been contaminated with a pathogen caused certain cases of gastrointestinal disease (outcome). If an exposure causes an outcome of interest, then persons known to have that exposure should be more likely to develop that outcome (this does not imply that the outcomes would all occur among those known to have the suspected causal exposure; there might be more than one causal exposure, or exposure events of which we are unaware). In analytical epidemiology we make inferences about whether an exposure has caused an outcome by calculating a **measure of association** based on such a comparison and then using statistical methods to assess the strength of the evidence this gives us.

Calculation of measures of association and associated statistical analyses is aided by cross-tabulation of outcomes with levels of exposure (a **contingency table**). In the simplest case we have an exposure with two possibilities (e.g. went swimming/did not go swimming) and an outcome which either occurred or did not (e.g. ill or not ill); this may be presented as a **two-by-two table** of counts, as shown in Table 22.2.

The **risk ratio** is the measure of association obtained by dividing the risk in the exposed by the risk in the unexposed. In a cohort study (see Chapters 23 and 24) as part of an outbreak investigation we obtain an estimate of risk from the attack rate. A risk ratio of one (RR = 1) indicates that there was no difference in risk between exposed and unexposed; there is no evidence that the exposure was the cause of the outcome. A risk ratio greater or less than one may arise by random chance when the true risk ratio is one; **significance tests** assess the likelihood of this. A risk ratio significantly greater than one (RR>1) indicates greater risk in those exposed; a risk ratio significantly less than one (RR<1) indicates lesser risk in those exposed.

Table 22.2 Example of a two-by-two table.

		Outcome		
		Ill	Not ill	Total
Exposure	Went swimming	a	b	a + b
	Did not go swimming	c	d	c + d
	Total	a + c	b + d	N

The risk ratio may be calculated from the two-by-two table using the formula:

$$RR = \frac{a/(a+b)}{c/(c+d)}$$

Different measures of effect may be appropriate in other types of study design. In case control studies (see Chapters 23 and 24) the information we obtain does not allow us to estimate risk in exposed and unexposed, but we can calculate another measure of association (the **odds ratio**) by comparing exposure between cases and controls; under certain circumstances the odds ratio approximates the risk ratio that would have been calculated if a cohort study had been done instead.

The **odds** is an alternative measure of probability. The odds of exposure is the number of persons with a particular exposure divided by the number of persons without that exposure. In a case control study we calculate an odds ratio by dividing the odds of exposure in cases by the odds of exposure in controls. The **odds ratio** may be calculated from a two-by-two table using one of these equivalent formulae:

$$OR = \frac{(a/c)}{(b/d)} = \frac{ad}{bc}$$

Interpretation of the direction and magnitude of the odds ratio is similar to that described above. However in many situations the odds ratio will give an overestimate of the risk ratio. Understanding when the odds ratio approximates the risk ratio requires consideration of the nature of the underlying population from which cases and controls are sampled, the method of sampling controls, and the frequency of the disease.

Other measures of effect with similar interpretation to the risk ratio are the prevalence ratio, the **rate ratio**, and the **hazard ratio**. The **prevalence ratio**, which may be calculated in **cross-sectional studies** (see Chapters 23 and 24), is the ratio of the prevalence of a disease among persons with a particular exposure divided by the prevalence of that disease among persons without that exposure. Persons with a longer duration of disease are more likely to be captured at a single point in time and may differ in their exposure profile to the totality of persons with the disease, and so prevalence ratios require careful interpretation.

♦ The **rate ratio** is an alternative to the risk ratio which is calculated in cohort studies where subjects enter and leave the study at different times. In this situation a rate is an estimate of the probability of occurrence of the outcome obtained by dividing the number of new outcome events during a period by the sum of the individual follow-up periods falling within that period (a **person–time denominator**). The rate ratio is the rate in the exposed divided by the rate in the unexposed. Interpretation is similar to that for the risk ratio. The hazard ratio is the measure of association typically calculated in **survival analysis**, where the focus of the analysis is on the time to a particular outcome (such as from onset of disease to death) and is interpreted similarly to the risk ratio and rate ratio.

♦ The **attributable risk** (AR) is the difference in risk of an outcome between persons with a given exposure and those without. It gives an indication of the additional risk to those with the exposure (if the exposure truly causes the outcome). Attributable risk may be adjusted for confounding and presented with confidence intervals as with other epidemiological measures. When the prevalence of an exposure in the wider population is known, it is possible to calculate an estimate of the overall population-level impact of an exposure called the **population attributable risk** (PAR), which is obtained by multiplying the prevalence of the exposure by the attributable risk.

22.4.1 Interpreting associations

Demonstrating a significant association between an exposure and an outcome is only the first step towards determining whether the exposure causes the outcome. Alternative explanations to be routinely considered include confounding (see below) and bias. Bias is the epidemiological term describing weaknesses in study procedures for the selection of participants or the ascertainment of information that may lead to distortion of the results; the likelihood of bias depends on the study design and methods.

The epidemiologist Austin Bradford Hill compiled a list of guiding principles for assessing whether an association between exposure and outcome is compatible with causation (Hill 1965). The evidence for causality is more compelling if one or more of the following are true.

♦ **Temporal relationship**: the time of development of the outcome is known and does not occur before the exposure (causality is ruled out if the outcome truly occurs before the time of exposure).

♦ **Strength**: there is a strong association (the measure of association is far from one).

♦ **Dose–response relationship**: greater exposure is associated with greater frequency of the outcome and vice versa.

♦ **Consistency**: the association is observed in different populations or types of study.

♦ **Plausibility:** there is a plausible biological mechanism whereby the exposure could cause the outcome.

♦ **Consideration of alternate explanations**: other possible explanations have been taken into account but ruled out.

♦ **Experiment**: there is experimental evidence showing the exposure can cause the outcome.

♦ **Specificity**: the association is only observed between the exposure and a particular outcome.

♦ **Coherence**: the finding does not conflict with other scientific knowledge, and/or other comparable causal associations are known to exist.

22.4.2 Confounding: matching, stratified analysis, standardization

When a study population consists of individuals who differ in a variable other than the exposure and the outcome (as commonly occurs in observational studies), an association seen in the data as a whole may sometimes differ from the associations that would have been seen if the data were analysed separately for groups defined by that variable, a phenomenon known as **confounding**. This may arise when associations exist between the third variable and both the exposure and the outcome variables; a **confounding variable** may be identified by considering the possibility of (or examining the data for) such associations. It is important to plan to collect data on possible confounding variables in the design of a study. Not all variables with a relationship with both the exposure and outcome variables should be regarded as confounders; there may be variables which represent an intermediate step in the chain of events between exposure and outcome, which should not be treated as confounding variables.

Confounding is an important issue in epidemiological studies which, if not addressed, may lead to serious errors of inference. Variables which commonly introduce confounding include age and sex. There are a number of ways of addressing confounding in the design and analysis of epidemiological studies:

- restriction (restricting recruitment to the study to those with a particular characteristic),
- matching (see below),
- randomization (in a randomized controlled trial, randomly allocating participants to different intervention groups, which balances both known and unknown confounding variables),
- stratified analysis (see below),
- standardization (adjusting measures such as incidence or prevalence in different groups using information from a standard population), and
- regression models (more advanced statistical methods).

Such methods may not eliminate all confounding; the interpretation of analytical findings should consider the possibility of **residual confounding**.

22.4.3 **Matching**

Matching is a method (most commonly used in case-control studies) where a balance of possible confounding variables between groups is achieved by the deliberate choice of subjects in a comparison group. For example, in a case-control study, a control may be selected for each case that shares certain characteristics with that case (**individual matching**). Alternatively, controls may be selected such that the proportions in each group with a given characteristic are equal (**frequency matching**). Individually matched (but not necessarily frequency-matched) studies must use specific analytical methods that take account of matching (see below). Matching may lead to increased **efficiency** (more precise estimates of measures of association) if there is strong confounding, but is not always desirable. Incorrect choice of matching variables (**overmatching**) may increase the complexity of recruitment without increasing efficiency, and in some circumstances may reduce the efficiency of the study.

22.4.4 **Stratified analysis**

Stratified analysis is the calculation of separate measures of effect for each level (or stratum) of a third variable and comparison of these to the overall measure of association. Where the measures of association are similar across levels of the third variable but different from the overall measure of association (which suggests confounding), it is usual to calculate an overall weighted average measure of association that is adjusted for confounding by the third variable (**Mantel–Haenszel analysis**).

22.4.5 **Effect modification**

Stratified analysis may also reveal differences in measure of association across strata of the third variable. This may indicate that the third variable modifies the effect of the exposure on the outcome in some way (**effect modification**). For example, vaccination may reduce the effect of exposure to an infectious disease on the risk of developing that disease, such that stratified analysis by vaccination status reveals different risk ratios. Effect modification may have a useful epidemiological interpretation; for example, it may imply that certain subgroups are at greater risk of disease caused by a particular exposure. Statistical tests for effect modification include the **Woolf** and **Breslow–Day tests of heterogeneity**. It is inappropriate to use Mantel–Haenszel methods when effect modification is present.

22.5 **Hypothesis testing**

Statistical tests are often used in data analysis to distinguish potentially important differences between groups from chance variation arising from random sampling or other factors. It is important in planning a study to have a clear question, an understanding of the data required to answer the question (in terms of both the number of observations required and the exposure/outcome/confounder/effect modifier variables to be recorded) and a plan of analysis using statistical methods appropriate to the study design.

The statistical tests most commonly used in health protection analysis take an approach called **null hypothesis testing**. This requires us to define two mutually exclusive hypotheses of interest and then use the data to calculate a **test statistic** which helps us to decide between the two hypotheses. For example, we can calculate a test statistic known as a **chi-squared statistic** from a two-by-two table. The two hypotheses are:

+ the **null hypothesis** (in an outbreak investigation, the null hypothesis would be that the true risk ratio or odds ratio is one; in other words, that there is no association between the exposure and the outcome), and

+ the **alternative hypothesis** (that the risk ratio or odds ratio is different from one; in other words, that there is an association).

Many common statistical tests (parametric tests) assume that we can describe the probabilities of the different possible values of the test statistic when the null hypothesis is true using a probability distribution such as the normal distribution. This assumption allows us to use statistical tables or software to estimate the probability of the measure of association we have observed (or one more extreme) if there was no association between exposure and outcome. If this probability (known as the **p value**) is below a pre-specified threshold (conventionally less than 0.05), then we reject the null hypothesis and accept the alternative hypothesis, concluding that there is an association, which is said to be **statistically significant**. If the p value is above the threshold, we are unable to reject the null hypothesis and cannot conclude that there is an association.

Null hypothesis testing is not an intuitive process and p values are frequently misunderstood. A p value greater than 5% does not prove that there is no association; the study may have been too small to detect an association. The p value is not the probability that the null hypothesis is true; it is a probability derived under the condition of the investigation that the null hypothesis is true. A statistically significant finding may be unimportant from a clinical or public health perspective; it is important also to consider the strength of association and other factors in its interpretation.

It is important to choose the p value threshold prior to analysis and to understand its implications. A 5% threshold implies that, on average, in one out of every 20 comparisons the null hypothesis will be rejected when it is true (a **type I error**). An analysis that examines multiple possible associations (**multiple testing** or **'data dredging'**) is therefore at greater risk of such an error. A number of methods exists for correcting p values for multiple testing, such as the **Bonferroni** and **Benjamini–Hochberg** corrections.

A study may fail to reject the null hypothesis when the alternative hypothesis is true (**type II error**). In planning a study, it is important to recruit enough participants to minimize the risk of a type II error, while at the same time not wasting resources by recruiting too many participants.

This is done by considering a number of factors, in particular the desired probability of detecting a true association where one exists (the **power** of the study; it is conventional to choose 80–90%), the likely magnitude of the association to be detected (stronger associations will be easier to detect), the study design (including how participants were sampled and whether the groups under comparison are of equal size or not), the intended analysis, the available time and resources, and the expected rate of non-response or refusal. A number of software tools, formulae, and rules of thumb exist to assist with estimation of the required minimum sample size for a particular analysis.

22.6 Confidence intervals

When interpreting means, proportions, measures of association, or standardized measures that have been calculated from random samples from a population, it is often helpful to calculate a range of values (a **confidence interval**) that we are confident will include the true population measure. A wide confidence interval suggests considerable uncertainty about the true population measure, possibly because of a small sample size; for measures of association, if the confidence interval is wide enough to include one, it suggests that the association is not significant. Confidence intervals with different probabilities of including the true population value may be constructed; most commonly 95% confidence intervals are constructed. Confidence intervals provide more information than p values and should be reported routinely.

22.7 Advanced statistical methods

Multivariable models such as multiple linear regression, logistic regression, Poisson regression, Cox regression, and others are useful for examining the relationship between multiple exposure variables and the outcome variable simultaneously, adjusting for confounding, assessing possible effect modification, and testing hypotheses. In general, the choice of the appropriate model depends on the nature of the outcome variable; for example, logistic regression is commonly used for analyses of binary outcomes.

There are also many other advanced statistical methods for analysing spatial, time series, survival, or complex survey data. In recent years Bayesian statistical methods have found an important place in epidemiological analysis.

While health protection specialists may not be experienced in these advanced techniques, close cooperation with statistical colleagues will enable more detailed studies and analyses to be done.

22.8 Conclusions

Good understanding of statistics and epidemiology is essential, if not critical for health protection practice. The majority of health protection interventions/control measures require good and robust evidence, but not all study designs, especially randomized controlled trials (RCTs), are feasible in the investigation and management of common health protection situations. Therefore, descriptive epidemiology and analytical studies, especially case-control and cohort studies, are more appropriate and common tools; and a good grasp of the measures of association and causation is important. This chapter provided a foundation in basic descriptive and analytical epidemiology, relevant statistical and epidemiological methods and tests, plus hypothesis testing appropriate for health protection practitioners.

References

Bradford Hill A. 1965. The environment and disease: association or causation? *Proceedings of the Royal Society of Medicine*, **58**: 295–300. http://www.edwardtufte.com/tufte/hill

Further reading

Bland JM. 2000. *An Introduction to Medical Statistics.* 3rd edition. Oxford: Oxford Medical Publications.

Bruce N, D Pope, D Stanistreet. 2008. *Quantitative Methods for Health Research: A Practical Interactive Guide to Epidemiology and Statistics.* London: John Wiley & Sons.

Doll R, A Bradford Hill. 1952. A study of the aetiology of carcinoma of the lung. *BMJ,* **2:** 1271–86.

Greenhalgh T. 2014. *How to Read a Paper: The Basics of Evidence-based Medicine.* 5th edition. London: John Wiley and Sons.

Harris M, G Taylor. 2014. *Medical Statistics Made Easy.* 3rd edition. Banbury: Scion Publishing.

Schesselman JJ. 1982. *Case-control Studies—Design, Conduct, Analysis.* Oxford: Oxford University Press.

Epi/Stats software package(s)

Centers for Disease Control and Prevention (CDC). n.d. *Epi Info 7—The essential free software tool for public health practice.* http://wwwn.cdc.gov/epiinfo/7/index.htm

Chapter 23

Conducting epidemiological studies in health protection

Sam Ghebrehewet, Paul Cleary, Merav Kliner, and Ewan Wilkinson

OVERVIEW

After reading this chapter the reader will be familiar with:
- the different types of study designs,
- how to conduct studies relevant for health protection practice,
- when each study design would be most appropriate, and
- the practical applications in health protection.

23.1 Introduction to epidemiological and analytical studies in health protection

Epidemiology is the study of the distribution and determinants of health-related states or events (including disease), and the application of this study to the control of diseases and other health problems (World Health Organization 2015). It is fundamental to many aspects of health protection by, for example, identifying risk factors for diseases or identifying interventions that work.

This chapter outlines epidemiological study designs that may be applied in incidents, outbreaks, and other infectious or environmental health protection situations. Epidemiological study designs may be divided into descriptive, observational, or experimental designs. Experimental designs fall outside everyday health protection practice and are not discussed in detail in this chapter.

23.2 Descriptive study designs

Descriptive studies are designed to answer 'place, person, and time' questions about the distribution of a disease, and may generate hypotheses of the possible cause or of risk factors for a particular disease in a population. Descriptive studies may be at the level of the individual (e.g. case reports or case series) or of the population (e.g. ecological studies).

In health protection practice, descriptive studies provide invaluable information for the timely investigation and management of incidents and outbreaks. They can also provide relevant information for planning healthcare services and preventive or educational programmes. They have a limited role in determining causal associations between exposures and outcomes, but may identify causal hypotheses to be tested using other study designs.

23.2.1 Case reports

A case report is the detailed account of the investigation and management of one patient with a novel or unusual disease or other outcome, which aims to present the main features of clinical or public health interest. Case reports may include contributions from clinicians, public health specialists, epidemiologists, veterinarians, microbiologists, toxicologists, environmental researchers, and scientists, along with a summary of relevant literature and consideration of implications for clinical or public health practice.

Case reports may describe:

♦ the first case of a new disease,

♦ a previously unreported cause of disease,

♦ a new mode of transmission of infectious diseases (within or between species),

♦ use of novel diagnostic technology,

♦ use of innovative disease control measures, and

♦ lessons learned for current practice.

Example of a case report: Flavell S, M Eder, R Beaton, L John. 2013. Extensively drug resistant Tuberculosis in a HIV-infected patient in a UK hospital. *International Journal of STD and AIDS*, **24(1): 63–66**

This was the first published case of extensively drug resistant tuberculosis (TB) and HIV co-infection in the UK. The patient required a complex anti-tuberculous treatment regimen combined with anti-retroviral medication, and experienced multiple complications. The case report outlined the patient's course and highlighted the complexities of managing drug-resistant TB in HIV-infected individuals, including difficulties in achieving compliance with treatment, drug toxicity, and potential public health risks.

23.2.2 Case series

A case series is a description of a group of similar patients. A clear case definition is required and recruitment methods should aim to minimize selection bias (where key exposures affect the likelihood of inclusion, leading to an unrepresentative sample), which may arise in a number of ways. For example, referral bias occurs when cases with a particular exposure are more likely to be referred to the particular health services where cases are recruited.

Example of a case series: Bwaka MA, MJ Bonnet, P Calain, et al. 1999. Ebola hemorrhagic fever in Kikwit, Democratic Republic of the Congo: clinical observations in 103 patients. *Journal of Infectious Diseases*, **179(Suppl. 1): S1–S7**

A clinical case series of 103 Ebola patients provided detailed demographic and disease features for affected individuals in the largest urban outbreak up to that time since the first recognition of Ebola in 1976. One key observation was the mean incubation period of Ebola of 6.1 (range 1–21) days.

23.2.3 Cross-sectional studies

Cross sectional studies aim to identify exposures and/or outcomes in populations at single points in time.

23.2.3.1 Prevalence studies

Prevalence studies (or surveys) describe the existence of disease or other factors in a population at a given point in time and provide information about the overall magnitude of a health problem. The prevalence of a disease at a given point in time (point prevalence) may be defined as:

$$\text{Prevalence} = \frac{Number\,of\,cases\,of\,disease\,at\,given\,point\,in\,time}{Number\,in\,population\,at\,risk\,at\,given\,point\,in\,time}$$

Prevalence is often best presented as cases per 10,000 or 100,000 population. For example: *there were 1,500 hepatitis C positive individuals per 100,000 population in Anytown in mid-2016*. Prevalence may be calculated for different subgroups of a population; for example, for groups defined by age, sex, education, occupation, socio-economic status, or ethnic group.

Key considerations in planning and reporting prevalence studies include, as a minimum:

♦ the rationale for the study,

♦ a clear statement of the aims and objectives of the study,

♦ clear identification of the study population and the time period of the study,

♦ procedures relating to eligibility, sampling, and recruitment of participants (and how bias was minimized),

♦ determination of the minimum sample size required, and whether this was achieved, and

♦ clear description of the study methods, including information to be collected, clinical or laboratory methods, and statistical analysis.

Prevalence studies may be logistically easier to conduct than other study designs, but require cautious interpretation, as they assess exposures at the same point in time that the outcome is determined, when the exposures that were present prior to the development of the outcome are most relevant and may have been different. Exposures identified at the same time as the outcome may sometimes have resulted from the outcome (reverse causality). Prevalence studies may also be affected by survival bias, which may occur in any study when cases are recruited from those existing at a point in time ('prevalent' or surviving cases).

Prevalent cases may differ in factors such as severity or treatment received from newly diagnosed cases ('incident' cases). Non-response bias occurs when cases who respond to the invitation to participate differ in important characteristics from those who do not.

Example of a prevalence study: Public Health England. 2012 *English National Point Prevalence Survey on Healthcare Associated Infections and Antimicrobial Use, 2011: Preliminary data.* **London: Health Protection Agency**

This study found that, in late 2011, 6.4% of patients in acute hospitals had an infection acquired in a healthcare setting, and described the types of infection and possible risk factors. The prevalence of healthcare-associated infections was lower than that described in a previous similar survey.

23.2.4 Ecological (also known as correlational) studies

In ecological studies, the units of observation are populations (e.g. the populations of different geographical areas). Disease occurrence and exposures are compared between populations at a given point in time. Ecological studies are often feasible using existing routine data sources, which reduces the costs of investigation.

Ecological studies may suggest or support hypotheses of causation, but require cautious interpretation. As with prevalence studies, the temporal sequence between exposure and outcome may not be clear. It is more difficult to control for confounding in ecological studies, and so associations that are apparent at the population level may not apply at the individual level; incorrectly drawing conclusions about individuals from ecological studies is known as the ecological fallacy. For example, rates of heart disease are higher in wealthier countries. However, it would be incorrect to conclude from this that wealthier people are more likely to develop heart disease; in fact, in wealthier countries, the opposite is true.

> **Example of an ecological study: Maheswaran RT, T Pearson, SD Beevers, et al. 2014. Outdoor air pollution, subtypes and severity of ischemic stroke—a small-area level ecological study.** *International Journal of Health Geographics*, **13: 23**
> ....
> Data from a stroke register for 1995 to 2007 were examined for all cases of first stroke occurring in parts of South London. Concentrations of the air pollutants PM_{10} (particulate matter up to 10 μm in size) and NO_2 (nitrogen dioxide) were modelled for a number of geographical areas. The study concluded that there was no evidence of association between outdoor PM_{10} and NO_2 concentrations and ischaemic stroke.

23.3 **Analytical studies**

Analytical studies can be categorized into (1) observational studies and (2) interventional (or experimental) studies.

Observational studies can identify or assess possible risk factors for or causes of disease by comparing different groups. They may suggest causality by demonstrating that an exposure and an outcome occur together more commonly than would be expected by chance (in other words, that there is an association between the exposure and the outcome), but further evidence is required to support a conclusion of causality. The two most commonly applied types of observational studies are cohort studies and case-control studies, which are used frequently in health protection to identify likely causes of ill health.

23.3.1 **Case-control studies**

A case-control study compares exposures of interest between individuals who have a disease (cases) and individuals who do not have the disease but are otherwise comparable in terms of background exposures (controls).

Case-control studies are an efficient way of studying rare outcomes or diseases, or of studying outcomes where multiple exposures are of interest. They may be undertaken as part of outbreak investigations, particularly when the population at risk is unknown, and can be conducted quickly and with limited resources.

Information on exposure is recorded for a number of cases (ideally determined by sample size estimation). Choosing the optimal method of control selection may be difficult, but is crucial to the validity of the study. Controls are ideally recruited from a random sample of the source population of the cases; where this is not feasible, controls are sometimes recruited from other accessible sources, such as friends or neighbours of cases. In a traditional case-control study, controls are recruited after all the outcomes have occurred; in a density case control study, one or more controls are recruited for each case from those free of disease at the time of identification of the case. To control for confounding, it may sometimes be necessary to recruit controls who are similar to cases in terms of confounding variables (matching). In some circumstances it is necessary to recruit more than one control per case to increase the power of the study. The analysis of case-control studies typically compares the odds of exposure in cases to those in controls, summarized as an odds ratio.

Case-control studies are prone to a number of biases, including selection bias and recall bias. Recall bias refers to the problem of more accurate and complete reporting of exposures by cases than by controls, which may lead to incorrect conclusions about associations.

Example of a case-control study: Hungerford D, P Cleary, S Ghebrehewet, et al. 2014. Risk factors for transmission of measles during an outbreak: matched case-control study. *Journal of Hospital Infection,* **86(2): 138–43**

During a large outbreak of measles in England, a case-control study was conducted which recruited 55 cases and 55 controls, matched for age and geography. Data on exposures in the two weeks before illness were collected via questionnaire. Three factors were associated with measles: incomplete/partial vaccination for age, being too young for vaccination, and hospital attendance, illustrating the importance of timely vaccination of individuals, and the importance of prompt isolation of cases during attendance at healthcare settings.

Key factors to be considered in planning a case-control study include:
- clear aims and objectives,
- hypotheses to be tested,
- clear case definition,
- data to be collected: information for the case definition; information on exposure, confounder, and effect modifier variables,
- clear methods for selection of controls,
- sample size estimation,
- clear process and methods for collecting information,
- statistical analytical methods, and
- consideration of the effect of bias.

23.3.2 Cohort studies

Whereas case-control studies compare exposures between cases of disease and healthy controls, cohort studies involve following up defined groups and comparing the frequency of outcomes between groups with different exposure status. Cohort studies may be conducted prospectively (where follow-up begins before outcomes have developed) or retrospectively (where exposure information for a defined group of participants is ascertained retrospectively, e.g. from occupational records). Cohort studies are often conducted rapidly as part of outbreak investigations, particularly where a defined group is affected. Larger or longer-term cohort studies may be expensive to conduct and logistically complex. The analysis of cohort studies typically involves comparing the risk of outcomes between those exposed and those not exposed, summarized as a relative risk. Case-cohort studies are an efficient alternative to cohort studies where the comparison group for cases is sampled from those initially at risk (even if those selected later become cases).

Prospective cohort studies provide information on the temporal sequence of exposure and outcomes, but are prone to particular types of bias, such as non-response bias and bias due to loss to follow-up.

Example of a cohort study: Wensley A, L Coole. 2013. Cohort study of a dual-pathogen point source outbreak associated with the consumption of chicken liver pâté, UK, October 2009. *Journal of Public Health,* **35(4): 585–89**
....

This investigation of an outbreak of *Campylobacter* and *Salmonella* infection affecting 59 guests attending a conference included a retrospective cohort study. A questionnaire was distributed to all guests after the conference to identify what participants had eaten and whether or not they had had symptoms. A strong association was found between illness and consumption of chicken liver pâté, suggesting this was the most likely cause of the outbreak.

Key factors to consider when planning a cohort study include:
• identifying appropriate source population,
• determining appropriated sample size,
• having a clear definition of groups to be followed,
• having a clear and detailed method of follow-up,
• taking account of possible change of exposure overtime,
• determining duration of follow-up,
• having a clear and unambiguous definition of disease/outcome, and
• planning ahead for dealing with loss to follow-up.

23.3.3 Choosing an appropriate study in incidents or outbreaks

In an incident or outbreak, it is not always easy to determine the nature and detail of the investigation required for public health management (Figure 23.1). Detailed descriptive epidemiology is a prerequisite, and may be sufficient to inform public health action. If further investigation is considered, the likely benefit to the investigation and the use of available resources should be assessed.

23.3.4 Sample size estimation and power

An epidemiological study should recruit sufficient individuals to test the hypotheses of interest. A number of methods exist for estimating the required sample sizes for epidemiological studies. However, in situations such as outbreak investigations, recruitment may be constrained by circumstances such as availability of time or the available number of cases, in which case it is important to consider the power of the study to test the hypotheses of interest when considering whether an analytical study is likely to be informative.

Sample size estimation and power are determined by similar factors, such as the strength of association and the frequency of disease in the comparison group. If an exposure is likely to be strongly associated with an outcome, then planning a study with a small sample size may be justifiable, and correspondingly a study with likely low recruitment may have adequate power to detect the association. For example, it may be estimated that a cohort study with six cases and six controls could detect a risk ratio of ten with 80% power when only 10% of those not exposed developed the outcome. Estimates of the expected strength of association may be derived from literature review, a pilot study, or expert opinion.

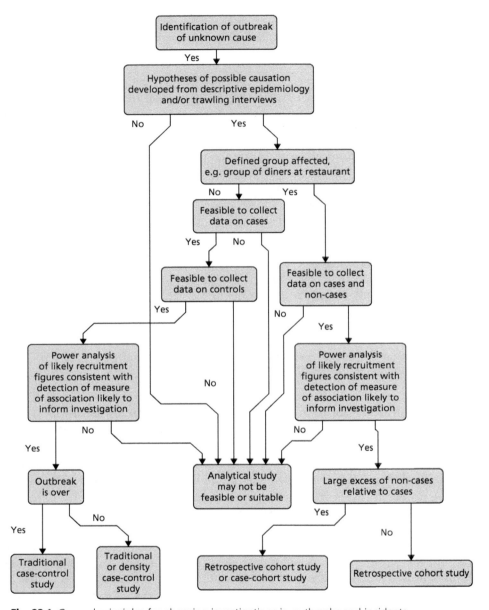

Fig. 23.1 General principles for choosing investigations in outbreaks and incidents

There are a number of other factors to be considered when estimating the required sample size for an epidemiological study, or for estimating the power of a study with a fixed sample size, such as the p value threshold to be applied in statistical tests of the study hypotheses and the number of statistical tests required. The lower the p value threshold, the larger the sample that is required. It is conventional to use 0.05 as the threshold in outbreak investigations; however, as multiple statistical tests are often required in outbreak investigations, it is important to consider the issue of multiple testing (see Chapter 22) in interpretation of the results.

23.4 **Interventional studies**

Interventional (or experimental) studies assess the effect of an intervention, in the simplest case by comparing outcomes between a group allocated to receive the intervention and a comparison group which receives no intervention or a dummy intervention (placebo).

In a randomized controlled trial (RCT), study participants are randomly allocated to intervention and control groups, which reduces the effect of selection bias and confounding. Blinding of RCTs reduces information bias (differential accuracy in reporting between comparison groups): in a single-blind RCT, participants do not know to which group they have been allocated; in a double-blind RCT, allocation is concealed from both participants and investigators.

A well-conducted RCT is a more robust means of testing a causal hypothesis than an observational study, as it reduces the effects of both bias and confounding and demonstrates the temporal sequence between exposure (here the intervention) and outcome. However, RCTs may need to be large or lengthy to demonstrate small effects, or may need to recruit from multiple centres, and they may therefore be costly and complex to run. RCTs may not be ethical or feasible for some research questions. Bias may occur in RCTs from non-compliance with interventions or loss to follow-up. In some circumstances the intervention applied to one group will have an effect on the control group (contamination); for example, an intervention to reduce smoking in one group may lead to reduced smoking in the control group if there is social interaction between the groups. Randomized controlled trials sometimes exclude key groups from recruitment, such as the elderly, which reduces the generalizability of results.

> **Example of RCT: Wilde JA, JA McMillan, J Serwint, et al. 1999 Effectiveness of influenza vaccine in health care professionals: a randomized trial.** *Journal of the American Medical Association*, 281(10): 908–13
>
> In this double-blind RCT, 264 hospital-based healthcare professionals without chronic medical problems were randomly assigned to receive either an influenza vaccine or a control intervention (meningococcal or pneumococcal vaccine, or placebo). Active weekly surveillance for illness was conducted during each influenza season. Vaccine efficacy against serologically defined infection was 88% for influenza A (95% CI 47–97%) and 89% for influenza B (95% CI 14–99%).

23.5 **Systematic reviews**

Systematic reviews are regarded as secondary research, as they summarize other published and non-published studies (primary research). They review all the research papers on a given topic, and, using agreed methods, summarize the results to give a more robust result than any one paper can (see Chapter 24). They are the study of choice when investigating the effectiveness of an intervention where a number of experimental (or possibly observational) studies have been published, e.g. 'How effective are antibiotics for preventing meningococcal infections?'

Key steps

♦ Undertake a comprehensive literature review, with predetermined protocol, defined search strategy with strict inclusion and exclusion criteria.

♦ Identify all studies undertaken on the topic (including unpublished studies): studies with positive findings are more likely to be submitted and published in a peer-review journal.

- Ensure published papers listed on electronic databases (e.g. Medline or Pubmed) as well as unpublished papers are included. Without this, the systematic review can be affected by publication bias.

- Review the methods of each study, identifying flaws in the study design that may affect the results. The quality of the methods is taken into consideration when interpreting the data and making conclusions.

- Compare studies: if included studies are similar in their methods and outcomes (homogeneous) comparison is easier. If they differ (heterogeneous), it is still possible to pool the results, but the differences must be taken into account, which may dilute the result.

- Present data from relevant studies descriptively, by summarizing the results of the included studies. Alternatively, outcomes from the relevant studies can be combined together in a meta-analysis, a statistical summary, with significance levels, taking into consideration the size of the individual studies and the size of the effect found in each study.

Practical issues

- Carrying out a systematic review to agreed standards, even on a topic with a small number of papers, can be time-consuming and should not be undertaken lightly.

- Searching first for any systematic review already published on the topic of interest may save resources. The Cochrane Library publishes high-quality systematic reviews on a wide range of topics.

- If a systematic review has not been undertaken on a topic, and there is a need for one, suggestions can be made to the relevant Cochrane group to develop a protocol (Cochrane Infectious Diseases Group 2014).

- Each step in a systematic review must be carried out by two people to reduce the risk of bias.

Example of a systematic review: Zalmanovici Trestioreanu A, A Fraser, A Gafter-Gvili, et al. 2011. Antibiotics for preventing meningococcal infections. *Cochrane Database of Systematic Reviews,* 10(8): CD004785

This systematic review of RCTs investigated the effectiveness of different antibiotics for eradication of *Neisseria meningitidis.* Two review authors independently appraised the quality and extracted data from the 24 included trials. Using meta-analysis, ciprofloxacin, rifampin (rifampicin), minocycline, and penicillin proved effective at eradication one week after treatment, when compared individually with placebo. Rifampin, ciprofloxacin, and penicillin proved effective at one to two weeks. Rifampin was also effective up to four weeks after treatment but resistant isolates were seen. The authors concluded that using rifampin during an outbreak may lead to the circulation of resistant isolates, therefore, ciprofloxacin, ceftriaxone or penicillin should be considered.

23.6 Other studies that have application to health protection

While most of the studies that are undertaken in health protection are quantitative, involving statistical analysis, there is a need for more frequent use of qualitative studies to understand knowledge, attitudes, and beliefs that affect the implementation of health protection programmes and responses. Similarly, operational research can be used to demonstrate service strengths and gaps, enabling quality improvements to be identified, implemented, and evaluated.

23.6.1 Qualitative study

Qualitative studies can provide an in-depth insight into perceptions, beliefs, and understanding of professionals and the general public. They generally involve asking participants questions to explore a situation or problem, but can also include group discussions, observation, and reflective field notes. Participants can be chosen at random, or purposively if there is a specific group of people of interest. There are many different approaches, including the following:

♦ *Thematic analysis* synthesizes common patterns (or themes) in responses to answer a question.

♦ *Grounded theory* constructs a theory based on the data that have been collected and analysed, potentially leading to further investigations.

♦ *Ethnographic research* aims to understand what people do, based on observation in a real-world setting.

♦ *Phenomenology* investigates how individuals experience situations.

The benefits of qualitative studies include hypothesis generation and improved understanding of processes and beliefs affecting health. However, results may be influenced by the beliefs or perceptions of researchers; proof of association or causation is difficult.

> **Example of a qualitative research: Wiley KE, SC Cooper, N Wood, et al. 2015. Understanding pregnant women's attitudes and behavior towards influenza and pertussis vaccination.** *Qualitative Health Research*, **25(3): 360–70**
>
> ....
>
> Semi-structured interviews explored pregnant women's perspectives on influenza vaccination during pregnancy and postpartum pertussis vaccination. Women were concerned about potential risks to their infants' health before their own. They viewed pertussis as a threat to the baby and were thus more likely to intend to vaccinate against pertussis. Framing of vaccination information toward protection of the baby might help increase vaccine uptake among pregnant women.

23.6.2 Operational study

Operational research can provide insights into how a programme (prevention, care, or treatment) is working, and how it can be improved. It has been defined as 'the search for knowledge on interventions, strategies, or tools that can enhance the quality, effectiveness, or coverage of programmes in which the research is being done' (Zachariah et al. 2009: 711). Operational research provides decision-makers with information to enable them to improve the performance of programmes, focuses on factors that are under the control of programmes, and seeks to improve processes, quality, outputs and outcomes (including cost-effectiveness), and sustainability (WHO 2007).

In operational research, the research questions are generated by identifying the constraints and challenges encountered during the implementation of a programme. The answers provided to these questions should have direct, practical relevance to solving problems and improving health-service delivery. As far as possible, existing data collected for management and monitoring of the programme are used.

Example of an operational research: Sikhondze W, T Dlamini, D Khumalo D. et al. 2015. Countrywide roll-out of Xpert° MTB/RIF in Swaziland: the first three years of implementation. *Public Health Action* **5(2): 140–46.**
....

A countrywide roll-out Xpert° MTB/RIF machines between June 2011 and June 2014 for testing tuberculosis specimens, and 93% of the tests were successful, and of these, 14% detected Mycobacterium tuberculosis and 12% showed rifampicin resistance. However, poor scores were obtained with equipment use and maintenance, internal audit, and process control. The authors concluded that countrywide roll-out of Xpert in Swaziland has been successful, although operational issues have been identified and need to be resolved.

23.7 Choosing a study design

Choosing a study design is not always a straightforward decision. Multiple factors dictate the design required for a specific situation, or question, at a specific time, including available resources, reason for the study (e.g. control of disease, responding to the need for legal action, or addressing community perceptions of the risk in a particular situation, political pressures), timescale, capacity, and capability of the investigators. Furthermore, the appropriateness of the study to answer the question raised (Box 23.1), and inherent limitations (Table 23.1) will influence the choice.

Box 23.1 When to use different study designs in health protection*

Measuring effectiveness and safety of interventions

+ intervention studies: RCTs, and
+ systematic reviews.

Hypothesis testing—does an intervention make a difference

+ experimental studies: randomized controlled trial (RCT), and
+ observational studies (e.g. cohort study, case-control study).

Hypothesis generation—identifying risk factors for diseases

+ descriptive epidemiology, and
+ observational studies: cohort study, case control study.

Other ways of identifying patterns of disease

+ cross-sectional (incidence and prevalence) studies, and
+ correlation and ecological studies.

Learning more about rare conditions or exposures

◆ case reports, case series, and
◆ observational studies: case-control, cohort study.

Assessing the process of service delivery

◆ operational research.

Assessing the acceptability of services

◆ qualitative studies.

*These are general guiding principles; therefore there will be some exceptions to the classification.

Table 23.1 Limitation of study designs used in health protection

Study	Limitations			
	Selection bias	**Recall bias**	**Loss to follow–up**	**Confounding**
Survey (cross–sectional)	++	++	–	++
Case–control	+++	+++	–	++
Cohort	++	–	++	++
RCT	+	–	++	–

Notes: – Non–existent (if done appropriately); + Low; ++ Medium; +++ High

23.7 **Conclusions**

Health protection practice requires an understanding of the different epidemiological study designs and their application and limitations. Descriptive and observational studies (including case-control and cohort) are most frequently used in health protection practice, as they can provide essential information without the need for complex studies. Descriptive studies should not be undervalued, as they often provide information as important as that provided by analytical studies, but requiring fewer resources. Careful study design and interpretation of study findings can provide invaluable information to inform public health action.

References

Bwaka MA, MJ Bonnet, P Calain, et al. 1999. Ebola hemorrhagic fever in Kikwit, Democratic Republic of the Congo: clinical observations in 103 patients. *Journal of Infectious Diseases*, **179**(Suppl. 1): S1–S7.

Cochrane Infectious Diseases Group. 2014. *Prospective Authors*. http://cidg.cochrane.org/prospective-authors (accessed 8 March 2016).

Flavell S, M Eder, R Beaton, L John. 2013. Extensively drug resistant tuberculosis in a HIV-infected patient in a UK hospital. *International Journal of STD & AIDS*, **24**(1): 63–66.

Hungerford D, P Cleary, S Ghebrehewet, et al. 2014. Risk factors for transmission of measles during an outbreak: matched case-control study. *Journal of Hospital Infection*, **86**(2): 138–43.

Maheswaran RT, SD Pearson, MJ Beevers, et al. 2014. Outdoor air pollution, subtypes and severity of ischemic stroke—a small-area level ecological study. *International Journal of Health Geographics*, **13**: 23. doi:10.1186/1476-072X-13-23.

Public Health England (PHE). 2012. *English National Point Prevalence Survey on Healthcare Associated Infections and Antimicrobial Use, 2011: Preliminary Data*. London: Health Protection Agency. https://www.gov.uk/government/uploads/system/uploads/attachment_data/file/331871/English_National_Point_Prevalence_Survey_on_Healthcare_associated_Infections_and_Antimicrobial_Use_2011.pdf (accessed 8 March 2016).

Sikhondze W, Dlamini T, Khumalo D. et al., 2015. Countrywide roll-out of Xpert® MTB/RIF in Swaziland: the first three years of implementation. *Public Health Action*, **5**(2): 140–46.

Wensley A, L Coole. 2013. Cohort study of a dual-pathogen point source outbreak associated with the consumption of chicken liver pâté UK, October 2009. *Journal of Public Health*, **35**(4): 585–89.

World Health Organization (WHO). 2015. *Epidemiology*. http://www.who.int/topics/epidemiology/en/ (accessed 8 March 2016).

WHO. 2007. *Guide to operational research in programs*. http://www.who.int/hiv/pub/toolkits/Operational%20Research%20Folder%20-%20FINAL.pdf (accessed 8 March 2016).

Zachariah, R, Harries AD, Ishikawa N., et al. 2009. Operational research in low-income countries: what, why, and how? *Lancet Infectious Diseases*, **9**(11): 711–17. doi:10.1016/S1473-3099(09)70229-4.

Zalmanovici Trestioreanu A, A Fraser, A Gafter-Gvili, et al. 2011. Antibiotics for Preventing Meningococcal Infections. *Cochrane Database of Systematic Reviews*, **10**(8): CD004785.

Further reading

Doll R, A Bradford Hill. 1952. A study of the aetiology of carcinoma of the lung. *BMJ*, **2**: 1271–86.

Higgins J, S Green. 2011. *Cochrane Handbook for Systematic Reviews of Interventions*. http://handbook.cochrane.org/ (accessed 8 March 2016).

Hopewell S, K Loudon, MJ Clarke, et al. 2009. Publication bias in clinical trials due to statistical significance or direction of trial results. *Cochrane Database of Systematic Reviews*, **1**:MR00000.

Reeve NF, TR Fanshawe, TJ Keegan, et al. 2013. Spatial analysis of health effects of large industrial incinerators in England, 1998–2008: a study using matched case–control areas. *BMJ Open*, **3**: e001847.

Chapter 24

Using evidence to guide practice in health protection

Merav Kliner, Ewan Wilkinson, and Sam Ghebrehewet

> **OVERVIEW**
> ....
> After reading this chapter the reader will be familiar with:
> • the hierarchy of evidence and its application in health protection,
> • the frameworks used to critically appraise evidence and summarize the quality of evidence, and
> • the process of turning evidence into policy, and some of the barriers and drivers that may help or hinder that process.

24.1 Introduction to evidence in health protection: why it is needed?

Decisions taken when working in health protection can have a significant impact on many people. Therefore, these decisions need to be evidence-based, to maximize the benefit and minimize harm for individuals and populations. In addition, decisions can be high profile, such as in the *E.coli O157* outbreak at Godstone Farm in 2009 (Independent Investigation Committee 2010). Therefore, it is paramount that any investigation/action/decision made, is able to withstand scrutiny.

There are a wide range of interventions used in health protection, from sophisticated medical products such as immunizations and antibiotics to advising on managing contaminated land. No one type of study design will be suitable to investigate the impact of every health protection intervention. These study designs have been outlined and discussed in Chapter 23.

24.2 Hierarchy of evidence

There are a well-recognized hierarchy of evidence (Figure 24.1). This was developed to support the biomedical model of health, and recognizes the importance of evidence provided by randomized controlled trials (RCTs), while valuing observational studies less.

The utility of the hierarchy of evidence has limitations because it does not provide an assessment of the relevance of the study design or the methodological approach adopted. As outlined in Chapter 23 ('Conducting studies in health protection'), an appropriate study design should be used to find the answer to the question posed. According to the hierarchy, an RCT gives a higher level of evidence than a cohort study, but there are times where a cohort study is more appropriate.

Table 23.1 in Chapter 23 outlines which study design may be more appropriately used to answer different questions. Therefore, in health protection the hierarchy of evidence is not typically followed.

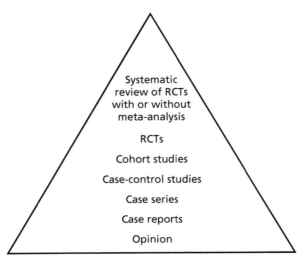

Fig. 24.1 Hierarchy of evidence

Reproduced with permission from Akobeng (2005) Copyright © 2005 BMJ Publishing Group Ltd & Royal College of Paediatrics and Child Health. All rights reserved.

24.3 **Undertaking studies in health protection**

There are many challenges to undertaking studies in health protection. Large interventional studies (such as RCTs) can be expensive. Therefore, they are generally funded by industry, as the company may gain significant financial benefit from proving that their intervention works. These include drugs or vaccines with a large number of users (e.g. diabetes, influenza vaccine), or diseases where small numbers of people require expensive drugs (e.g. HIV, hepatitis C). Other areas subject to substantial amounts of research are those with political backing. HIV, TB, and malaria research predominate in Africa and other resource-poor settings, funded through public health programmes such as the Global Fund to Fight AIDS, Tuberculosis and Malaria.

Where there is a smaller financial incentive, there is usually less funding for studies (e.g. antibiotic chemoprophylaxis in meningococcal disease). Funding for public health research in areas that are less attractive to industry is difficult to obtain. This is one, but not the only reason that some key health protection interventions are based on limited evidence from small observational studies, such as cohort or case-control studies, or studies using data that have already been collected as part of surveillance (see Chapter 21), such as ecological studies.

24.4 **Assessing the methodological quality**

It is important that any study is well conducted, using robust study methodology. The quality of individual papers can be considered by critical appraisal, where a framework is used to systematically assess the methodological approach taken by the researchers, focusing on the inherent issues of bias for that study design, as outlined in Chapter 23. The framework most commonly used in public health is CASP (critical appraisal skills programme), which provides detailed frameworks for each study design (Critical Appraisal Skills Programme 2013). The AMSTAR (Assessment of Multiple SysTemAtic Reviews) tool can be used to critically appraise systematic reviews and meta-analysis (Shea et al. 2007). These tools ask a number of questions to guide the assessor to read the paper with a critical eye, and help them identify flaws that may affect the applicability of the paper.

Critical appraisal takes time and practice, but understanding the strength and flaws of a study is vital if/when consideration is given to using the results to guide practice.

24.5 Assessing the quality of a body of evidence

Assessing the overall quality of a body of evidence is important when it is collated to inform policy, for example in a systematic review or as part of guideline development. The Grading of Recommendation Assessment, Development and Evaluation (GRADE) Working Group has developed a system for assessing the quality of all the evidence on a subject area in a transparent manner (Table 24.1) (GRADE Working Group 2004). It clearly separates the assessment of the quality of evidence from the strength of the recommendation. The quality assessment should then be presented alongside the effect size (strength of recommendation) to indicate clearly the quality of the underlying evidence to readers of the systematic review or guideline.

This approach starts with rating the study design. The assessor should rate: RCTs as high quality; observational studies as low quality; and any other evidence (such as case reports) as very low quality. The quality rating is then downgraded or upgraded upon consideration of set criteria. Downgrading means that quality assessment drops by one or more level (e.g. from high to moderate or low) and upgrading means that quality assessment increases by one or more points (e.g. from low to moderate or high). Five criteria are important.

♦ **Risk of bias within studies:** are the study methodologies sound? (Bias is a systematic error in a study which can lead to an incorrect estimation of the outcome. Studies which reduce the risk of bias more effectively are more likely to yield results that are closer to the truth.)

♦ **Directness of results**: are the studies investigating the correct question in the correct population?

♦ **Consistency of results**: are the results of the studies constant and not significantly different?

Table 24.1 GRADE criteria for downgrading and upgrading quality assessment

Criteria	Downgrade if:	Upgrade if:
Risk of bias	Serious (1 level) or very serious (2 levels) limitation to study quality	All plausible confounders would have reduced the effect (1 level)
Indirectness of results	Some (1 level) or major (2 levels) uncertainty about directness	NA
Inconsistency of results	Important inconsistency (1 level)	Evidence of a dose response gradient (1 level)
Precision	Imprecise or sparse data (1 level)	Strong (1 level) or very strong (2 levels) evidence of association (Relative risk: >2 or <0.5; or >5 or <0.2 respectively) based on evidence from 2+ studies with no plausible confounders
Reporting bias	High probability of reporting bias (1 level)	NA

Source: data from GRADE Working Group. Grading quality of evidence and strength of recommendations. British Medical Journal, Volume 328, pp. 1490, Copyright © 2004 BMJ Publishing Group Ltd.

- **Precision**: what are the studies' power and confidence intervals? (see Chapters 22 and 23)
- **Risk of reporting (publication) bias**: are there any missing studies from the systematic review, i.e. are there any other studies conducted but not published?

The outcome of GRADE is an assessment of the quality of evidence rated as high, moderate, low, or very low. These are defined as:

- high quality: further research is unlikely to change the confidence of the estimate of effect,
- moderate quality: further research is likely to change the confidence in the estimate of effect, and may change the size of the effect,
- low quality: further research is very likely to change the confidence in the estimate of effect, and may change the size of the effect, or
- very low quality: the current estimate of effect is very uncertain.

24.6 **The limits of evidence**

While it is important that the available evidence is used, it will not always be possible to answer the public health question with the available evidence. In such situations it is important to find what evidence is available and then undertake a risk assessment using reason, logic, and experience to reach the 'best' conclusion. It is advisable to record your thoughts, discussions, and references so that you can re-evaluate the process later if necessary.

24.7 **Turning evidence into policy**

As research can be difficult to undertake in health protection, policy may be based on limited evidence and expert consensus. Where possible, policy should be based on the synthesis of this evidence, undertaken in a transparent manner as above. Transparency in guideline development ensures that the influence of these factors on policy is clearly documented and justified.

Tools have been developed to facilitate groups to reach evidence-based recommendations for policies and guidelines. Developing and Evaluating Communication strategies to support Informed Decisions and practice based on Evidence (DECIDE) have developed an Evidence to Decision Framework to help people move from a body of evidence to recommendations or decisions (DECIDE 2014). This is a continuation of work undertaken by the GRADE Working Group. The framework aims to assist decision makers to have structured and transparent discussions about the benefits and harms of each intervention, and to ensure that all relevant evidence and influencing factors are considered as part of the decision-making process. An online version of the framework has been developed to aid decision makers (GRADE/DECIDE 2014).

The framework starts with framing the question and providing background information such as outlining the problem, the population, and summarizing the research evidence. The next step is then asking a series of questions that will facilitate making a judgement, such as size and certainty of the desirable and undesirable anticipated effects, societal value placed on the effect, consideration of the resource implications, impact on health equity, acceptability to stakeholders, and feasibility of implementation. A decision can then be made taking into account all the issues discussed above. The framework suggests four types of recommendation:

- recommend the intervention (strong recommendation in favour of the intervention),
- suggest the intervention (weak, conditional, discretionary, or qualified recommendation in favour of the intervention),
- suggest against the intervention (weak, conditional, discretionary, or qualified recommendation in favour of the comparison), or
- recommend against the intervention (strong recommendation in favour of the comparison).

24.8 **Factors that may influence policy development and implementation**

As stated above, there are a number of factors besides just the evidence that may influence policy development and subsequent implementation. Issues such as societal value placed on the outcome of disease, resource implications, acceptability to the population, understanding and beliefs of professionals and society, and the political landscape may all have an impact.

There is likely to be a wide range of understanding and opinions in both the public and professionals about a condition, its cause, and control measures, which can influence the translation into policy and its implementation. When health professionals are united and providing leadership, the public is more likely to become well informed and follow the advice of the professionals, which may then influence political decisions. Leadership, media support, and backing by interested parties (including industry, pressure groups, politicians, and members of the public) all contribute to successful development and implementation of policy. These individuals or groups can sway policy, either driving it forwards or obstructing the development or implementation of evidence-based policy.

Table 24.2 provides some examples of how policy development and implementation is influenced by other factors. A good example of a successful translation of evidence into policy is smallpox eradication, where the four key components: evidence, professional conviction, public commitment, and political will were all united and resulted in the development and successful implementation of a policy. In contrast, other public health policies have had less successful development and implementation due to varying levels of professional, public, and political commitment or will.

Table 24.2 Examples of influencing factors on policy development and implementation*

	Smallpox eradication	Global polio eradication	Improving air quality through active transport	Incinerators for managing waste
Essential elements required for policy development and implementation				
Supporting evidence	Strongly supportive	Strongly supportive	Strongly supportive	Moderately supportive
Health professional conviction	Strongly supportive	Moderately supportive	Strongly supportive	Weakly supportive
Public commitment	Strongly supportive	Weakly supportive	Weakly supportive	Strong opposition
Political will	Strongly supportive	Weakly supportive	Moderately supportive	Moderately supportive
Current position				
Policy position	Strong global policy	Strong global policy (WHO 2014)	National policy (Department of Transport 2011)	EU and national policy (Defra 2013)
Implementation	Completed, disease eradicated	Partially implemented, resurgence of disease	Patchy; future of Local Sustainable Transport Fund beyond 2016 unclear.	Implemented despite sustained opposition

*The examples and the ratings are based on the authors' experience and personal judgements. Therefore, they are subject to the evidence reviewed at the time the chapter was drafted, plus they do not represent any organizational views or position.

24.9 **Assessing the quality of policy**

As described above, policy development is a complex process, but gratifying when done well. However, policy development can vary in its methodological approach, as is the case for individual studies. Therefore policy in itself should be critically appraised before it is followed, to reassure the user that the process of policy development has been transparent, and that the methods used are robust. One tool that is used to critically appraise policy is the AGREE II tool (Brouwers et al. 2010). This tool appraises guidelines against 23 criteria across six domains: scope and purpose, stakeholder involvement, rigour of development, clarity of presentation, applicability, and editorial independence.

24.10 **Conclusions**

Assessing the methodological quality of single papers and a body of evidence is very important before implementing the recommendations made on the basis of that evidence, to reduce the risk of incorrect advice being given.

Health protection policy should be based on the evidence, while understanding the strengths and flaws of the body of evidence. Policy development also needs to consider the wider political and social context to understand barriers and facilitators to its development and implementation. Policies in themselves should be critically appraised to ensure that rigorous methods have been adopted when considering implementing their recommendations.

References

Akobeng A. 2005. Understanding randomised controlled trials. *Archives of Disease in Childhood*, **90**: 840–44.

Brouwers M, ME Kho, GP Browman, et al. 2010. AGREE II: Advancing guideline development, reporting and evaluation in healthcare. *Canadian Medical Association Journal*, **182**: E839–42.

Critical Appraisal Skills Programme. 2013. *Making Sense of Evidence*. http://www.casp-uk.net/ (accessed 8 March 2016).

DECIDE. 2014. *DECIDE (2011–2015): Developing and Evaluating Communication Strategies to Support Informed Decisions and Practice Based on Evidence*. http://www.decide-collaboration.eu (accessed 8 March 2016).

Department for Environment, Food & Rural Affairs (Defra). 2013. *Incineration of Municipal Solid Waste*. London: Defra.

Department of Transport. 2011. *Creating Growth, Cutting Carbon: Making Sustainable Local Transport Happen*. https://www.gov.uk/government/publications/creating-growth-cutting-carbon-making-sustainable-local-transport-happen (accessed 8 March 2016).

GRADE Working Group 2004. Grading quality of evidence and strength of recommendations. *BMJ*, **328**: 1490.

GRADE/DECIDE, 2014. *Interactive Evidence to Decision Framework*. http://ietd.epistemonikos.org/#/login (accessed 8 March 2016).

Independent Investigation Committee. 2010. *Review of the Major Outbreak of* E. Coli O157 *in Surrey, 2009: Report of the Independent Investigation Committee*. London: Health Protection Agency. https://www.gov.uk/government/uploads/system/uploads/attachment_data/file/342361/Review_of_major_outbreak_of_e_coli_o157_in_surrey_2009.pdf (accessed 5 April 2016).

Shea BJ, JM Grimshaw, GA Wells, et al. 2007. Development of AMSTAR: a measurement tool to assess the methodological quality of systematic reviews. *BMC Medical Research Methodology*, **7**(10). doi:10.1186/1471-2288-7-10.

World Health Organization (WHO). 2014. *Polio Eradication Initiative*. http://www.emro.who.int/polio/about/ (accessed 8 March 2016).

Further reading

Cochrane Collaboration. 2011. *Cochrane Handbook for Systematic Reviews of Interventions*. http://community.cochrane.org/handbook (accessed 8 March 2016).

Chapter 25

Quality assurance and audit

Amal Rushdy and Sam Ghebrehewet

OVERVIEW

....

After reading this chapter the reader will be familiar with:
• the definitions of clinical audit, clinical governance, and quality assurance,
• the audit cycle, the steps in the audit cycle, and the application of clinical audit in health protection,
• the difference between clinical audit, research, evaluation, and surveillance, and
• the identification and prioritization of audit topics, factors to consider in implementing change, and importance of re-audit.

25.1 Introduction to quality assurance and audit

The origins of quality assurance and audit in health protection practice lie in healthcare, both in the UK and elsewhere, with its foundations in patient safety, improving outcomes, and good clinical governance (Black 1992; Donaldson and Scally 1998; Vincent 2006). Quality assurance and audit are fundamental parts of health protection practice and service delivery.

It is important to define what is meant by these terms before further explaining what they mean for health protection practice.

25.2 Definitions and relationships

Quality assurance is an overall concept that encompasses the systems we have for improving quality. These systems include clinical governance (definition below) systems in healthcare and health protection, and quality improvement tools that are used to improve practice, the most common being 'clinical' audit (Maxwell 1984; Donabedian 2003; World Health Organization 2006; USA Public Health Quality Forum 2008). Clinical audit and clinical governance are more clearly defined in the UK (Donaldson and Scally 1998; NICE 2002). These definitions are given below and adapted for health protection in Box 25.1. It can be seen from these definitions that clinical governance, quality assurance, and clinical audit are intrinsically linked.

♦ Quality assurance in healthcare has been defined as 'all actions taken to establish, protect, promote, and improve the quality of health care' (Donabedian 2003, pp. xxiii–xxiv). In today's NHS, quality in healthcare looks at five dimensions of safety, effectiveness, patient experience, caring, and leadership (CQC 2013).

♦ Clinical governance has been defined as 'a system through which (NHS) organizations are accountable for continuously improving the quality of their services and safeguarding high standards of care by creating an environment in which excellence in clinical care will flourish' (Donaldson and Scally 1998). The focus for clinical governance is rightly on improving quality and builds on years of quality initiatives such as clinical audit and clinical effectiveness in the health sector (Boaden 2008). It integrates different approaches to quality improvement.

Box 25.1 Definitions adapted for health protection from healthcare definitions

Quality assurance in health protection

All actions taken to establish, protect, promote, and improve the quality of health protection service delivery for individuals and populations.

Health protection governance

A system through which health protection teams and organizations are accountable for continuously improving the quality of their services and safeguarding high standards of service delivery by creating an environment in which excellence in health protection for individuals and populations will flourish.

Health protection audit

A quality improvement process that seeks to improve individual and population health and health outcomes through systematic review of service delivery against explicit criteria and the implementation of change.

♦ Clinical audit has been defined as 'a quality improvement process that seeks to improve patient care and outcomes through systematic review of care against explicit criteria and the implementation of change' (NICE 2002, p. 1).

All audit should be (Morrell and Harvey 1999):

♦ led by professionals,
♦ regarded as an educational process,
♦ part of routine practice,
♦ based on standards,
♦ used to improve outcomes of care,
♦ inclusive of management in the process and outcome,
♦ confidential at individual patient/practitioner level, and
♦ informed by patient views.

Clinical audit is a tool for quality improvement and involves measurement against standards that can be based on any quality component or dimension. It is a key component of clinical governance and any quality assurance or improvement system.

Audit is not the only tool for assessing the quality of services or identifying areas for improvement. Other methods such as service evaluation and reviews are also useful tools in the quality assurance tool kit (Ovretveit 1998; Faculty of Public Health 2002, 2004; World Health Organization 2005; Brophy et al. 2008). However, these are not considered further in this chapter.

25.3 Health protection audit

The above definitions naturally focus on healthcare and patients. Are they applicable to health protection? There is relevance for health protection practice where the definitions are adapted to apply to individuals (cases and contacts), populations, and other aspects of health protection service and delivery where quality and quality improvement are essential to deliver safe, effective, and efficient services.

This chapter substitutes 'health protection' in the definitions for 'clinical', and 'heath protection service' for 'healthcare'. The main focus is health protection audit, with a brief look at quality assurance and improvement.

Health protection audit is about improving the quality of service delivery for the population. It is a key tool for service improvement at all levels of practice, locally and nationally.

25.3.1 Audit versus research, evaluation, routine surveillance

Audit is not research or service evaluation. Smith (1992) writes that 'research is concerned with discovering the right thing to do; audit with ensuring it is done right'. There are good tools to assist in differentiating between audit and research, evaluation, surveillance, and routine health protection/public health activity (Health Research Authority 2013). Examples of health protection questions that illustrate the differences between audit, research, evaluation, and surveillance are given in Table 25.1. The key for audit is that it measures against a predetermined standard/best practice and asks whether it is being followed.

25.3.2 Audit cycle

Audit is a cyclical activity that has a series of well-defined steps known as the audit cycle (Ovretveit 1998; Ruthven and Ashmore 2008).

25.3.2.1 Steps in the audit cycle (Ruthven and Ashmore 2008)

- select audit topic (in consultation—involve team, partners, stakeholders),
- identify best practice,
- agree criteria and standards (based on evidence/best practice),
- collect data (criteria measurement),
- analyse data (against the standards),
- preliminary report and recommended changes (in consultation—involve team, partners, stakeholders; also informed by root cause analysis of gaps),
- implement necessary changes,
- conduct re-audit (repeat previous four steps), and
- write final report and share learning (plus making recommendations for future audit including adjustment of standards as required).

Table 25.1 Audit, research, evaluation, surveillance

Examples of health protection study questions	Suggested study method
1. Do people's health beliefs about TB influence the completion of TB treatment?	Research (testing a hypothesis)
2. Are service standards on control and prevention of TB being followed?	Audit (measuring against standards)
3. What are the demographic characteristics of cases of multi-drug-resistant TB?	Surveillance (descriptive analysis of surveillance data)
4. Do we have the required services for the effective control and prevention of TB in the district?	Service evaluation (evaluation)

25.3.3 **Why is audit important?**

Fundamentally audit is about improving quality. An audit should not be undertaken if the purpose is not to improve quality.

On an individual, team, or local partner level, it enables individuals and teams to reflect systematically on their own practice and continually improve the service they are delivering. It can provide assurance that in critical areas of a service, the service is performing well and using the best available evidence. It also enables teams to review services jointly with partners to ensure the best health protection outcomes.

Nationally, audit may be part of the professional requirements and appraisal for health protection specialists. There is also an association between clinical audit and good governance; organizations that had audit embedded were also those that demonstrated good governance mechanisms (National Audit Office 2007). Organizations involved in healthcare and health improvement outcomes are expected to undertake audit as part of good governance. This is a requirement from national monitoring bodies such as the Care Quality Commission (2010).

25.3.4 **Audit in health protection**

Audit can be applied to most if not all aspects of health protection practice.
These include:

- surveillance and epidemiology,
- advice, including case management,
- incident and outbreak response,
- emergency preparedness and response,
- business and continuity,
- environmental public health functions,
- education and training,
- partnership working/stakeholders engagement,
- information governance,
- health and safety, and
- operational activities supporting practice (records management, on call, training, standard operating procedures).

25.3.5 **Audit topics and prioritization**

Audit topics can be determined by local or national needs and certain triggers may lead to undertaking an audit. Some examples are given in Table 25.2; however, this is not an exhaustive list. Health protection teams or their organization may also have an annual audit programme of topics that staff are asked to participate in.

Several tools exist to help with developing and implementing audit.

A. The Health Quality Improvement Partnership (HQIP) (2012a) has developed many tools, one of which is a prioritization tool to help determine which audits to undertake when there is limited time and resources.

B. A useful tool to determine if this audit will be successful (available at http://www.clinicalaudit-tools.com/) asks five questions of a proposed audit: relevance, priority, ease of data collection, accuracy of data, and the possibility of resulting change.

C. Quality indicators for audit (HQIP 2012b) are useful as a checklist when planning an audit.

Table 25.2 Determining audit topics

Need for audit	Health protection examples
'Must-do' determined nationally either mandatory external or internal	Audit of advice on prescribing of antibiotics, emergency planning audit
New guidelines developed recently—have they been implemented well?	Disease-specific audit, outbreak control plan standards audit
In response to a major incident	Chemical incident emergency response audit
Adverse incident or complaint about case/incident management or advice given indicating an area of potential concern	Disease-specific audit or a case event review audit
Areas of high risk, high volume, or high-cost activity	High risk—emergency planning audit High volume—Healthcare Acquired Infection; gastro-intestinal; other notifiable infections audit High cost—out-of-hours on-call standards audit
Effective working with partners—disease guidelines or service standards	Antenatal screening (hepatitis B) audit, TB audits
Variation in practice—specific audits identified through monitoring or concerns	Hepatitis A case management; E.Coli O157 audits
Recent changes leading to need for assurance on safety of service, e.g. moving offices/organizational change	On-call audit, acute service standards audit

Using an audit proposal form available from the local audit lead or department for each audit also acts as a checklist, helps clearly to outline what is proposed, and can be used for reference for future audits. It usually includes the topic, the aims of the audit, proposed methods including data collection, how results will be analysed, presentation of results, and re-audit plans.

25.3.6 Planning an audit

Audit projects are best planned with a multi-disciplinary team and a defined lead for each project. Ideally, in each health protection team there is an audit lead or experienced colleagues who can advise and support the audit. Involve team members, partners, and stakeholders. Audit projects do not usually require ethics approval (HQIP 2011).

25.3.7 Evidence base and best practice

Clear guidelines and best practice in the topic area of the audit may be available, or, if not, these can be found through a literature search. It may also be that it is an area with no clear agreed best practice. In this case, standards would need to be developed and agreed by the local team before starting the audit. This is particularly true in environmental public health practice. A review prior to the audit may be undertaken to see what 'good practice' there is amongst teams to inform the development of standards. Lessons learnt during health protection practice may also help inform the development of best practice guidance for future audits (Kipping et al. 2006).

25.3.8 Audit criteria and standards

Once best practice has been identified, the criteria to be measured and the standard to be met need to be agreed. Definitions of these with health protection examples are given in Table 25.3.

Table 25.3 Definitions with health protection examples

	Definition	Health protection examples	
Criterion to be measured	A defined and measurable item in the health protection service which describes quality and can be used to assess it; should be evidence/best practice based	*Salmonella cases who are food handlers should be advised about exclusion criteria (food poisoning guidelines)*	*Suspected cases of measles should have their MMR status recorded on the case record*
Standard to be met	Describes the level of health protection service to be achieved for any particular criterion	*100% of food handlers who are cases of Salmonella are advised about exclusion criteria (food poisoning guidelines)*	*100% of suspected measles cases have their MMR status recorded on the case record*

Source: data from Morrell C and Harvey G. The Clinical Audit Handbook. London: Ballière Tindall, Copyright © 1999 Elsevier Ltd.

25.3.9 Audit data collection

There are some simple rules for audit data collection (Ashmore et al. 2011):

♦ collect only data relevant to the audit criteria,

♦ collect minimum data required to meet the aims of the audit,

♦ maintain confidentiality of individual cases and professionals,

♦ calculate the sample size before data collection to ensure that results are meaningful and that the sample is representative, and

♦ pilot the data collection tool first before embarking on the full audit.

There are online tools to help with data collection on the Clinical Audit Tools website (http://www.clinicalaudittools.com/).

25.3.10 Data analysis and presentation

Analysis should be focused on finding out if the standards have been met and identifying areas for improvement. Simple charts and graphs and use of percentages are often all that is needed. Qualitative data can be thematically analysed but will be more subjective. Analysis and presentation of results should also focus on what is being done well as well as highlighting areas for improvement. The results should be shared with those who contributed to the data collection. Areas for improvement can be further analysed to look for underlying causes. This assists in developing plans for improvement and can be done in consultation when the initial results are shared and from analysis of any qualitative information collated during the audit.

More on the methodology of audit can be found on the HQIP website and in Ashmore et al. (2011).

25.3.11 Implementing changes

Not all audits reveal a need for change. However, the National Institute for Clinical Excellence (NICE 2002) recommends that at least 80% of audits should reveal a need for change, otherwise unnecessary audits are being done.

Deviation in practice from the standards should be identified by the audit and an action plan developed to address them. Actions need to be developed and agreed with those participating in the audit, relevant stakeholders, and management. Each action should have a named owner and a timescale for achievement. The action plan needs to be managed and monitored to ensure that steps have been taken towards improvement.

Feedback of results alone can sometimes be effective, but change is more likely if it forms part of change processes (NICE 2002). The ease of implementing changes depends on a number of factors. Morrell and Harvey (1999) describe these as including:

♦ the culture,

♦ existing systems and structures,

♦ the learning environment,

♦ resources for change,

♦ those involved in changing their practice,

♦ use of change agents that empower others, are enthusiastic about the change, facilitate the audit actions, and

♦ innovators that readily embrace new initiatives.

With the long history of audit in healthcare, there is also much published on the culture surrounding audit, especially barriers and enablers to undertaking and completing the audit cycle, that may be of relevance to individual teams or organizations (Johnston et al. 2000). The following can be helpful but are not essential to carry out a successful audit (NICE 2002):

♦ good leadership,

♦ a supportive organizational environment,

♦ structures and systems to support audit (such as training in audit, audit leads, tools to facilitate audit),

♦ a well-managed audit programme,

♦ addressing a range of audit issues important to both staff and the organization, and

♦ giving adequate attention to all stages of audit.

Improving quality after an audit can include a range of actions from providing training for staff to updating protocols and guidelines and developing and implementing new procedures.

25.3.12 **Re-audit or completing the audit**

After changes have been implemented, there is further data collection and analysis to complete the first audit cycle and to measure changes to the standards for improvement. It is at this stage that many audits fail to be completed as the re-audit is not carried out and improvements are not measured and may not be sustained.

Dixon and Pierce (2011) suggest that these measurements should be repeated at appropriate time intervals until the desired improvements have been made, an applicable standard is achieved, and sustainable change is embedded.

25.3.13 **Audit report**

Audit reports are an integral part of the audit cycle. They provide evidence for the quality of the audit project and the quality improvement actions and measurement. They allow the methods to be recorded so that the audit may be repeated at a later time or place. Templates for audit reports and how to write a good audit report are available on the HQIP website.

25.3.14 **Resources for audit**

Resources available within health protection may include reports of completed audits, templates for audit proposals, reports, and audit data collection forms. These can be accessed through organizational intranets, designated national and local health protection audit leads, and colleagues with an interest in audit. Local hospital audit departments can also help in audits with NHS partners. See 'Further reading'.

25.4 **Quality assurance and improvement**

The definition on quality assurance given in this chapter encompasses all that is done to drive and improve quality. There is a narrower definition, where quality assurance is about ensuring that quality requirements are being met with a focus on compliance rather than improvement.

Taking the wider approach, quality assurance involves a range of activities closely interlinked with good governance and measurement for improvement (Franks 2001).

These activities are well described elsewhere and for health protection are summarized in Hawker et al. (2012).

There are three aspects briefly to consider here; self-assessment, peer review, and quality improvement methods other than audit.

In health protection, individuals, teams, and organizations should have a clear view on 'what good looks like' and teams should be able to self-assess themselves against these, both seeing what they are doing well and looking for areas for improvement. The assessment can cover the core functions of a team and its quality standards and governance arrangements or focus on particular areas for improvement such as partnership working.

Teams and departments may also participate in peer review with other similar teams to see how they compare against best practice, share learning on good practice, and make improvements where necessary. Peer review can also be undertaken with or involve partners looking across a system.

There are a variety of quality improvement tools and methods for making and sustaining improvements for quality, including Plan Do Study Act (PDSA) cycles, process redesign, and others, as appropriate, which can be found on the NHS Improving Quality website (http://www.nhsiq.nhs.uk/capacity-capability/nhs-change-model/improvement-methodology.aspx).

25.5 **Conclusions**

Although specific literature on clinical audit and quality assurance in relation to health protection is sparse, the principles of audit and quality assurance programmes in healthcare apply to health protection with minimal adaptation. Audit still needs further embedding in health protection practice, particularly in terms of completing the full audit cycle with re-audit. Every aspect of health protection practice would benefit from embedding the audit culture to continuously improve service quality and safety.

References

Ashmore S, T Ruthven, L Hazelwood. 2011. Stage 2. Measuring performance. In *New Principles of Best Practice in Clinical Audit*, edited by R Burgess. London: Radcliffe.

Black N. 1992. Research, audit and education. *BMJ*, **304**: 698–700.

Boaden R, G Harvey, C Moxham, et al. 2008. *Quality Improvement: Theory and Practice in Healthcare.* Coventry: NHS Institute for Innovation and Improvement.

Brophy S, H Snooks, L Griffiths. 2008. *Small-Scale Evaluation in Health—A Practical Guide.* London: Sage.

Care Quality Commission (CQC). 2010. *CQC Guidance about Compliance: Essential Standards of Quality and Safety.* London: CQC.

CQC. 2013. *A New Start: Consultation on Changes to the Way CQC Regulates, Inspects and Monitors Care, June 2013.* Newcastle: CQC.

Dixon N, M Pearse. 2011. *Guide to Using Quality Improvement Tools to Drive Clinical Audits.* London: Health Quality Improvement Partnership.

Donabedian A. 2003. *An Introduction to Quality Assurance in Health Care.* Oxford: Oxford University Press.

Donaldson L, G Scally. 1998. Clinical governance and the drive for quality improvement in the new NHS in England. *BMJ,* **317**: 61–65.

Faculty of Public Health (FPH). 2002. *Good Public Health Practice: Standards for Organisations with a Public Health Function: Governance in Public Health Departments, Employing Organisations and Partner Organisations.* London: FPH.

FPH. 2004. *Public Health Audit Toolkit: Clinical Governance Function Audit.* London: FPH.

Franks AJ. 2001. Clinical governance as a restructuring of quality assurance processes: shifting the focus from corporate to clinical action. *British Journal of Clinical Governance,* **6**: 259–63.

Hawker J, N Begg, I Blair, et al. 2012. *Communicable Disease Control and Health Protection Handbook,* 3rd edition. London: John Wiley & Sons.

Health Quality Improvement Partnership (HQIP). 2011. *Ethics and Clinical Audit and Quality Improvement—A Guide for NHS Organisations.* http://citeseerx.ist.psu.edu/viewdoc/download?doi=10.1.1.457.4981&rep=rep1&type=pdf (accessed 8 March 2016).

HQIP. 2012a. *Clinical Audit Programme Guidance.* http://www.hqip.org.uk/resources/hqip-clinical-audit-programme-guidance/ (accessed 8 March 2016).

HQIP. 2012b. *Criteria and Indicators of Best Practice in Clinical Audit.* http://www.hqip.org.uk/resources/hqip-criteria-and-indicators-of-best-practice-in-clinical-audit-guidance/ (accessed 8 March 2016).

Health Research Authority. 2013. *Defining Research.* London: HMSO.

Johnston G, IK Crombie, HTO Davies, et al. 2000. Reviewing audit: barriers and facilitating factors in closing the audit loop. *Quality in Health Care,* **9**: 23–36.

Kipping RR, S Hamilton, M Roderick, et al. 2006. Developing audit standards required for outbreaks of communicable diseases—lessons from a mumps outbreak. *Journal of Public Health,* **28**: 347–50.

Maxwell R. 1984. Quality Assessment in health. *BMJ,* **288**: 1470–72.

Morrell C, G Harvey. 1999. *The Clinical Audit Handbook.* London: Balliere Tindall & Royal College of Nursing.

National Audit Office. 2007. *Improving Quality and Safety—Progress in Implementing Clinical Governance in Primary Care: Lessons for the New Primary Care Trusts. A report by the Comptroller and Auditor General.* London: HMSO.

National Institute for Clinical Excellence (NICE). 2002. *Principles of Best Practice in Clinical Audit.* Abingdon: Radcliffe Medical Press.

Ovretveit J. 1998. *Evaluating Health Interventions.* Maidenhead: Open University Press.

Ruthven T, S Ashmore. 2008. Clinical audit: a guide for nurses. *Nursing Management,* **15**(1): 18–22.

Smith R. 1992. Audit and Research. *BMJ,* **305**: 905.

USA Public Health Quality Forum. 2008. *Consensus Statement on Quality in the Public Health System.* USA: Department of Health and Human Services.

Vincent C. 2006. *Patient Safety.* London: Churchill Livingstone.

Walshe K. 2007. Understanding what works—and why—in quality improvement: the need for theory-driven evaluation. *International Journal for Quality in Health Care,* **19**: 57–59.

World Health Organization (WHO). 2005. *What are the Advantages and Limitations of Different Quality and Safety Tools for Health Care?* Geneva: WHO.

WHO. 2006. *Quality of Care: A Process for Making Strategic Choices in Health Systems.* Geneva: WHO.

Further reading

Clinical Audit Tools. http://www.clinicalaudittools.com/ (accessed 8 March 2016).

Clinical Audit Support Centre (CASC). http://www.clinicalauditsupport.com/ (accessed 8 March 2016).

Health Quality Improvement Partnership (HQIP). http://www.hqip.org.uk (accessed 8 March 2016).

NHS Improving Quality. http://www.nhsiq.nhs.uk (accessed 8 March 2016).

Section 6

New and emerging health protection issues

Chapter 26

New and emerging infectious diseases

Alex G. Stewart, Sam Ghebrehewet, and Peter MacPherson

OVERVIEW

After reading this chapter the reader will be familiar with:
- the concepts of new and emerging infections,
- the technological, environmental, human, and microbiological factors associated with emerging infections,
- the public health response to new and emerging infections, and
- the UK Detection, Assessment, Treatment, Escalation, Recovery, i.e. the 'DATER' strategy for dealing with epidemic and pandemic influenza and its application for new and emerging infections.

26.1 Introduction to emerging infectious diseases

The field of infectious disease is not static, but shows continuous change, with the significance of some diseases fluctuating (scarlet fever) or decreasing (polio), while that of others gains prominence (Ebola virus, Zika virus). An emerging disease is a known disease that is rapidly increasing in incidence or geographic range (Morse 1995) (e.g. human immunodeficiency virus (HIV)), while a new disease is one that has not previously been recorded (Nipah, severe acute respiratory virus (SARS)).

Many human pathogens emerge and may cause epidemics, become unstably adapted, re-emerge periodically, and eventually become endemic, but retain the potential for future outbreaks (van Doorn 2014). HIV, probably the greatest recent global infectious threat, originated as a zoonosis from non-human primates (Sharp and Hahn 2011).

Between 1940 and 2004, 335 events recording new or emerging infectious diseases were identified. Global patterns, unlikely due to chance, were dominated by zoonoses (60%), of which the majority (72%) originated in wildlife (SARS, Ebola), with evidence that the threat of emergence of new disease is increasing (Jones et al. 2008). As sources, bats host more zoonotic viruses per species than rodents (Luis et al. 2013). They are worldwide sources of high viral diversity and high-profile zoonotic viruses, including coronaviruses (SARS, Middle East respiratory syndrome (MERS), with camel-to-human transmission demonstrated; Memish et al. 2014), Ebola and Marburg haemorrhagic fever viruses, Nipah and Hendra viruses, rabies and rabies-related lyssaviruses (O'Shea et al. 2014; Tee et al. 2009).

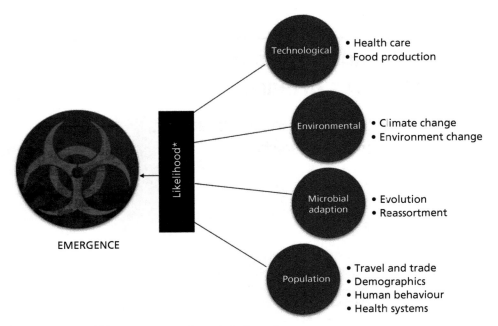

Fig. 26.1 Factors driving emergence of new infectious diseases

*Likelihood of acquisition and transmission depends on the presence or absence of favourable circumstances regarding host, agent, and environment plus concurrence of sources, pathways, and receptors.

The factors driving changes in infectious disease significance can be classified several ways (Figure 26.1). Jones et al. (2008) noted that the origins of emerging infections were significantly correlated with socio-economic (human population density and human population growth), environmental (latitude, rainfall), and ecological (wildlife host species richness) factors.

In this chapter, we adopt a pragmatic, but not definitive, approach; our classification is intended to bring a structure that public health professionals may find helpful in systematizing their approaches for prevention and control as well as anticipation of potential future impact. It is worth noting the various factors may interact in complex manners (Alexander et al. 2015; WHO 2015).

Factors that increase the risk of emergence may be remembered by the acronym TEMP— technology, environment, microbiology, people—although we approach these in a different order, from the global to the microscopic:

♦ Technological changes,

♦ Environmental:

  • climate change, and

  • environmental change and land use, including increasing urbanization;

♦ Microbial adaptation.

♦ People:

  • global travel and trade,

  • population change,

  • human behaviour,

  • changes in health-care and public health services, and

  • migration resulting from development programmes.

26.2 **Factors influencing the occurrence and spread of new and emerging infections**

26.2.1 **Environmental**

26.2.1.1 **Climate change**

There is no doubt that climate change will have major consequences on the transmission patterns of infectious diseases. Its wide-ranging impact will influence other factors, including local ecology, trade, travel, land use, population change and movement, population behaviour and microbial adaptation (dengue in South America and Asia due to warmer and wetter climate with more breeding sites for Aedes mosquitoes).

26.2.1.2 **Environmental change and land use**

Climate change affecting weather patterns, rainfall amounts, harvests, and resulting food scarcity and famine may lead to increasing outbreaks of new and emerging infections by increasing human–animal contact and allowing hitherto unknown micro-organisms access to suitable hosts. Environmental change, even when not driven by climate change, is an important influence on infectious disease (Table 26.1).

Nipah virus infection was first identified in an outbreak in Malaysia in 1998 (Chua 2010). Pigs were the intermediate hosts between the reservoir in fruit bats and the local population because new pig farms were sited in previously untouched jungle beside bat colonies. Fruit bat saliva dropping on the pigs led to entire herds dying from infections. Illness spread first to the pig farmers, then to the slaughterers and out into the community.

Table 26.1 Examples of environmental changes leading to increases in infections

Disease	Change	Examples of change	Potential route of exposure
Malaria	Water supplies	Increased precipitation, irrigation, canals, dams	Increased mosquito breeding sites
	Agriculture	Increased use of insecticides	Changing vector resistance, altered faunal balance
Malaria, trypanosomiasis, yellow fever	Land use	Deforestation	Increased numbers of breeding sites, vectors, exposed people
Lyme disease	Use of environment	Increased recreational use and commercial development of forests	Increased exposure to ticks
Dengue	Flooding	Storms increasing standing water (e.g. in discarded tyres, containers)	New urban breeding sites for mosquitoes
Infectious gastrointestinal diseases	Urbanization	Migration due to crop failures from decreased rural precipitation	Poor sanitation

Source: data from Wilson ML, Ecology and infectious disease. In: Aron JL and Patz JA (eds.) (2001) Ecosystem Change and Public Health: A Global Perspective. Baltimore: Johns Hopkins University Press, pp. 283–324. Copyright © 2001 The Johns Hopkins University Press.

26.2.2 **People**

26.2.2.1 Global travel and trade

Global travel continues to increase. In 2012 more than a billion tourists travelled outside their countries' borders, and this trend is expected to increase at 4–5% yearly (UNWTO 2014). The resulting potential exposure of susceptible individuals to new or emerging infectious diseases is huge.

The speed of spread may be related to the speed of travel: in medieval Europe, plague took three to five years to cross Europe: nowadays, few places are further than 24hrs apart. Three important consequences of the expansion of the global transport network are (Tatem et al. 2006):

♦ infectious diseases can spread rapidly, causing pandemics: swine flu 2009 (York and Donis 2013), cholera (Piarroux and Faucher 2012),

♦ invasion of vectors: *Aedes albopictus* mosquito moving into Mediterranean countries (eggs in car tyres, Lucky bamboo plants; adults in transport) and *Aedes aegypti* into Georgia, the Russian Federation and Madeira (Portugal), enabling the transmission of dengue and chikungunya (van den Berg et al. 2013), and

♦ importation of vector-borne pathogens into areas with potential vectors: malaria into Greece (Gougoutsi et al. 2014).

As well as tourist travel, people movements related to disasters and war can lead to the unexpected emergence of infections in previously unaffected population: outbreaks of poliomyelitis, measles, and cutaneous leishmaniasis due to the civil war in Syria (Sharara and Kanj 2014); cholera imported into Haiti from Nepal after the earthquake (Eppinger et al. 2014).

Similarly, global movements in traded goods can lead to unexpected emergence of infections: a large *E.coli* outbreak in Germany from Egyptian fenugreek seeds (Goodridge et al. 2012; EFSA 2011); goods, including vehicles and tyres, transported by sea-freight across global distribution chains, have led to outbreaks of dengue and chikungunya (van den Berg et al. 2013).

New and emerging infections are not limited to their initial geographical origins, but can affect susceptible populations who travel. With conducive environmental and social mixing conditions, organism and host-response characteristics and susceptible populations, the introduction of an infection into new populations can rapidly result in endemicity: West Nile Virus, first detected in North America in 1999, has since spread across the continental United States and Canada (CDC 2014).

26.2.2.2 Population change

The world is becoming increasingly urbanized, with the most rapid changes in low-and-middle income countries. Crowded, unsanitary urban conditions are highly conducive to the spread of infections. Farms are moving closer to urban centres, lifespans lengthen, and chronic disease leads to increased susceptibility to opportunistic infections (e.g. listeria). Overall, human population density is a common, significant, independent predictor of emerging infection events (Jones et al. 2008).

26.2.2.3 Human behaviour

Cultural practices (e.g. hugging as a greeting, close contact with corpses during funeral customs, eating wild animals ('bush meat')) have contributed to the spread of Ebola, particularly in West Africa (Nielsen et al. 2015). The Western interest in leisure in the countryside helps propagate Lyme disease by exposing people to the vector (*Ixodes* ('hard') ticks), which occasionally bite humans instead of deer, the animal reservoir of the disease (Donohoe et al. 2015).

Changes in personal and community sexual and drug-use practices have exposed many individuals to bloodborne viruses (HIV, hepatitis B, hepatitis C), and given rise to outbreaks in previously uninfected groups.

Nipah virus outbreaks have occurred without intermediate hosts. In 2004 in Bangladesh, infections arose from drinking contaminated date palm sap, which is a sugary drink popular with children. It is sold by society's poorest. It is also popular with fruit bats, which produce copious amounts of urine and foul the sap with the virus, thus leading directly to human cases as new palms are tapped for their sap (Luby 2013).

26.2.2.4 Changes in health care and public health services

In the 1990s there was a large-scale outbreak of diphtheria in the independent states which made up the former Soviet Union. Following the dissolution of the Soviet Union in 1991, the previously strong childhood immunization programme fragmented, adding a large number of susceptible children to the many susceptible adults. Deteriorating socio-economic conditions and high population movement only compounded these risk factors to produce the first large-scale diphtheria epidemic in industrialized countries in 30 years (Vitek and Wharton 1998).

26.2.2.5 Migration resulting from development programmes

As well as fleeing war, people from low-and-middle income countries migrate to new destinations (Relman et al. 2010) to seek fresh opportunities, and better living and working conditions. Such movement is usually from high-infection incidence to low-infection incidence countries, and infections can be carried from home to the host community: hepatitis A outbreaks have been initiated by non-immune migrants, with resulting secondary spread (Heywood et al. 2007); reactivation of TB or late presentation of infection with *Strongyloides* or *Schistosoma species* after many years in the host country are well-documented but not always easily recognized (McCarthy et al. 2013).

26.2.3 Impact of technology

Bovine spongiform encephalopathy (BSE), a disease of cattle, was first reported in the United Kingdom in 1986. It was caused by cattle being fed the remains of other cattle (meat and bone meal) which was contaminated from sheep with scrapie that were processed in the same slaughterhouse. In addition, the reduced temperature during the rendering process contributed to the spread of the disease in the UK. Human consumption of food derived from cattle contaminated with the BSE prion led to human cases of variant Creutzfeldt– Jakob disease (vCJD), a rare and fatal human neurodegenerative condition, first described in 1996 (WHO 2012).

HIV and hepatitis C were spread in the UK in the 1970s and 1980s through unscreened blood transfusion and blood products (Penrose 2015).

Anisakis larvae ingested in raw (but not frozen) sushi or herring can cause gastrointestinal disease (Nawa et al. 2005). With increasing global fish movements for food, farming, and sport fishing as well as human-driven habitat changes, it is likely that other wild fish pathogens will emerge into the human population.

26.2.4 Microbial adaptation

The majority (54%) of pathogens involved in emerging infection events are bacteria, including newly developed drug-resistant strains (tuberculosis, carbapenemase producing *Enterobacteriaceae* (CPE)) or *rickettsia*, many of which show changes and adaptation over time. Viruses and prions account for 24% of emerging organisms, protozoa (11%), fungi (6%), and helminths (3%) (Jones et al. 2008).

Major influenza epidemics show no predictable periodicity or pattern, and all differ from one another. Pandemics (global epidemics) arise through changes in virus subtypes, due to genetic reassortment with animal influenza A viruses: 1918 Spanish flu, antigenic subtype H1N1; 1957

Asian, H2N2; 1968 Hong Kong, H3N2; 2009 Swine, H1N1 (Kilbourne 2006). However, human-to-swine transmission of influenza viruses is far more common than the reverse, and is fundamental to developing diversity in influenza viruses in pigs (Nelson and Vincent 2015). Outbreaks of avian influenza in poultry have raised global public health concerns due to their contribution to the 1918 pandemic, their effect on poultry populations, their potential to cause serious disease in people, and their pandemic potential.

26.3 Public health response to new and emerging infections

Zoonotic infections represent an increasing and very significant threat to global health. Zoonotic pathogens from wildlife accounted for 52% of all emerging infection events from 1990–2000, and showed an increasing trend over time (Jones et al. 2008). The importance of understanding the factors that intensify contact between wildlife and humans cannot be underestimated and demands improved collaboration between the veterinary, environmental and farming communities, and human health professionals. This 'One Health' approach to zoonotic infections, which addresses the connections between health and the wider environment has been formalized in the One Health Initiative, and encourages cooperation in the development of integrated solutions for complex problems that impact the health of animals, humans, and the planet (Breitschwerdt 2014).

The UK responsive strategy developed following the 2009 influenza pandemic provides a good approach: Detection, Assessment, Treatment, Escalation and Recovery ('DATER') (NHS 2013). Communication is an integral part of each section, internally, externally, nationally, and internationally.

The DATER strategy could be adopted as a framework to identify and deal with new and emerging diseases, as its components provide a more practical approach than the screening, assessment, and communication framework.

26.3.1 Detection

New infectious diseases are often identified many years after breaching the species barrier (Heymann and Dar 2014). There is an ongoing need to remain alert for novel, unexpected, or particularly severe clinical presentations, to use syndromic surveillance (surveillance of symptoms rather than diagnoses) for early identification of potential outbreaks, to confirm infections by laboratory investigations, and coordinate national scanning of any source of intelligence which might suggest new or emerging issues. In northeastern Brazilian states, a 20-fold increase in the prevalence of microcephaly in newborns in 2015 compared to previous years (PAHO 2015) within nine months of emergence of an outbreak of Zika virus disease demonstrated the value of routine surveillance systems in identifying emerging infectious threats to public health. Zika infection (a Flaviviral infection) had previously ocurred sporadically in Africa, SE Asia, and Oceania, but in 2015 a widespread epidemic began in south and central America. Transmission is primarily by *Aedes* mosquitoes (predominantly day-biters often found in urban environments), but mother to foetus infection and sexual transmission have been described. At the time of writing, WHO has declared the cluster of newborn neurological disorders linked to the Zika virus outbreak in South and Central America and the Pacific to be a Public Health Emergency of International Concern (WHO 2016), and considerable scientific efforts have been mobilized to improve understanding and surveillance, and to reduce Zika virus transmission.

Internet-based syndromic surveillance systems offer novel means of monitoring conditions of public health concern, including emerging infectious diseases. They have good equivalence with traditional approaches and are logistically and economically appealing. However, they are not alternatives, but extensions of traditional surveillance systems (Milinovich et al. 2014). Nevertheless, global resources to counter disease emergence are poorly allocated, with the majority of the scientific and surveillance effort focused on countries from where the next important emergence is least likely to originate (Jones et al. 2008).

26.3.2 **Assessment**

Each new infectious situation should have a formal or informal risk assessment with regard to infectivity, spread, susceptibility, impact, and response. In the UK, the formal assessment is coordinated through and communicated by the Human and Animal Infections and Risk Surveillance (HAIRS) group.

26.3.3 **Treatment**

Prevention, control, and treatment should be as complete as possible at both the individual and population levels.

26.3.4 **Escalation**

Diseases do not consider borders or resources: an international focus is important. Trust needs to be developed to enable effective, meaningful collaboration between countries, allowing the rapid detection of potential pandemic infections and early public health action. Inter-country collaboration should be based upon the International Health Regulations and encouraged in a way that acknowledges the benefits of sharing biological material as well as establishing equitable, collaborative research partnerships. The One Health approach provides such a means (McCloskey et al. 2014). The international response to SARS benefited from such an approach (Vonga et al. 2013).

26.3.5 **Recovery**

Lessons of coordination, identification, infrastructure, and capacity can and should be applied, not forgotten (Vonga et al. 2013) and communicated widely.

26.4 **Conclusions**

Recent problems, such as the emergence of Ebola in West Africa in 2014–15, have raised the profile of new and emerging infections. The systematic assessment of intelligence, gathered across a wide range of issues (covering **T**echnology, **E**nvironment, **M**icrobiology, **P**eople) is vital to enable a timely and coordinated response. Public health action depends on a robust infrastructure that enables early signs to be detected, recognized, assessed, and communicated to the relevant operational agencies and decision makers. Globally equitable investment before emergence is a preventive measure that will save lives, money, materials, and avoid a lot of suffering and frustration.

References

Alexander KA, CE Sanderson, M Marath, et al. 2015. What factors might have led to the emergence of Ebola in West Africa? *PLOS Neglected Tropical Diseases*. doi:10.1371/journal.pntd.0003652

Breitschwerdt EB. 2014. Bartonellosis: one health perspectives for an emerging infectious disease. *ILAR Journal*, **55**(1): 46–58.

Centers for Disease Prevention and Control (CDC). 2014. *West Nile Virus. Final Annual Maps & Data for 1999–2013*. http://www.cdc.gov/westnile/statsMaps/finalMapsData/index.html (accessed 8 March 2016).

Chua KB. (2010). Epidemiology, surveillance and control of Nipah virus infections in Malaysia. *Malaysian Journal of Pathology*, **32**(2): 69–73.

Donohoe H, L Pennington-Gray, O Omodior. 2015. Lyme disease: Current issues, implications, and recommendations for tourism management. *Tourism Management*, **46**: 408–18.

Eppinger M, T Pearson T, Koenig SSK, et al. 2014. Genomic epidemiology of the Haitian cholera outbreak: a single introduction followed by rapid, extensive, and continued spread characterized the onset of the epidemic. *mBio*, 5(6): e01721.

European Food Safety Authority (EFSA). 2011. *Tracing seeds, in particular fenugreek (Trigonella foenum-graecum) seeds, in relation to the Shiga toxin-producing E. coli (STEC) O104:H4 2011 Outbreaks in Germany and France. Question No EFSA-Q-2011-00817*. http://www.efsa.europa.eu/en/supporting/pub/176e.htm (accessed 8 March 2016).

Goodridge LD, JT LeJeune, L Beutin. 2012. What was the source of the 2011 outbreak of *Escherichia coli* in Germany and France? In *Case Studies in Food Safety and Authenticity*, edited by J Hoorfar. Oxford: Woodhead Publishing, pp. 43–54.

Gougoutsi A, DE Karageorgopoulos, A Dimitriadou, et al. 2014. Severe Plasmodium vivax malaria complicated with acute respiratory distress syndrome: a case associated with focal autochthonous transmission in Greece. *Vector Borne Zoonotic Diseases*, 14(5): 378–81.

Heymann D, OA Dar. 2014. Prevention is better than cure for emerging infectious diseases. *BMJ*, 348: g1499.

Heywood P, J Cutler, K Burrows, et al. 2007. A community outbreak of travel-acquired hepatitis A transmitted by an infected food handler. *Canadian Communicable Disease Report*, 33(11): 16–22.

Jones KE, NG Patel, MA Levy, et al. 2008. Global trends in emerging infectious diseases. *Nature*, 451: 990–993.

Kilbourne ED. 2006. Influenza pandemics of the 20th century. *Emerging Infectious Diseases*, 12(1): 9–14.

Luby SP. 2013. The pandemic potential of Nipah virus. *Antiviral Research*, 100(1): 38–43.

Luis AD, DTS Hayman, TJ O'Shea, et al. 2013. A comparison of bats and rodents as reservoirs of zoonotic viruses: are bats special? *Proceedings of the Royal Society Series B: Biological Sciences*, 280: 20122753

McCarthy AE, LH Weld, ED Barnett, et al. 2013. Spectrum of illness in international migrants seen at GeoSentinel clinics in 1997–2009, Part 2: Migrants resettled internationally and evaluated for specific health concerns. *Clinical Infectious Diseases*, 56(7): 925–33.

McCloskey B, O Dar, A Zumla, et al. 2014. Emerging infectious diseases and pandemic potential: status quo and reducing risk of global spread. *Lancet Infectious Diseases*, 14(10): 1001–10.

Marx PA, C Apetrei, E Drucker. 2004. AIDS as a zoonosis? Confusion over the origin of the virus and the origin of the epidemics. *Journal of Medical Primatology*, 33(5–6): 220–26.

Memish ZA, M Cotten, B Meyer, et al. 2013. Human infection with MERS coronavirus after exposure to infected camels, Saudi Arabia, 2013. *Emerging Infectious Diseases*, 20(6): 1012–15.

Milinovich GJ, GM Williams, ACA Clements, et al. 2014. Internet-based surveillance systems for monitoring emerging infectious diseases. *Lancet Infectious Diseases*, 14(2): 160–68.

Morse SS. 1995. Factors in the emergence of infectious diseases. *Emerging Infectious Diseases*, 1(1): 7–15.

Nawa Y, C Hatz, J Blum. 2005. Sushi delights and parasites: the risk of fishborne and foodborne parasitic zoonoses in Asia. *Clinical Infectious Diseases*, 41(9): 1297–1303.

Nelson MI, AL Vincent. 2015. Reverse zoonosis of influenza to swine: new perspectives on the human-animal interface. *Trends in Microbiology*, 23(3): 142–53.

NHS. 2013. *Operating Framework for Managing the Response to Pandemic Influenza*. Leeds: NHS England.

Nielsen CF, S Kidd, ARM Sillah, et al. 2015. Improving burial practices and cemetery management during an Ebola virus disease epidemic—Sierra Leone, 2014. *Morbidity and Mortality Weekly Report*, 64(01): 20–27.

O'Shea TJ, PM Cryan, AA Cunningham, et al. 2014. Bat flight and zoonotic viruses. *Emerging Infectious Diseases*, 20(5): 741–45.

PAHO 2015. *Epidemiological Alert: Neurological syndrome, congenital malformations, and Zika virus infection. Implications for public health in the Americas*. http://www.paho.org/hq/index.php?option=com_docman&task=doc_view&Itemid=270&gid=32405&lang=en (accessed 8 March 2016).

Penrose GW. 2015. *The Penrose Enquiry Final Report.* Edinburgh: APS Group Scotland.

Piarroux R, B Faucher. 2012. Cholera epidemics in 2010: respective roles of environment, strain changes, and human-driven dissemination. *Clinical Microbiologt and Infection,* **18**(3): 231–38.

Redford KH, W Adams, GM Mace. 2013. Synthetic biology and conservation of nature: wicked problems and wicked solutions. *PLoS Biology,* **11**(4): e1001530.

Relman DA, ER Choffnes, A Mack. 2010. *Infectious Disease Movement in a Borderless World: Workshop Summary.* Dulles, VA: National Academies Press.

Sharara SL, SS Kanj. 2014. War and infectious diseases: challenges of the Syrian civil war. *PLoS Pathogens,* **10**(11): e1004438.

Sharp PM, BH Hahn. 2011. Origins of HIV and the AIDS pandemic. *Cold Spring Harbour Perspectives,* **1**(1): a006841.

Tatem AJ, DJ Rogers, SI Hay. 2006. Global transport networks and infectious disease spread. *Advanced Parasitology,* **62**: 293–343.

Tee KK, Y Takebe, A Kamarulzaman. 2009. Emerging and re-emerging viruses in Malaysia, 1997–2007. *International Journal of Infectious Diseases,* **13**(3): 307–18.

UNWTO. 2014. *UNWTO Annual Report 2013.* Madrid, Spain: World Tourism Organization (UNWTO).

van den Berg H, R Velayudhan, M Ejov. 2013. *Regional Framework for Surveillance and Control of Invasive Mosquito Vectors and Re-emerging Vector-borne Diseases 2014–2020.* Copenhagen: WHO Regional Office for Europe.

van Doorn HR. 2014. Emerging infectious diseases. *Medicine (Abingdon),* **42**(1): 60–63.

Vitek CR, M Wharton. 1998. Diphtheria in the former Soviet Union: reemergence of a pandemic disease. *Emerging Infectious Diseases,* **4**(4): 539–50.

Vonga S, M O'Leary, Z Feng. 2013. Early response to the emergence of influenza A(H7N9) virus in humans in China: the central role of prompt information sharing and public communication. *Bulletin of the World Health Organization,* **92**(4): 303–308.

World Health Organization (WHO). 2012. *Variant Creutzfeldt–Jakob Disease.* World Health Organization fact sheet. http://www.who.int/mediacentre/factsheets/fs180/en/ (accessed 8 March 2016).

WHO. 2015. *Global Alert and Response. Factors that Contributed to Undetected Spread of the Ebola Virus and Impeded Rapid Containment.* http://www.who.int/csr/disease/ebola/one-year-report/factors/en/ (accessed 8 March 2016).

WHO. 2016. *WHO statement on the first meeting of the International Health Regulations (2005) (IHR 2005) Emergency Committee on Zika virus and observed increase in neurological disorders and neonatal malformations.* http://www.who.int/mediacentre/news/statements/2016/1st-emergency-committee-zika/en/ (accessed 8 March 2016).

Wilson ML. 2001. Ecology and infectious disease. In *Ecosystem Change and Public Health: A Global Perspective,* edited by JL Aron, JA Patz. Baltimore: Johns Hopkins University Press, pp. 283–324.

York I, RO Donis. 2013. The 2009 pandemic influenza virus: where did it come from, where is it now, and where is it going? *Current Topics in Microbiology and Immunology,* **370**: 241–57.

Chapter 27

New and emerging environmental hazards and situations

Alec Dobney and Greg Hodgson

OVERVIEW

After reading this chapter the reader will be familiar with:
- the impact of new and emerging environmental hazards/situations such as commercial waste fires,
- emerging industrial processes (e.g. shale gas exploration and extraction) and their potential impact on environment and public health, and
- new technologies (nanotechnology) with their possible environmental and human health impacts.

27.1 Introduction to emerging environmental hazards

Environmental public health scientists and those working in the field of health protection are constantly challenged to respond to new or poorly understood hazards. Practitioners might also be required to address previously well-characterized hazards that either increase in magnitude or re-emerge in different situations. For example, a recent case of a well-characterized industrial chemical 2, 4-dinitrophenol (DNP), used in the manufacture of dyes and wood preservatives, has been unlawfully promoted as a 'fat burner' or 'slimming aid', even though the chemical is known to be unfit for human consumption and illegal for use in foodstuffs (FSA 2012). These situations can present a variety of challenges in determining the associated public health risks and how these risks can be mitigated and communicated to the public. They can present new pathways and routes of exposure and may have a limited or emerging evidence base on which to determine the risk.

Many tools have been developed to try to anticipate and take account of new developments that have the potential to become important in the future, whether these result in a new and emerging threat or a positive health outcome (Cabinet Office and Government Office for Science 2014). Horizon scanning is one such example of a fundamental first step in identifying and examining potential threats, opportunities, and likely developments including, but not restricted to, those at the margins of current thinking and planning. It may explore novel and unexpected issues as well as persistent problems or trends. This creates an evidence-based approach to identifying new threats and opportunities, which can complement the more traditional expert-driven identification of new issues (PHE 2014).

Developing technological advances and new and emerging industrial processes can raise difficult questions for the public health practitioner, especially where research and health-related evidence is lacking. In these cases public health science has a key role in undertaking risk assessments and risk communication, and in providing the most accurate available scientific evidence and advice. There are multiple new and emerging environmental hazards that the reader should be aware of; the significance of exposures in utero and to mixtures of chemicals, the increase in allergic diseases, and the potential for exposures to result in epigenetic changes are areas of growing concern. It is, however, beyond the scope of this chapter to address all these topics.

The following examples described in this chapter consider aspects of new and emerging environmental hazards with regard to: how well-characterized hazards can change or increase in magnitude; how new environmental processes can bring about both perceived and potential risks; and how data generation from new technologies can often outpace scientific understanding related to the determinants of health.

27.2 Commercial waste fires—a well-characterized hazard changing or increasing in magnitude

Fire hazards within the UK are generally well understood; however, an increased number of incidents occurred in the UK during 2012–14 related to the way large volumes of waste material were being stored on sites, making these fires significantly more difficult to extinguish. Fires extended over many days and in some cases even months (Wyre Forest DC 2013). Changes in the UK waste legislation over this period, such as landfill tax charges along with market influences, resulted in some companies stockpiling waste at their sites, increasing the risk of fires (WISH 2014). There were multifarious reasons for each incident; however, they were connected by the complexities the fires brought to the local emergency services, health agencies, and others in managing and tackling such incidents.

Fires at waste sites can involve large volumes of waste burning for prolonged periods, in uncontrolled conditions, which can potentially have impacts on local communities, including local residents and adjacent businesses. The nature of the material is typically large bales of high calorific material destined to be processed into refuse-derived fuel. The bales are often stacked on top of each other across open hard standings or tightly compacted within large warehouses, making it difficult for emergency services to gain access. The fires are usually deep-seated and extremely difficult to extinguish. The combination of the material type involved and combustion conditions can release large plumes of black smoke, a complex mixture of particulate matter and irritant gases. Light and disused industrial sites are generally preferred as waste storage facilities and as such have led to the increased potential for public health impact because they are often located in close proximity to residential areas.

The management of these incidents has increasingly become resource intensive for both the local emergency services and the health community. Public health practitioners are often called upon to be represented at multi-agency Strategic Coordinating Groups (SCG) and Tactical Coordinating Groups (TCG) or to attend the Scientific and Technical Advice Cell (STAC). Due to the protracted nature of these fires, advice from public health scientists is sought in regard to estimating the impact on public health by undertaking risk assessments, estimating the exposure to members of the public, and supporting risk communication, including the formulation and coordination of public health messages throughout the incident response. It often requires public health scientists to undertake comparative risk assessments for the different fire management strategies and work with partner agencies to influence a strategy that poses least risk to public health. This is then followed by working closely with the Recovery Coordinating Group, where established, to ensure that public health continues to be considered while the site is returned to normal operations or rendered safe. Generally, protracted waste fire incidents last for approximately three to six months (Cabinet Office 2013). Site restoration and clean-up can sometimes take even longer depending on insurance or litigation issues, and further risk assessments might be required around residual wastes remaining at the site.

The Waste Industry Safety and Health Forum (WISH) and the Environment Agency have produced new guidance for waste and recycling sites 'Reducing Fire Risk at Waste Management Sites' and 'Fire Prevention Plans' for storing combustible waste at permitted sites, respectively (WISH 2014; EA 2015). Their subsequent actions recognize the emerging issues and subsequent interventions that can come about from what can be a well-characterized hazard that has increased or changed in magnitude to present a different or emergent threat.

27.3 New emerging industrial processes: shale gas exploration and extraction

Shale gas is a natural gas found in shale formations, a fine-grained sedimentary rock derived from decay of organic matter in the Carboniferous period. Estimations indicate the UK shale gas reserve could be as large as 150 billion cubic metres (bcm) compared to a 2–6 bcm estimate of undiscovered UK gas resources for onshore conventional petroleum (DECC 2015). The extraction or production of natural gas from shale differs from conventional forms of gas and oil extraction from defined reservoirs or traps where the hydrocarbon (the gas or oil) has migrated from the source rock. In the case of shale gas, the extraction is considered unconventional as the gas is obtained directly from the source rock.

To extract shale gas, the usual approach involves the drilling of a number of horizontal wells in different directions from a single well pad to target potential reserves of gas at depths typically more than 1000 m below the surface. This is followed by fracture stimulation technology, commonly referred to as fracking, to enhance the natural fractures and recover gas from rocks with low permeability. Hydraulic fracturing involves pumping water into the rock at high pressures, creating small fractures and allowing the gas to escape and be collected at the well bore. The flowback water which returns to the surface is comprised of a high-pressure mixture of methane and other gases, water, brine, solids, minerals, hydrocarbons, and low levels of naturally occurring radioactive materials. Large quantities of water are required for the process, often resulting in concerns around the capacity at water treatment facilities to treat waste water. Chemicals are often added to the water to increase the efficiency of the process, resulting in a mixture known as hydraulic fracturing fluid. In the US a wide variety of chemicals has been used, including known endocrine disruptor chemicals and chemicals which can impact the immune or nervous system. Operators in the UK will disclose publicly the chemical additives they use and undertake risk assessments to determine their suitability for use as components of hydraulic fracturing fluid.

The exploration and development of shale gas in the UK is subject to the Department of Environment and Climate Change (DECC) licences, local authority planning consent, and Environmental Permitting and Health and Safety Executive (HSE) Regulations. Exploration for shale gas is currently underway in the UK; however, the industry is in its infancy, with very few exploratory wells drilled (DECC 2015).

Public concern has been centred on the uncertainties around the emerging technologies used to extract what, until recently, were considered uneconomic hydrocarbon deposits. Technologies such as hydraulic fracturing have previously been used in conventional hydrocarbon extraction in the UK but have only recently started to be adapted and applied to exploration for shale gas. Publications from other countries, most notably the US, report that drilling for, and extraction of shale gas using hydraulic fracturing, has the potential adversely to impact the environment and human health (OCMOH 2012; AEA Technology 2012). However, caution is required when extrapolating experiences from other countries to the UK since the mode of operation, underlying geology, and regulatory environment are likely to be different (PHE 2014). Concerns have been raised around a range of potential and perceived hazards. As a public health practitioner, the key role here is effectively to communicate risk to the public, contextualizing the scientific evidence available.

Some of the public health concerns include the potential health effects linked to emissions to atmosphere and ground and surface waters, and the treatment of waste and flowback water. It has been noted in several UK reviews that water pollution, both ground and surface, has occurred in the US (RS and RAE 2012). Key to preventing this occurring in the UK is good well integrity (well design and construction) *and* procedures to manage and prevent spills. In the UK, the Environment Agency will not permit developments to take place within proximity of an aquifer that is used as a potable source. If commercial-scale shale gas developments are to be considered viable, it is important to determine how best to evaluate health issues prior to operation. There are a number of potential tools and methods that could look at the health impact of shale gas extraction and related activities (e.g. human health risk assessment, environmental impact assessments, strategic environmental assessments, or health impact assessments).

There is, to date, little peer-reviewed research looking at the effects on populations around fracking sites, but experiences from countries with commercial-scale operations, such as the US, demonstrate that good on-site management and strong regulation of all aspects of the operations are essential to minimize the impacts on the environment as a whole, including public health. The currently available evidence indicates that the potential risks to public health from exposure to the emissions associated with shale gas extraction, in the UK, are low if the operations are properly run and regulated (PHE 2014).

27.4 Keeping pace with material technology: nanotechnology

New materials and products are constantly being developed and introduced to the marketplace. Providing suitable controls, regulatory and otherwise, to ensure adequate protection of human health from novel materials is therefore an ongoing challenge (RCEP 2008). Nanotechnology is one source of such materials. Nanotechnology is the manipulation of matter at the atomic, molecular, and supramolecular levels, often defined as relating to a size range between 1 and 100 nanometres (nm) (1 nm is a millionth of a millimetre—a human hair is between 20,000 and 200,000 nm). Nanomaterials can be engineered as particles, rods and 'fullerene' balls, as well as wires and tubes, which can be many thousands or millions of nanometres in length, and sheets (e.g. graphene). At the nanoscale, materials can have markedly different optical, electrical, and magnetic properties and behaviours. Nanomaterials can be engineered to be incredibly strong but very light—e.g. carbon nanotubes (hollow tubes of graphene) are, on a mass basis, over 100 times stronger than steel and 30 times stronger than Kevlar (Chang et al. 2010). These properties are being exploited to produce novel structures and systems for myriad different applications, including electronics, optical, and imaging technologies, 'self-cleaning' textiles, antimicrobial domestic cleaning products, construction materials, medical diagnostic tools and treatments, pharmaceuticals, foods, skincare products, and cosmetics. Individual members of the public can be exposed to nanomaterials either directly through use of a consumer product containing nanomaterials (e.g. use of sunscreen containing titanium dioxide nanoparticles) or potentially via release of nanomaterials into the environment at the end of a product life cycle.

Alongside the huge potential benefits of nanomaterials are some uncertainties and concerns regarding their possible environmental and human health impacts (Royal Society 2004; RCEP 2008). The development and incorporation of good-quality, independent scientific information has to be central to the design of appropriate public health communications for individuals potentially exposed to nanoparticles (Cox et al. 2003). Research has shown that the general mechanisms by which many nanoparticles exert their toxic effects appear similar to those of larger particles.

However, it does appear that nanoparticles, following entry into the body, might reach parts inaccessible to larger particles (e.g. transported to the brain along the olfactory nerve; Oberdörster et al, 2004). There also remain significant concerns regarding nanofibres, arising from reported toxicological similarities between carbon nanotubes and asbestos. The International Agency on Research on Cancer has recently declared that one form of carbon nanotubes is 'possibly carcinogenic to humans' (Grosse et al. 2014). Such concerns have prompted calls for strict controls on exposures within the workplace (HSE 2013; NIOSH 2013).

These concerns have led to the rapid development of a specialized branch of toxicology called 'nanotoxicology'. Global funding for nanosafety has also increased significantly; for example, the EC has spent many €100 million funding this area. At an international level the Organisation for Economic Co-operation and Development (OECD) has a programme of work related to nanotechnology, including the production of dossiers on hazard identification for 14 common nanomaterials and the updating of standard toxicity testing guidelines to ensure they are appropriate for nanomaterials.

In the UK the main legislation covering nanomaterials is the EU REACH regulations (Registration, Evaluation, Authorisation, and restriction of Chemicals), which came into force on 1 June 2007. These apply to substances, including nanomaterials, manufactured in or imported into the EU and require those who place chemicals on the market (manufacturers and importers) to be responsible for understanding and managing the risks associated with their use. Another piece of legislation covering products containing nanomaterials is the EU Cosmetics Directive, which limits the uses of certain nanomaterials in various products.

It is important to recognize that the majority of the nanomaterials which currently dominate the global market have either been in use for many years (e.g. carbon black) or are nano-sized versions of materials that have been in use for decades (e.g. titanium dioxide and zinc oxide). More sophisticated third- and fourth-generation nanomaterials may represent a further step change in functionalities and properties, with concomitant challenges in relation to risk assessment and regulation (RCEP 2008).

27.5 Conclusions

Environmental public health scientists and those working in the field of health protection are constantly challenged to respond to new and emerging environmental hazards or to address well-characterized hazards that either increase in magnitude or re-emerge in different situations. The environmental public health environment is crowded with complex problems demanding our attention. It is impossible to devote sufficient clinical, research, and advocacy energies to all of these problems at once. Public health professionals and environmental public health scientists have to choose which health issues take priority. As such, these situations can present a variety of challenges in determining the associated public health risks and how these risks can be mitigated and communicated to the public, sometimes in the light of a limited or an emerging evidence base.

References

AEA Technology. 2012. *Support to the Identification of Potential Risks for the Environment and Human Health arising from Hydrocarbons Operations involving Hydraulic Fracturing in Europe.* Report for the European Commission DG Environment. Didcot: AEA.

Cabinet Office (CO). 2013. *Emergency Response and Recovery: Non Statutory Guidance Accompanying the Civil Contingencies Act 2004.* London: Cabinet Office.

CO and Government Office for Science. 2014. *The Futures Toolkit—Tools for Strategic Futures for Policy Makers and Analysts.* https://www.gov.uk/government/uploads/system/uploads/attachment_data/file/328069/Futures_Toolkit_beta.pdf (accessed 8 March 2016).

Cox P, J Niewöhner, N Pidgeon, et al. 2003. The use of mental models in chemical risk protection: developing a generic workplace methodology. *Risk Analysis*, **23**, 311–24.

Department of Energy and Climate Change (DECC). 2015. *Regulatory Roadmap: Onshore Oil and Gas Exploration in the UK Regulation and Best Practice*. https://www.gov.uk/government/publications/regulatory-roadmap-onshore-oil-and-gas-exploration-in-the-uk-regulation-and-best-practice (accessed 27 April 2016).

Environment Agency (EA). 2015. *Fire Prevention Plans version 2 March 2015*. https://www.gov.uk/government/uploads/system/uploads/attachment_data/file/415262/LIT_10105.pdf (accessed 27 April 2016).

Food Standards Agency (FSA). 2012). *Warning about 'fat-burner' substances containing DNP*. http://www.food.gov.uk/news-updates/news/2012/5371/dnp-warning (accessed 8 March 2016).

Grosse Y, D Loomis, K Guyton, et al. 2014. Carcinogenicity of fluoro-edenite, silicon carbide fibres and whiskers, and carbon nanotubes. *Lancet Oncology*, **15**(13): 1427–28.

Health and Safety Executive (HSE). 2013. *Using Nanomaterials at Work—Including Carbon Nanotubes (CNTs) and Other Biopersistent High Aspect Ratio Nanomaterials (HARNs)*. Publication HSG272. London: HSE. www.hse.gov.uk/pubns/books/hsg272.pdf (accessed 8 March 2016).

National Institute for Occupational Safety and Health (NIOSH). 2013. *Current Intelligence Bulletin 65— Occupational Exposure to Carbon Nanotubes and Nanofibres*. DHHS (NIOSH) Publication Number 2013–145. Atlanta, GA: NIOSH. www.cdc.gov/niosh/docs/2013-145/pdfs/2013-145.pdf (accessed 8 March 2016).

Oberdörster G, Z Sharp, V Atudorei, et al. 2004. Translocation of inhaled ultrafine particles to the brain. *Inhalation Toxicology*, **16**(6–7): 437–45.

Office of the Chief Medical Officer of Health (OCMOH). 2012. *Chief Medical Officer of Health's Recommendations Concerning Shale Gas Developments in New Brunswick*. New Brunswick Department of Health.

Public Health England (PHE). 2014. *Review of the Potential Public Health Impacts of Exposures to Chemical and Radioactive Pollutants as a Result of Shale Gas Extraction*. Didcot: PHE.

Royal Commission on Environmental Pollution (RCEP). 2008. *Novel Materials in the Environment: The Case of Nanotechnology*. Cm 7468.

Royal Society (RS) and Royal Academy of Engineering (RAE). 2004. *Nanoscience and Nanotechnologies: Opportunities and Uncertainties*. London: RS and RAE. https://royalsociety.org/~/media/Royal_Society_Content/policy/publications/2004/9693.pdf (accessed 8 March 2016).

RS and RAE. 2012. *Shale Gas Extraction in the UK: A Review of Hydraulic Fracturing*. London: RS and RAE.

Waste Industry Safety and Health Forum (WISH). 2014. *WASTE 28 Reducing Fire Risk at Waste Management Sites*. http://www.hse.gov.uk/waste/wish-guidance.htm (accessed 8 March 2016).

Wyre Forest District Council. 2013. *Fire at Lawrence Recycling & Waste Management, Kidderminster*. http://www.wyreforestdc.gov.uk/community-wellbeing-and-environment/emergencies/lawrences-fire-june-2013.aspx (accessed 8 March 2016).

Chapter 28

Global disasters and risk reduction strategies

Virginia Murray, Amina Aitsi-Selmi, and Alex G. Stewart

OVERVIEW

After reading this chapter the reader will be familiar with:
- the United Nations International Strategy on Disaster Reduction (UNISDR),
- the Sendai Framework, which aims to prevent new and reduce existing disaster risk through the implementation of an integrated and inclusive approach to strengthening resilience,
- non-catastrophic disasters both infectious (e.g. congenital rubella syndrome) and non-infectious (e.g. iodine deficiency), and
- the need for a systems approach response and the synergy that can be realized between public health and global disaster risk reduction (DRR).

28.1 Introduction to global disaster risk

In 2009 the UNISDR defined disaster as:

A serious disruption of the functioning of a community or a society involving widespread human, material, economic or environmental losses and impacts, which exceeds the ability of the affected community or society to cope using its own resources.

UNISDR added that

Disasters are often described as a result of the combination of: the exposure to a hazard; the conditions of vulnerability that are present; and insufficient capacity or measures to reduce or cope with the potential negative consequences. Disaster impacts may include loss of life, injury, disease and other negative effects on human physical, mental and social well-being, together with damage to property, destruction of assets, loss of services, social and economic disruption and environmental degradation.

(UNISDR 2009)

Hazards can include latent conditions that may represent future threats and can have different origins:

♦ natural: geological (e.g. earthquakes, volcanoes), hydro-meteorological (e.g. floods, droughts), biological epidemics and pandemics (e.g. outbreaks of cholera, Ebola),

♦ induced by human processes: environmental degradation (e.g. deforestation, mining) and technological hazards (e.g. chemical spills, IT failures).

Vulnerability to catastrophic disasters is increasing as more people inhabit high-risk areas. Since 1970, the world's population has grown by 87%. At the same time, the proportion of people living in flood-prone river basins has increased by 114% and on cyclone-exposed coastlines by

192%. Rapid urbanization and the growth of megacities (urban area with >10 million inhabitants) increase exposure to natural hazards; the global population living in informal settlements is currently estimated at approximately one billion, many of whom live in hazard-prone areas, and this is growing by 40 million people annually.

Disasters affect human lives by causing injury and resulting in long-term impact, as well as destroying lives and livelihoods:

- 1.7 million people killed globally 2000–12,
- more than 2.9 billion of the world's approximate seven-billion population affected, and
- an estimated US$1.7 trillion of damage sustained in >10,000 events (UNISDR 2012).

Disasters and some of the hazards that trigger them require an all-hazards approach. They are endogenous to society and disaster risk arises when hazards interact with the physical, social, economic, and environmental vulnerabilities of populations.

The number, scale, and cost of disasters are increasing, although, with early warning, improved building codes, and other DRR interventions, the number of deaths from these events appears to be reducing. Climate change is expected to increase the frequency and intensity of the most severe weather-related hazards. Furthermore, events that transcend national, geographical, social, and economic boundaries are more common as a result of globalization and highly interdependent economic supply chains.

28.2 **International frameworks and national implementation**

Following several decades of work, three landmark UN agreements were adopted in 2015, offering an opportunity for convergence between them:

- the Sendai Framework for Disaster Risk Reduction (adopted on March 18 2015; UN 2015a),
- Sustainable Development Goals (September) (UN 2014) which will follow on from the Millennium Development Goals of 2000–15, and
- climate change agreements through the United Nations Framework Convention on Climate Change (UNFCCC) (December) (UN 2015b).

The Sendai Framework was adopted by 187 UN member states in March 2015. This framework has an explicit focus on people and their health. Its aim over the next 15 years is:

> The substantial reduction of disaster risk and losses in lives, livelihoods and health and in the economic, physical, social, cultural and environmental assets of persons, businesses, communities and countries.
>
> (UN 2015a: 12)

To achieve this outcome, the Sendai Framework states the following goal:

> Prevent new and reduce existing disaster risk through the implementation of integrated and inclusive economic, structural, legal, social, health, cultural, educational, environmental, technological, political and institutional measures that prevent and reduce hazard exposure and vulnerability to disaster, increase preparedness for response and recovery, and thus strengthen resilience.
>
> (UN 2015a: 12)

Achieving this goal, the implementation and follow-up of this framework require the creation of a conducive and enabling environment as well as 'the enhancement of the implementation capacity and capability of developing countries' (UN 2015a: 12). Seven global targets have been agreed to support the assessment of progress, including reducing global disaster mortality, the number of affected people, disaster damage to critical infrastructure and disruption of basic services, including health facilities, and substantially increasing the availability of and access to multi-hazard early warning systems and disaster risk information and assessments to communities by 2030.

In the Sendai Framework, public health issues were agreed as priorities for local, national, regional, and global partners, and included enhancing resilience of national health systems, developing the capacity of health workers in understanding disaster risk and applying and implementing DRR approaches in health work; improving training capacities in disaster medicine; and supporting and training community health groups in DRR approaches in health programmes, in collaboration with other sectors, as well as through the International Health Regulations (2005) (Box 28.1).

National mechanisms to implement international frameworks are key. In many countries this is via civil contingency mechanisms (see Chapter 3). The UK was the first country to volunteer to be peer reviewed on its disaster preparedness, by international representatives (UNISDR 2013). The review confirmed that the UK had achieved a high level of preparedness, helping national

---

Box 28.1 Health/public health issues identified in the Sendai Framework for Disaster Risk Reduction 2015–2030

- ✦ Enhance the resilience of national health systems, including by integrating disaster risk management into primary, secondary and tertiary health care, especially at the local level; developing the capacity of health workers in understanding disaster risk and applying and implementing disaster risk reduction approaches in health work; and promoting and enhancing the training capacities in the field of disaster medicine; and supporting and training community health groups in disaster risk reduction approaches in health programmes, in collaboration with other sectors, as well as in the implementation of the International Health Regulations (2005) of the World Health Organization (paragraph 30(i)).

- ✦ People with life threatening and chronic disease, due to their particular needs, should be included in the design of policies and plans to manage their risks before, during and after disasters, including having access to life-saving services; (paragraph 30(k)).

- ✦ Enhance cooperation between health authorities and other relevant stakeholders to strengthen country capacity for disaster risk management for health, the implementation of the International Health Regulations (2005) and the building of resilient health systems; (paragraph 31(e)).

- ✦ Promote the resilience of new and existing critical infrastructure, including water, transportation and telecommunications infrastructure, educational facilities, hospitals and other health facilities, to ensure that they remain safe, effective and operational during and after disasters in order to provide live-saving and essential services (paragraph 33(c)).

- ✦ Establish a mechanism of case registry and a database of mortality caused by disaster in order to improve the prevention of morbidity and mortality; (paragraph 33(n)).

- ✦ Enhance recovery schemes to provide psychosocial support and mental health services for all people in need; (paragraph 33(o)).

Reproduced from *Sendai Framework for Disaster Risk Reduction 2015–2030*, by United Nations Office for Disaster Risk Reduction, Geneva, © 2015 United Nations. Reprinted with the permission of the United Nations. Available from: http://www.wcdrr.org/uploads/Sendai_Framework_for_Disaster_Risk_Reduction_2015-2030.pdf, 01 Oct. 2015.

and regional authorities to respond to a variety of disruptive challenges with effective and coordinated crisis management. In many respects, the UK resilience approach showed state-of-the-art innovations, including large-scale use of science to support policy. Close links between the Civil Contingencies Secretariat, the Department of Health, and Public Health England have led to policies and practices such as the Heatwave and the Cold Weather Plans, used across the UK. Monitoring tools for the implementation of recommended measures (e.g. within the health system) have also been established.

The only other country so far to be assessed by peer review is Finland. Proposals are now in place to make this tool widely available for individual countries.

28.3 **Public health aspects**

DRR activities are wide and aim to reduce the impact of disasters on loss of life, injury, or other health consequences, as well as the wider socio-economic-environmental determinants of health, including property damage, loss of livelihoods and services, social and economic disruption, and environmental damage. To build knowledge that can be useful, in this broad, complex landscape, science should be considered in its widest sense to include the natural, environmental, social, economic, health, and engineering disciplines. Scientific capacities should also be interpreted broadly, to include all relevant resources and skills, whether scientific or technical.

Science clearly underpins much health and public health practice, and over the last two decades in many places, evidence-based health and policy movements have grown, leading to improved outcomes for people (Aitsi-Selmi et al. 2015).

28.3.1 **Non-catastrophic disasters**

Not all situations that fit the UNISDR definition of disaster are catastrophic; some are quiet, largely unnoticed, and yet have devastating consequences, needing coordinated and concerted effort on a global scale. We give two examples of major public health disasters: one, an infection; the other, environmental.

28.3.1.1 Communicable disease hazard: congenital rubella

Rubella is a viral infection which spreads from person-to-person through sneezing and coughing. In the early twentieth century, the link between rubella intrauterine infections causing foetal damage, foetal loss, and birth defects (Congenital Rubella Syndrome (CRS)) was largely unrecognized. Rubella was common, mostly infecting children. Outbreaks of rubella are public health disasters: in the 1960s an epidemic swept the world. In the United States alone, approximately 11,000 babies died and 20,000 babies were born with CRS.

A vaccine became available in 1969. The number of countries using rubella-containing vaccine in their national immunization programmes continues to grow, from 83 (44% of 190 World Health Organization (WHO) Member States) in 1996 to 130 (67% of 194) in 2009.

Rubella has been eliminated in the WHO Americas Region, with less than 1 case of CRS per 100,000 births. Their experiences were turned into guidance to support elimination elsewhere. Lessons include:

♦ High-level commitment and partnerships are essential,
♦ Link political commitment with technical strategies,
♦ Use proven surveillance tools,
♦ Recognize outstanding performance by individual countries, and
♦ Provide ongoing training for surveillance staff.

The WHO European Regional Office has targeted the elimination of CRS. However, CRS still affects an estimated 110,000 infants in developing countries each year (Southgate et al. 2013).

28.3.1.2 Environmental hazard: iodine deficiency

The global problem of iodine deficiency disorders (IDD) is caused by dietary deficiency of iodine (Iodine Global Network http://www.ign.org/). While goitre is easily visible, the most devastating disorders are cretinism (characteristic severe mental and growth retardation) and disorders of pregnancy (infertility, miscarriages, low birth weight). All are preventable with a minute daily quantity of iodine, starting before and in early pregnancy, but needed throughout life (Bath et al. 2013). Cretinism remains the commonest preventable cause of mental disability at the global scale. Much international effort by governments, community organizations, health and development agencies and professionals, and salt and food producers has been put into ensuring access to iodized salt in every community. Although about 30% of the world still lives in iodine-deficient regions, much has been achieved. Gross cretinism has largely disappeared, but moderate and mild iodine deficiency still lead to preventable brain damage, with individual and social impacts and consequent diminished material and economic prospects. Questions remain about the role of environmental factors in iodine ecology (Stewart et al. 2003) and the integration of environmental science, including clearer understanding of the pathway of iodine through the environment into the diet, and policy could further improve prevention (Johnson et al. 2003).

28.4 Synergy between public health and DRR: an evidence-based approach

Examples of public health science and DRR working together include taking a health systems approach to embed the management of risk and response to disasters throughout the system, knowledge-sharing through disaster risk management fact sheets, and research into the mental health impacts of disasters and their treatment through psychosocial approaches. Others include joint risk assessments, vaccination, and control of infectious diseases related to disasters, and data collection to provide evidence of the impact on and vulnerability of those with chronic diseases following disasters.

28.4.1 The value of the health systems approach

WHO's 64th World Health Assembly (2011) resolved to strengthen national emergency and disaster management capacities and the resilience of health systems. Health systems can be defined as the structured and interrelated work of all agencies contributing to health within a country, including efforts to influence determinants of health, as well as more direct health-improving activities.

Lessons identified from disasters have not always been collated effectively; essential experience has been forgotten. A holistic health system approach to disaster management has neither been practised nor evaluated (Bayntun 2012). However, the disaster management literature identifies how a strengthened health system can promote resilience and efficient recovery following disasters (Bayntun et al. 2012).

An example of a health-systems-specific issue is power outages. Extreme events (e.g. flooding, strong winds) threaten critical infrastructure. Electricity is the most vital infrastructure service because, without it, most other services will not function, but the impact of power outages on health is poorly understood. They impact access to healthcare, the maintenance of front-line services, and the challenges of community care. In Japan, 65% of disaster base hospitals (hospitals that give disaster support to other hospitals) considered electricity to be their most vital lifeline;

in addition to laboratories, imaging and sterilization, 60% felt that key services (e.g. emergency surgery, haemodialysis) would stop without generator power. Most hospitals have generator backup for eight hours but, in longer power outages, could face limited and difficult fuel supplies, particularly if transportation and communication services are also disrupted (Okamoto and Suginaka 2013).

28.4.2 Disaster risk management fact sheets

To address significant impacts on people's health, including loss of life, WHO/UNISDR and the Health Protection Agency (predecessor to Public Health England) developed a series of Disaster Risk Management for Health Fact Sheets (WHO 2012), written as an introduction for health workers engaged in disaster risk management and for multi-sectoral partners to consider how to integrate health into their disaster risk management strategies.

Disaster risk management is placed in the context of multi-sectoral action, and focuses on the generic elements which apply across various health domains, including potential hazards, vulnerabilities of a population, and their wider public health and cross- and inter-sectoral capacities. On two sides of one sheet, an easy-to-read document addresses key points, including why the topic is important, health risks, and risk management considerations. References and further reading are provided. Issues addressed include chemical safety; child health; climate risk management; communicable diseases; people with disabilities and older people; mass casualty management; mass fatalities/dead bodies; mass gatherings; mental health; non-communicable disease; nutrition; radiation emergencies; safe hospitals prepared for emergencies and disasters; sexual and reproductive health; and water, sanitation, and health. Although each fact sheet is a stand-alone, since all health domains are interlinked, each should be read as part of one complete set.

28.4.3 Mental health impacts following disasters

Requirements to enhance psychosocial support and mental health services for everyone in need are included in the Sendai Framework. Member States have agreed to: 'Enhance recovery schemes to provide psychosocial support and mental health services for all people in need' (paragraph 33(o)).

Extreme events and disasters can cause great stress (e.g. triggering short-term fear of death and mental health disorders) (Williams and Drury 2011). People's abilities to rebuild, recover, and adapt following disasters are determined by their own physical, psychological, and social characteristics, and the characteristics of support received. Primary stressors inherent in many disasters include injuries sustained or witnessing someone die. Secondary stressors, such as a lack of financial assistance, the gruelling process of submitting an insurance claim, parents' worries about their children, and continued lack of infrastructure, can manifest their effects shortly after a disaster and persist for extended periods of time, hence should not be overlooked (Lock et al. 2012). There is a clear difference between distress and mental disorders following a disaster. The thresholds are difficult to define; the pathways are complex and need further research.

28.5 Conclusions

In order to reduce disaster risk and public health impacts, there is a need to address existing challenges and prepare for future ones by focusing on: monitoring, assessing, and understanding disaster risk; sharing such information and how it is created; strengthening disaster risk governance and coordination across relevant institutions and sectors and the full and meaningful participation of relevant stakeholders at appropriate levels. In addition, there is a need for focusing on: investing in the economic, social, health, cultural, and educational resilience of individuals, communities, and countries and in the environment, also through technology and research;

enhancing multi-hazard early warning systems, preparedness, response, recovery, rehabilitation, and reconstruction. The recent Zika virus outbreak and its effects on pregnant women around the world is another reminder that challenges are continuously emerging (PHE 2015). The devastating sequelae of the West African Ebola outbreak of 2014 are a similar, more sombre reminder.

To support the capacity development and knowledge transfer requests by UN member states to support their own national capacity, there is a need to enhance international cooperation between developed and developing countries and between states and international organizations.

The Sendai Framework for Disaster Risk Reduction provides the mandate for this work, particularly in its linking to the Sustainable Development Goals (September 2015) and the climate change agreements through the United Nations Framework Convention on Climate Change (UNFCCC) (December 2015).

References

Aitsi-Selmi A, K Blanchard, D Al-Khudhairy, et al. 2015. *UNISDR STAG 2015 Report: Science is Used for Disaster Risk Reduction.* http://preventionweb.net/go/42848 (accessed 8 March 2016).

Bath SC, CD Steer, J Golding, et al. 2013. Effect of inadequate iodine status in UK pregnant women on cognitive outcomes in their children: results from the Avon Longitudinal Study of Parents and Children (ALSPAC). *Lancet*, 382(9889): 331–37.

Bayntun C. 2012. A health system approach to all-hazards disaster management: a systematic review. *PLOS Currents Disasters*, 1. doi:10.1371/50081cad5861d

Bayntun C, G Rockenschaub, V Murray. 2012. Developing a health system approach to disaster management: a qualitative analysis of the core literature to complement the WHO toolkit for assessing health-system capacity for crisis management. *PLOS Currents Disasters*, 1. doi:10.1371/5028b6037259a

Johnson CC, FM Fordyce, AG Stewart. 2003. *Environmental Controls in Iodine Deficiency Disorders: Project Summary Report.* Commissioned Report. Keyworth, Nottingham: British Geological Survey.

Lock S, GJ Rubin, V Murray, et al. 2012. Secondary stressors and extreme events and disasters: a systematic review of primary research from 2010–2011. *PLOS Currents Disasters*, 1. doi:10.1371/currents.dis. a9b76fed1b2dd5c5bfcfc13c87a2f24f

Okamoto K, H Suginaka. 2013. Impact of prolonged electrical power failure on hospital function by a disaster. *Prehospital and Disaster Medicine*, 28: s45.

Public Health England (PHE). 2016. *Zika virus: updated travel advice for pregnant women.* https://www.gov.uk/government/news/zika-virus-updated-travel-advice-for-pregnant-women (accessed 27 April 2016).

Southgate RJ, C Roth, J Schneider, et al. 2013. *Using Science for Disaster Risk Reduction.* www.preventionweb.net/go/scitech (accessed 8 March 2016).

Stewart AG, J Carter, A Parker, et al. 2003. The illusion of environmental iodine deficiency. *Environmental Geochemistry and Health*, 25(1): 165–70.

UN. 2014. *UN Sustainable Development Knowledge Platform. Outcome Document—Open Working Group on Sustainable Development Goals.* http://sustainabledevelopment.un.org/content/documents/4518SDGs_FINAL_Proposal%20of%20OWG_19%20July%20at%201320hrs.pdf (accessed 8 March 2016).

UN. 2015a. *Sendai Framework for Disaster Risk Reduction 2015–2030.* http://www.wcdrr.org/uploads/Sendai_Framework_for_Disaster_Risk_Reduction_2015-2030.pdf (accessed 8 March 2016).

UN. 2015b. *Twenty-first Session of the Conference of the Parties and the Eleventh Session of the Conference of the Parties Serving as the Meeting of the Parties to the Kyoto Protocol.* UNFCCC COP 21/CMP 11.

United Nations International Strategy for Disaster Reduction (UNISDR). 2009. *Terminology.* http://www.unisdr.org/we/inform/terminology#letter-d (accessed 8 March 2016).

UNISDR. 2012. *Disaster impacts 2000–2012.* http://www.preventionweb.net/files/31737_20130312disaster20002012copy.pdf (accessed 8 March 2016).

UNISDR. 2013. *United Kingdom Peer Review Report 2013: Building Resilience to Disasters: Implementation of the Hyogo Framework for Action (2005–2015)*. http://www.unisdr.org/files/32996_32996hfaukpeerreview20131.pdf (accessed 8 March 2016).

World Health Organization (WHO), Public Health England (PHE), UNISDR. 2012. *Humanitarian Action. Disaster Risk Management for Health Fact Sheets.* http://www.who.int/hac/techguidance/preparedness/factsheets/en/ (accessed 8 March 2016).

WHO Europe. 2012. *Strengthening Health-system Emergency Preparedness. Toolkit for Assessing Health-system Capacity for Crisis Management. Part 1. User manual.* http://www.euro.who.int/__data/assets/pdf_file/0008/157886/e96187.pdf (accessed 8 March 2016)

Williams R, J Drury. 2011. Personal and collective psychosocial resilience: Implications for children, young people and their families involved in war and disasters. In D. T. Cook & J. Wall (Eds.), *Children and Armed Conflict: Cross-disciplinary Investigations.* Basingstoke, UK: Palgrave Macmillan, pp. 55–75.

Further reading

International Strategy for Disaster Reduction. 2007. *Guidelines for National Platforms for Disaster Risk Reduction.* http://www.unisdr.org/files/601_engguidelinesnpdrr.pdf (accessed 8 March 2016).

World Health Organization International Health Regulations. 2005. *Alert, Response, and Capacity Building under the International Health Regulations (IHR),* 2nd edition. http://www.who.int/ihr/publications/9789241596664/en/ (accessed 8 March 2016).

Chapter 29

Sustainability

Richard Jarvis, Angie Bone, and Alex G. Stewart

OVERVIEW

After reading this chapter the reader will be familiar with:
- the key definitions and principles of sustainability,
- the scope of sustainability and its relationship to health protection,
- the contribution of sustainability to the response to climate change and other global threats, and
- the practical actions that should be considered by individuals and groups.

29.1 Key concepts of sustainability in health protection

The concept of 'sustainable development' has gained attention in health protection in the last few years. The idea brings to the fore many issues that affect health and environmental quality now and in the future, linking very local issues and actions with the largest global problems, such as climate change.

There are various definitions of sustainable development. The simplest and most widely accepted definition comes from the World Commission on Environment and Development led by former Norwegian Prime Minister, Gro Brundtland:[1]

> Sustainable development is development that meets the needs of the present without compromising the ability of future generations to meet their own needs.

(WCED 1987)

The terms 'sustainable development' and 'sustainability' are often used interchangeably. Sustainability is the set of conditions that meet current need without compromising the ability of future generations to meet their own needs, while sustainable development is the plan of action required to achieve this.

This definition refers to meeting *needs*, which in public health terms includes the complex interaction of need, supply, and demand and how they apply to groups and populations. The definition also implies that there are limits to:

- resources available within the planet's ecosystem,
- the current state of technology available, and
- the ability of humans to organize themselves to address potential threats.

Sustainable development is usually described by the 'three pillars', which is the interaction of the economy, social equity, and the environment (WCED 1987) (Figure 29.1).

To achieve sustainability all three pillars must be addressed together. For example, an intervention that addresses economic development and the environment but not social equity will generate a viable situation, but may not be fair nor equitable.

There are a variety of perspectives on the relative importance of the three pillars and on the most effective and efficient path to sustainability. Several view Western capitalist economics as the

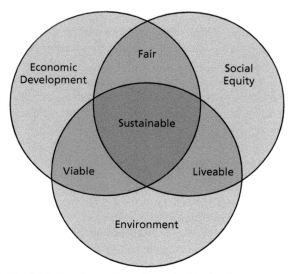

Fig. 29.1 The three pillars of sustainable development

underlying cause of most of the planet's problems and challenge the inclusion of the economy as a pillar. Nevertheless, these viewpoints still rely on some model of economy to achieve sustainability.

29.2 Health protection and public health as components of sustainable development

The relation of sustainable development to public health and health protection can be seen by examining each of the three pillars.

♦ **Environment**: polluting the environment creates source–pathway–receptor linkages with the potential directly to harm human health. Air pollution is a good example of the interaction of environmental sustainability with health protection. There is good evidence that the combustion of fossil fuels, especially from road traffic, releases fine particulates that increase cardiovascular morbidity and mortality (COMEAP 2010). In England, local authorities may designate Air Quality Management Areas as areas of special need due to high levels of atmospheric pollutants, and are required to make plans to improve air quality and take action to prevent its detrimental effects. Other perspectives of sustainable development go further, viewing humans as part of the environment and their health as part of the health of the environment.

♦ **Social equity**: fundamentally unequal societies cannot be sustainable societies, nor can they be healthy; communities that have high social cohesion tend to experience better overall health than those that do not. The evidence shows a direct association between socio-economic status and residence on or near areas of environmental degradation (WHO 2010) in a similar pattern to the association between socio-economic status and health.

♦ **Economy**: two major reports employed economic evaluation on areas of interest to public health. The first, the Wanless Report (2002), was the UK's first assessment of long-term healthcare funding arrangements. The second, the Stern Review (2006), was a review of the economics related to climate change. Despite these reports looking at very different areas, their results were surprisingly similar. Wanless recommended that public health needed investment now in order to prevent much greater healthcare costs later. Stern concluded that the cost of mitigating climate change would be far outweighed by the direct costs of the effects of climate change and attempts to adapt to its effects. Both concluded that it is more expensive to do nothing. Nevertheless, there is limited evidence to date of positive action resulting from these reports.

While links between the three pillars, health protection, and public health may initially appear opaque, it can be seen that sustainability is fundamental to protecting and improving health—in fact, without sustainable development there can be no public health. The importance of sustainable development in achieving good health has been recognized in the English health sector's Sustainable Development Strategy (NHS and PHE 2014).

29.3 **Sustainability and tipping points**

Sustainable development is a means to help humans survive and prosper as a species into the future. This assumes that some existential threat to human survival or life as we know it is coming into play.

Planet earth can be viewed as a closed ecosystem in which everything except solar and gravitational energy is finite. There are a very wide number of components of this ecosystem, such as living things, the chemical and physical environments. Within such systems, a change to one aspect often affects many other components. The Gaia Hypothesis, initially developed by J.E. Lovelock (1972, 1974) suggests that the planet has homoeostatic mechanisms in the same way that living organisms do. These mechanisms normally act to restore equilibrium when a change is made. However, they do not have limitless capacity to adjust and, like physiological mechanisms, may suddenly change to amplify rather than reduce the change once a certain limit is reached. The point at which the change takes place is known as the tipping point.

Tipping points are important because they can be used to predict how much damage we can do to the planet before it becomes irreversible. The first major publication in this area, *The Limits to Growth* (Meadows 1972) made predictions for potential tipping points in human population, industrialization, pollution, food production, and resource depletion using mathematical modelling. Updates have been published at regular intervals and the 40-year update (Bardi 2011) showed that the reality followed the 1972 predictions very closely.

Planetary tipping points are now combined into the wider idea of planetary boundaries as described by researchers at the Stockholm Resilience Centre (Table 29.1). Nine boundaries have been assessed to decide whether the tipping point has been reached or is close to being reached. It therefore defines a 'safe operating space' for humanity. The concept is further developed with a public health and economic perspective to reflect minimum human needs as the 'doughnut of social and planetary boundaries' (Raworth 2012).

It is clear from the planetary boundaries that have been exceeded or are likely to be exceeded in the near future, particularly climate change, that we are living way beyond our means.

Climate change is its own planetary boundary. It is beyond reasonable doubt that anthropogenic carbon emissions have changed the global climate. The general consensus is that global warming of 2°C is now inevitable, irreversible, and requires significant adaptation, as Stern predicts. This has been agreed internationally as a feasible target and is supported by an agreement to reduce carbon emissions be 80% by 2050. Climate change in excess of this (some models are now predicting warming of 4°C or more) would have a wide range of potentially catastrophic effects. These include but are not limited to sea-level rise, loss of agricultural land and desertification, increased frequency and intensity of extreme meteorological events, habitat loss, and increasing rate of mass extinctions. All of these effects compound trends against other planetary boundaries.

Meeting the challenge of climate change is the need and challenge of the current generation. We are already likely to have compromised future generations' abilities to meet their own needs. The consequence of not acting now is that the impacts will become immeasurably worse.

Table 29.1 Planetary boundaries

Planetary boundary	Description	Assessment of tipping point
Climate change	The global CO_2 concentration exceeded 400 ppb in 2014. It is likely to exceed tipping point in the near future. Loss of summer polar sea ice highly likely to be irreversible.	Increasing risk
Biosphere integrity (genetic and functional diversity)	Loss of biodiversity with extinctions. Anthropogenic extinction rates greater than at any time outside the four mass extinctions the planet has experienced.	**Genetic diversity** High risk **Functional diversity** Boundary not yet quantified
Land system change	Human-driven land uses are key contributors to loss of diversity.	Increasing risk
Fresh water use and global hydrological cycle	Beginning to have global level effects, including the availability of drinking water.	Safe
Bio-geochemical flows (nitrogen and phosphorus)	Reactive nitrogen and phosphorus released on large scale due to human activities.	High risk
Ocean acidification	Due to dissolved CO_2.	Safe
Atmospheric aerosol loading	Affects cloud formation and weather system behaviour.	Boundary not yet quantified
Stratospheric ozone depletion	Increases ground level UV exposure.	Safe
Chemical pollution and novel entities		Boundary not yet quantified

Source: data from Raworth K. *A safe and just space for humanity: Can we live within the doughnut?* Oxfam Discussion Papers (Oxford: Oxfam International, 2012), Copyright © 2012 Oxfam International, http://www.oxfam.org/sites/www.oxfam.org/files/dp-a-safe-and-just-space-for-humanity-130212-en.pdf, accessed 01 Oct. 2015; Stockholm Resilience Centre. (2015) *Quantitative evolution of the boundaries*, http://www.stockholmresilience.org/21/research/research-programmes/planetary-boundaries/planetary-boundaries/about-the-research/quantitative-evolution-of-boundaries.html, accessed 18 Nov. 2015.

Not all the planetary boundaries are moving in the wrong direction. In the 1970s it became apparent that stratospheric ozone production was decreasing and that 'holes' in the ozone layer had formed over the poles. There was concern that should this continue it would lead to raised ultraviolet light exposure with a wide variety of negative effects, including increasing incidence of human skin cancer. The cause was identified as anthropogenic chlorofluorocarbons (CFCs), mainly used as refrigerants, which migrate to the stratosphere and catalyse ozone (O_3) to oxygen (O_2). The solution was the global eradication of the use of CFCs as agreed in the 1987 Montreal Protocol. CFC use has dramatically reduced and ozone depletion has reversed. This demonstrates that where there is a clear threat, it can be possible to reach international agreement and to implement a global solution. Attempts to do the same with global warming still prove problematic despite 20+ years of international effort to agree a solution.

29.4 **The health co-benefits of sustainable development**

Actions to improve sustainability or to mitigate or adapt to climate change are often beneficial to health. Positive effects are called 'health co-benefits'.

A frequently described health co-benefit is the positive effect on cardiovascular health from reduced reliance on internal combustion engines for travel. Most trips in the UK are over relatively short distances—a few kilometres at most—and most take place in urban environments and in private cars (Department for Transport 2013). Changing the mode of transport to public mass transport (buses and trains) reduces the carbon dioxide emitted per trip. Changing it to cycling or walking almost eliminates the carbon burden, and has positive benefits in terms of cardiovascular morbidity and mortality through both exercise and reduced levels of fine particulate pollutants, improves mental health, and helps reduce obesity and rates of diabetes mellitus.

Changing our eating preferences and the agricultural practices that serve these preferences can have similar benefits. In the Western world we have a meat-rich diet and this contributes to cardiovascular problems and obesity, and is associated with a variety of cancers. It is also unsustainable in terms of the carbon burden, greenhouse gas emission, and the use of water and land associated with rearing food animals. In particular, cattle produce a lot of methane, which is a potent greenhouse gas, *and* their rearing is particularly carbon-intensive compared to vegetable or fruit growing. Where the ground is fertile enough to support it, growing vegetables and fruit is much more sustainable. If the Western world can change its dietary preferences away from meat and towards a more vegetable- and fruit-based diet it is likely to have health co-benefits in reducing obesity, and reducing both cardiovascular disease and a variety of cancers.

Household energy is a global problem, though for different reasons in the developing and developed world. Most cooking in the developing world is done using wood or kerosene and using makeshift or low efficiency stoves and this is associated with high particulate emissions. Changing to high-efficiency biomass-using stoves that are no more expensive to mass-produce would improve the fuel efficiency, help to move to sustainable fuel sources, and improve health by reducing fine particulates. In the developed world, addressing the problem of cold homes and fuel poverty through improved domestic energy efficiency improvements can have physical and mental health benefits, as well as reduce carbon emissions and contribute to developing a 'green' economy. In 2015, most electricity was still generated by burning fossil fuels (mainly coal) which is not only unsustainable in terms of exploiting fossil fuel resources and the release of carbon dioxide, but is also responsible for a high burden of disease associated with fine particulate emissions. Moving from fossil fuels to renewables for the bulk of electricity generation is key in combating climate change and would lead to major reductions in the burden of cardiovascular and respiratory disease worldwide.

29.5 **Practical local actions**

Most of what we can practically do as public health professionals occurs, and has effects, at the local level. Using the lens of the three pillars allows interventions to be designed that make public health action more sustainable, and/or maximizes the public health co-benefits of sustainable development. The power of groups to deliver sustainability from the ground up and influence decision makers and those in authority should not be underestimated.

Some such contributions of individuals and groups include:

♦ turning electrical devices off when not in use,

♦ reducing travel by using teleconferences and public transport,

♦ walking or cycling whenever possible,

♦ learning how to use the heating/air-conditioning system appropriately,

- reducing, reusing, and recycling materials,
- avoiding unnecessary printing by reading documents on-screen,
- using appliances as long as possible. Repair instead of replace,
- reducing water usage: showers instead of baths; avoiding leaving water running,
- making the most of local suppliers, especially for food, and
- using the stairs instead of the lift if appropriate and possible.

Ideas and solutions are likely to be locally specific, but most of the above can be implemented with minimal effort in every location. A few issues may be beyond an individual's control (e.g. travel policy), but most are not. It is not just about being green, but about balancing our needs to do business in the most economical way. All local organizations and agencies need targets to help focus on sustainability; everyone needs to ask themselves continually what they are doing to improve their contribution to sustainability.

Some specific examples include:

- **'Dr Bike' scheme**: on one of Public Health England's sites with several hundred staff, one staff member ran lunch-hour bike maintenance sessions, supporting and teaching maintenance. This kept more people cycling than otherwise, improving their health through exercise, saving money on transport, and reducing carbon emissions. Social contact improved as well as (work-place) community resilience as a result.
- Access to nature benefits physical and mental health; urban green infrastructure plays a key role in mitigating urban heat and flood risk, improving air quality and social cohesion. **London's Pocket Park programme** is creating or improving 100 areas of greenery, including play spaces, community orchards, green gyms, and wildlife gardens.
- **Sefton Air Quality Management Area**: Sefton is a coastal authority with its main route of access to the port of Liverpool on a steep hill controlled by traffic lights. Lorries leaving the port wait at the lights before accelerating uphill with cold, inefficient, engines, causing high levels of fine particulate and nitrogen oxide pollution. Sefton designated the junction an Air Quality Management Area, which enabled it to install sensors in the roadway to detect lorries (but not cars) before they reach the junction, and change the traffic lights accordingly. Lorries do not idle or accelerate. As a result, air quality has improved and noise has been reduced, to the benefit of the local population and commuters.

29.6 **Conclusions**

Sustainability is fundamental to protecting and improving health and relies on the conglomeration of small individual actions as well as actions by large industries and countries. Public health and health protection are intricately interlinked with all three pillars of sustainability (economic development, environment, social equity) and actions to improve health should support sustainability. Sustainable development can be achieved through meeting current needs without compromising the ability of future generations to meet their needs. While some factors that drive the planet towards irreversible damage are close to the point of no return, there is still much that can be achieved by concerted individual and corporate action.

Note

1. It is not incidental that Gro Brundtland was appointed to lead the World Commission on Environment and Development due to her strong background in science and public health. This emphasizes the importance of public health professionals being prepared to take on political and diplomatic leadership roles.

References

Bardi U. 2011. *The Limits to Growth Revisited*. New York: Springer.

COMEAP. 2010. *Mortality Effects of Long Term Exposure to Particulate Air Pollution in the UK*. London: Health Protection Agency. https://www.gov.uk/government/publications/comeap-mortality-effects-of-long-term-exposure-to-particulate-air-pollution-in-the-uk (accessed 8 March 2016).

Department for Transport. 2013. *National Travel Survey: 2013*. https://www.gov.uk/government/uploads/system/uploads/attachment_data/file/342160/nts2013-01.pdf (accessed 8 March 2016).

Lovelock JE. (1972). Gaia as seen through the atmosphere. *Atmospheric Environment*, **6**(8): 579–80.

Lovelock JE, L Margulis. (1974). Atmospheric homeostasis by and for the biosphere: the Gaia hypothesis. *Tellu, A*, **26**(1–2): 2–10.

Meadows D. 1972. *The Limits to Growth*. London: Signet. http://www.donellameadows.org/wp-content/userfiles/Limits-to-Growth-digital-scan-version.pdf (accessed 8 March 2016).

NHS and Public Health England (PHE). 2014. *Sustainable, Resilient, Healthy People & Places*. Cambridge: Sustainable Development Unit.

Raworth K. 2012. *A Safe and Just Space for Humanity: Can We Live within the Doughnut?* Oxfam Discussion papers. Oxford: Oxfam. http://www.oxfam.org/sites/www.oxfam.org/files/dp-a-safe-and-just-space-for-humanity-130212-en.pdf (accessed 8 March 2016).

Stern N. 2006. *The Economics of Climate Change. The Stern Review*. Cambridge: Cambridge University Press.

Stockholm Resilience Centre. 2015. *Quantitative Evolution of the Boundaries*. http://www.stockholmresilience.org/21/research/planetary-boundaries/planetary-boundaries/about-the-research/quantitative-evolution-of-boundaries.html (accessed 27 April 2016).

United Nations General Assembly. 2005. 2005 World Summit Outcome, Resolution A/60/1, adopted by the General Assembly on 15 September 2005.

Wanless D. 2002. *Securing our Future Health: Taking a Long-term View. Final Report*. London: HM Treasury.

World Commission on Environment and Development. 1987. *Our Common Future*. Oxford: Oxford University Press.

World Health Organization (WHO). 2010. *Environment and Health Risks: A Review of the Influence and Effects of Social Inequalities*. Copenhagen: WHO. http://www.euro.who.int/__data/assets/pdf_file/0003/78069/E93670.pdf (accessed 8 March 2016).

Further reading

Mcoy D. 2014. The science of anthropogenic climate change: what every doctor should know. *BMJ*, **349**: g5178.

Appendices

SIMCARDs for dealing with infectious diseases

Appendix 1.1

Concise SIMCARDs providing information on infections with public health significance in the UK

A1.1.1 **Avian Influenza SIMCARD**

(Not notifiable in the UK)
Respiratory infection caused by virus: avian influenza virus, relatively common strains
include H5N1, H7N7, H7N9, and H9N2.

		Yes/No
1	**Signs & Symptoms:** ■ Consistent with avian influenza (vary depending on viral strain or subtype). ■ Influenza-like illness (may be particularly severe in elderly, and individuals with underlying chronic medical problems): fever, cough, shortness of breath, myalgia, sore throat, coryzal symptoms, conjunctivitis, diarrhoea, vomiting, bleeding from gums, hypoxia, secondary bacterial and fungal infections.	
2	**Incubation Period & Infectivity:** ■ Incubation: 2–8 days (possibly up to 17 days). ■ Person-to-person not common and currently there is no evidence of easy person-to-person spread.	
3	**Mode of Transmission:** ■ Animal reservoirs: birds (especially wild water fowl: ducks, geese). May spread to farmed and domestic poultry, causing large outbreaks in birds. ■ Human infections with avian influenza (H5N1 and H7N9) predominantly associated with close contact with infected live or dead poultry, or person-to-person transmission by respiratory droplets.	
4	**Confirmation (diagnosis):** Clinical ■ Possible case: clinically compatible, with either a) close contact [<1m] with live or dead birds in area of world affected by avian influenza, or b) close contact with human case. ■ Probable: clinically and epidemiologically compatible; infection with influenza subgroup A has been made, but not fully subtyped. Laboratory ■ Confirmed: laboratory confirmed avian influenza, whether or not meets clinical/epidemiological criteria. ■ Nasopharyngeal swab; nasal aspirate or wash; oropharyngeal swab in viral culture media for real-time PCR detection of influenza A and subtyping (discuss with reference lab prior to sending). ■ In individuals with lower respiratory tract symptoms or signs, sputum or bronchioalveolar lavage specimen for PCR. ■ See UK investigation and management algorithm https://www.gov.uk/government/uploads/system/uploads/attachment_data/file/358675/Case_management_of_suspected_human_case.pdf	
5	**Action:** Early Detection; Treatment; Isolation and Infection Control: ■ Ensure implementation of infection control measures. ■ Staff: correctly fitted FFP3 respirator, gown, gloves, and eye protection. ■ Patient location: strict respiratory isolation, preferably in negative pressure room. ■ Establish travel and exposure history (bird contacts, including wild bird markets, poultry, domestic fowl; contact with confirmed or probable cases). ■ Undertake surveillance of close contacts for symptoms for 10 days. ■ Work with animal health authorities to control infection in bird populations. Prophylaxis (Vaccination/immunoglobulin/Antibiotics/Antivirals): ■ Antiviral therapy (e.g. Oseltamivir); supportive therapy as required. ■ Identify close contacts; arrange antiviral chemoprophylaxis (Oseltamivir): guidance: https://www.gov.uk/government/uploads/system/uploads/attachment_data/file/358674/Guidance_note_rationale_for_change_to_Ah7n9_prophylaxis_0.pdf	
6	**Report/Communication:** ■ National and international surveillance systems. ■ Probable media interest warrants preparation of proactive media statements with advice for public about risk of transmission.	
7	**Disease Trends, Clusters, and Significant Situations:** ■ Outbreaks have been associated with exposure to infected birds at wild poultry ('wet') markets in China and Hong Kong; occupational exposure to infected poultry. ■ Potential exists for pandemic spread. Therefore, following notification of first possible/probable case, incident management team should be established as a matter of urgency.	

A1.1.2 *Bacillus cereus* SIMCARD

(Not notifiable in the UK)
But notifiable if food poisoning is suspected.
Gastrointestinal infection caused by bacteria: *Bacillius cereus*.

		Yes/No
1	**Signs & Symptoms:** ■ Food poisoning caused by *B.cereus* can present with vomiting, abdominal pain, and diarrhoea. Symptoms may last 24 hours. ■ Rarely *B.cereus* may cause systemic infections, e.g. following contamination of medical devices by environmental spores.	

2	**Incubation Period & Infectivity:**
	■ *B.cereus* may produce 2 toxins:
	  ● Heat stable 'emetic' toxin may be formed in ingested food, causing vomiting after 3–6 hours (incubation period).
	  ● Heat labile toxin is produced from ingested bacteria in the gut, causing abdominal pain, diarrhoea, and possible vomiting after 6–24 hours of incubation.
	■ Infectivity: No person-to-person transmission.	

3	**Mode of Transmission:** ■ Food can be contaminated by spores from the environment. Spores survive normal cooking temperatures and then germinate in food stored at ambient temperatures. ■ Important reservoirs for foodborne outbreaks include pasta, meatballs and barbecue chicken. Reheated, precooked rice is particularly implicated. ■ Person-to-person transmission does not occur. Contamination of laundry and medical devices/preparations may occur from the environment and lead to infections in immunocompromised patients.	
4	**Confirmation (diagnosis):** Clinical ■ Many cases are presumptively diagnosed on the basis of symptoms and food exposure history. Laboratory ■ Send stool samples from suspected cases for bacterial culture, with appropriate clinical and food history. *B.cereus* may be cultured from suspect foods, but a quantitative bacterial count rather than just bacterial growth is necessary. ■ Rarely, *B.cereus* has been isolated from blood culture.	
5	**Action:** Early Detection; Treatment; Isolation and Infection Control: ■ Standard infection control precautions required. ■ Patient management: Supportive, Ciprofloxacin plus one or two further antibiotics (need multiple antimicrobials) under advice of infectious disease physician. ■ Follow standard investigation for a foodborne outbreak. ■ Recent food history from known suspected cases; look for other cases. Where possible, stool and food samples should be obtained and tested. ■ Suspect food outlets should be visited, and food preparation/environmental health investigations undertaken. ■ Screening of contacts is normally not indicated. Prophylaxis (Vaccination/immunoglobulin/Antibiotics/Antivirals): ■ Not applicable.	
6	**Report/Communication:** ■ Relevant public health bodies should be informed, including local communication departments, of any confirmed incidents or clusters. ■ Press holding statements should be prepared for clusters/outbreaks.	
7	**Disease Trends, Clusters, and Significant Situations:** ■ *B. cereus* food poisoning is a notifiable disease. ■ Any incident (cluster/outbreak) should be managed through an incident management team. ■ Potentially contaminated medical or feeding instruments need to be sampled and appropriate public health actions considered as soon as possible.	

A1.1.3 *Campylobacter* infection SIMCARD

(Not notifiable in the UK)
But notifiable if food poisoning is suspected.
Gastrointestinal infection caused by bacteria: *Campylobacter species [Campylobacter jejuni (common) and Campylobacter coli (less common)]*.

		Yes/No
1	**Signs & Symptoms:** ■ Diarrhoea, cramping, abdominal pain, fever. Diarrhoea may be bloody, and accompanied by nausea and vomiting. Illness typically lasts about one week. Some infected persons have no symptoms. ■ In immunocompromised persons, occasionally spreads to bloodstream, causing life-threatening infection. ■ Acute post-infective demyelination may develop, affecting peripheral nervous system (Guillain-Barré Syndrome), and/or the central nervous system (e.g. Miller-Fisher Syndrome).	
2	**Incubation Period & Infectivity:** ■ Incubation usually 2–5 days (range 1–11 days). ■ Infectivity: Infectious period lasts throughout infection; once symptoms have resolved, risk of transmission is low if good hygiene practised. Average duration of excretion 2–3 weeks (occasionally 2–3 months).	
3	**Mode of Transmission:** ■ Faecal oral route: organism lives in mammal gut, including livestock, pets (dogs, cats). ■ Transmission predominantly via contaminated food (raw or undercooked meat, especially poultry, unpasteurized milk or untreated water). ■ Person-to-person transmission occurs if hygiene is poor and/or the case is faecally incontinent.	
4	**Confirmation (diagnosis):** Laboratory ■ Culture of campylobacter in stool of infected person. (*Campylobacter jejuni* and *C. coli*) ■ Laboratories may use PCR for primary diagnosis. ■ PCR result should be confirmed by stool culture. ■ Strain identification may be requested from reference laboratory.	
5	**Action:** Early Detection; Treatment; Isolation and Infection Control: ■ Antibiotics unnecessary unless severe or prolonged illness. ■ Exclude symptomatic patients from work or school for 48 hours after symptoms resolve. ■ Advice on hand hygiene particularly after using the toilet, handling pets and before eating. ■ No microbiological clearance is required. ■ Liaise with local Environmental Health to investigate source of the infection. Prophylaxis (Vaccination/immunoglobulin/Antibiotics/Antivirals): ■ Not applicable.	
6	**Report/Communication:** ■ Unless there an indication of a cluster/an outbreak no further communication is required by the local public health/health protection team.	
7	**Disease Trends, Clusters, and Significant Situations:** ■ Through surveillance monitoring for clusters/outbreaks: instigate public health measures as indicated.	

A1.1.4 **Carbapenemase-producing Enterobacteriaceae (CPE) SIMCARD**

(Not notifiable in the UK)
Gastrointestinal colonization, occasionally systemic infection, caused by bacteria: carbapenemase-resistant *Enterobacteriaceae.*

		Yes/No
1	**Signs & Symptoms:** ■ Patients colonized with CPE: no specific signs or symptoms. Signs and symptoms of infection depend on the site infected.	
2	**Incubation Period & Infectivity:** ■ Some infections endogenous (patient already colonized). ■ Colonization (in lower bowel) probably occurs 2–4 days after exposure, on ward or in nursing home. ■ Infectivity: any colonized patients potentially infectious. Infected patients may also be infectious from wounds and pressure sores.	
3	**Mode of Transmission:** ■ Main reservoir: colonized patients, although environmental surfaces may become contaminated. ■ Transmission through poor staff hand hygiene, utensils and contaminated toilet areas.	
4	**Confirmation (diagnosis):** Laboratory ■ Screening: stool samples or rectal swabs plus any exit sites (e.g. urinary catheters, intravenous cannulae). ■ Laboratories use special techniques to isolate CPEs; requests must be clearly indicated on screening request form. ■ Take appropriate clinical samples when infection is suspected (rectal swab/stool sample).	
5	**Action:** Early Detection; Treatment; Isolation and Infection Control: ■ Few effective antibiotics; microbiological advice must be obtained. ■ Currently no effective regime for decolonization. ■ Depending on local guidelines, patients may be screened on admission to specific units, or on wards where patients have been exposed to a known case. ■ Screen patients hospitalized outside the UK or transferred from a unit with known CPE cases. ■ Isolate colonized patients; with increasing numbers of patients, ward cohorting with strict infection control is an alternative. ■ No indication to restrict discharge of colonized patients to nursing/residential homes. ■ When clusters occur affecting whole ward or unit, considerations include ward closure to admissions, restriction of discharges to other units/hospitals, more extensive screening. Prophylaxis (Vaccination/immunoglobulin/Antibiotics/Antivirals): ■ Not applicable.	
6	**Report/Communication:** ■ Share information about cases with NHS colleagues and external agencies as necessary. ■ Relevant public health bodies should be informed of any confirmed incidents or outbreaks, including local communications departments. ■ Press holding statements should be prepared for incidents/outbreaks.	
7	**Disease Trends, Clusters, and Significant Situations:** ■ CPE infections not formally notifiable, but laboratories in England report isolates to AMRHAI (Antimicrobial resistance and healthcare associated infections laboratory). ■ Any incident/outbreak should be managed through convening an incident management team or outbreak control team with public health involvement.	

A1.1.5 *Clostridium difficile* (*C. difficile*) SIMCARD

(Not notifiable in the UK)
Gastrointestinal infection caused by bacteria: *Clostridium difficile* (*C. difficile*),
*an anaerobic spore-forming bacterium widely distributed in the intestinal tract
of humans, animals, and in soil.*

		Yes/No
1	**Signs & Symptoms:** ■ Diarrhoea (mostly among elderly in hospital or nursing/residential homes. Also occurs in hospitalized patients on chemotherapy). ■ May rarely lead to pseudomembranous colitis and toxic megacolon.	
2	**Incubation Period & Infectivity:** ■ Incubation probably 48–72 hours, though some patients may be carriers before diarrhoea. ■ Infective while symptomatic; asymptomatic carriers may cause environmental contamination.	
3	**Mode of Transmission:** ■ Faecal-oral, via contaminated utensils, toilet areas, and staff, if inadequate hand hygiene. Spores remain viable in the environment for many months. ■ Reservoir is symptomatic/colonized patients, and contaminated environment.	
4	**Confirmation (diagnosis):** Laboratory ■ Detection of toxin in stool samples from symptomatic patients. ■ Current UK guidelines recommend 2-stage test, comprising a gluteraldehyde (GDH) or PCR test to screen samples for *C. difficile*, followed (if positive) by a toxin ELISA test.	
5	**Action:** Early Detection; Treatment; Isolation and Infection Control: ■ Isolate confirmed cases, either in dedicated side room or in isolation ward. Implement strict enteric precautions and infection control measures. Clean vacated bed space with chlorine-based disinfectant. ■ Following increased incidence in one or more wards: close ward(s) to new admissions; move all symptomatic patients to isolation rooms/unit if available or use affected ward as cohort ward; send positive stool samples for ribotyping to determine if true cluster; maintain strict infection control. ■ After outbreak, decontaminate affected wards with hydrogen peroxide vapour (HPV). ■ Standard therapy is 10 days oral metronidazole, plus fluid maintenance, monitoring of bowel function and abdomen (to detect signs of megacolon). Manage patients by multi-disciplinary team. Certain antibiotics (particularly cephalosporins, fluoroquinolones and clindamycin) associated with infection. Prophylaxis (Vaccination/immunoglobulin/Antibiotics/Antivirals): ■ Not applicable.	
6	**Report/Communication:** ■ Disease not notifiable in UK, but mandatory reporting system for hospital-acquired (>48hrs after admission) cases. ■ Within hospitals, cases should be recorded using regularly audited databases, for timely detection of periods of increased incidence. ■ Clusters or outbreaks in any setting should be reported as soon as identified to the relevant local Public Health officials in the UK.	
7	**Disease Trends, Clusters, and Significant Situations:** ■ *C. difficile* found in intestines of healthy people with no symptoms (about 3% adults, 2/3 babies); causes disease when normal gut bacteria flora disturbed, usually by antibiotic therapy. ■ >80% cases reported in over–65s. Immunocompromised patients also at risk. Children <2 years not usually symptomatic. ■ Strain typing required in investigation of clusters and outbreaks. ■ Ribotype strain 027 particularly associated with outbreaks and increased virulence.	

A1.1.6 **Creutzfeldt–Jakob Disease (CJD) SIMCARD**

(Not notifiable in the UK)

Human transmissible spongiform encephalopathies (TSEs) include *Creutzfeldt–Jakob Disease* (CJD); variant CJD; Kuru and fatal familial insomnia. Prion proteins (PrP) are believed to be the cause of vCJD.

		Yes/No
1	**Signs & Symptoms:** Symptoms and signs consistent with Creutzfeldt–Jakob disease ▪ Ataxia, with myoclonus in later disease. ▪ Personality change, dementia, often rapidly progressive, impaired memory. ▪ Visual disturbance leading to blindness. ▪ Loss of speech and movement. ▪ Repeated respiratory tract infections (pneumonia). ▪ Coma, death. ▪ (Individuals with new variant CJD younger when symptoms present; increased psychiatric symptoms, and slower course of disease progression).	
2	**Incubation Period & infectivity:** ▪ Incubation period: 15 months to >30 years. ▪ Infectivity: No known person-to-person transmission; but the risk from iatrogenic procedures remains.	
3	**Mode of Transmission:** ▪ Caused by neurological accumulation of abnormally-folded prion proteins. ▪ Infection may be: sporadic (about 90%); variant CJD, consumption of infected neurological tissue from cattle; iatrogenic CJD, exposed during medical and surgical procedures (e.g. corneal transplants, neurosurgical instruments pituitary glands, blood product transfusion); inherited.	
4	**Confirmation (diagnosis):** Clinical ▪ Define, probable or possible, categorized on basis of type of illness, results of laboratory investigations and clinical criteria (UK January 2010 Diagnostic Criteria (http://www.cjd.ed.ac.uk/documents/criteria.pdf)). Laboratory ▪ Definitive diagnosis requires neuropathological examination of brain tissue, usually post-mortem. ▪ In suspected cases, use NCJDRSU guidelines to investigate (http://www.cjd.ed.ac.uk/documents/investigations.pdf).	
5	**Action:** Early Detection; Treatment; Isolation and Infection Control: ▪ CJD invariably fatal; no therapies available to slow or reverse disease progression. ▪ Holistic supportive care required. ▪ Refer to UK guidelines (https://www.gov.uk/government/uploads/system/uploads/attachment_data/file/474338/CJD_public_health_action_new_case_301015.pdf) for public health action following report of new case, or increased risk. Objective: to prevent further transmission and ensure surveillance of persons at increased risk. ▪ Review GP records: identify all significant procedures in look-back period. Risks assess each procedure for CJD transmission (see guidance). ▪ Support providers to ensure contaminated instruments are removed from general use (following procedure look back and risk assessment). ▪ Work with providers to identify and agree management of patients possibly exposed and at increased risk. Prophylaxis (Vaccination/immunoglobulin/Antibiotics/Antivirals): ▪ Not applicable.	
6	**Report/Communication:** ▪ Reporting to national and international surveillance systems (e.g. UK: http://www.cjd.ed.ac.uk/surveillance.html). ▪ Clear communication with hospital infection control teams and general practitioners required for prompt, effective response.	
7	**Disease Trends, Clusters, and Significant Situations:** ▪ Potential exists for clusters of CJD related to contaminated medical and surgical instruments. ▪ UK: approximately half-a-million bovine spongiform encephalopathy (BSE) infected cattle entered the food chain prior to 1989 controls. By the end of 2012, 176 cases of variant CJD reported in the UK, all of whom had died. Incidence peaked in 2000.	

A1.1.7 **Cryptosporidiosis SIMCARD**

(Not notifiable in the UK)
But notifiable if food poisoning (definition includes water) is suspected.
Gastrointestinal infection caused by protozoa parasites:
Cryptosporidium hominis (humans), *C.parvum* (humans and animals).

		Yes/No
1	**Signs & Symptoms:** ■ Acute self-limiting diarrhoea, often with cramping abdominal pain. ■ In immunocompromised patients, particularly HIV, the infection has a prolonged and fulminant course.	
2	**Incubation Period & Infectivity:** ■ Incubation period between 1–12 days, average around 7 days. ■ Infectivity: symptomatic patients are infectious, and excretion of infective oocysts may continue for several weeks after symptoms resolve. Asymptomatic infections may occur. ■ Oocysts may remain infective for several months in moist environments.	
3	**Mode of Transmission:** ■ Water-borne from contaminated supplies; and person-to-person faecal-oral. Domestic cats and dogs may act as reservoirs. ■ Contamination of water supplies arises from catchment areas grazed by sheep or cattle, and subsequent use of untreated or inadequately treated water. ■ Inadequate hand hygiene at visitor farms may result in infection. Occasional outbreaks have been associated with swimming pools.	
4	**Confirmation (diagnosis):** Laboratory ■ Microscopy of faecal specimens demonstrating oocysts. ■ Occasionally, diagnosis is made from intestinal biopsy. ■ More sensitive antigen detection tests such as PCR may be available from a reference lab.	
5	**Action:** Early Detection; Treatment; Isolation and Infection Control: ■ No anti-protozoal treatment appropriate for immunocompetent individuals. ■ In household cases advise enteric precautions (hand washing; safe disposal of bodily excretions and contaminated materials; disinfection of all relevant facilities such as sink taps and toilet flush handles; and education and training on personal, domestic and environmental hygiene). ■ Exclusion of cases from school/workplace or other relevant setting for until 48 hours after resolution of symptoms. Clearance samples not required. ■ Cases should not use swimming pools for 2 weeks after end of symptoms. Investigate illness in family contacts. ■ Clusters may be associated with contaminated water supplies, farm visits, or specific locations such as nurseries or swimming pools. If water supply-related, epidemiological investigations involving mapping of cases and working with water supply companies will be required. ■ Boil water notices may be necessary. Prophylaxis (Vaccination/immunoglobulin/Antibiotics/Antivirals): ■ Not applicable.	
6	**Report/Communication:** ■ Not notifiable, but cases should be reported to local public health bodies for further investigation.	
7	**Disease Trends, Clusters, and Significant Situations:** ■ CCDC and Health Protection Teams at PHE through surveillance measures to monitor for clusters/outbreaks and instigate public health measures as indicated.	

A1.1.8 **Diphtheria SIMCARD**

(Notifiable in the UK)

Respiratory (occasionally skin) infection caused by bacteria: *Corynebacterium diphtheria; C. ulcerans;* and *C. pseudotuberculosis.*

		Yes/No
1	**Signs & Symptoms:** ▪ Usually asymptomatic or mild; occasionally severe upper respiratory tract infection, localized skin infection or systemic infection. Bacterial exotoxin can damage other organs. ▪ Initial symptoms frequently non-specific (low-grade fever, malaise, headache), resembling viral upper respiratory tract infection. ▪ Sore throat with pharyngitis, dysphagia and hoarseness, with pseudomembrane (develops locally during infection, e.g. limited to the tonsils, or extending throughout the tracheo-bronchial tract, giving classic bull neck appearance). ▪ Cutaneous diphtheria: indolent, poorly healing ulcers covered with grey membrane, frequently co-infected with other pathogens—e.g. *Staphlycoccus aureus.*	
2	**Incubation Period & Infectivity:** ▪ Incubation period usually 2–5 days (range 2–10). ▪ Without antibiotics, patients can be a source of infection for 2–6 weeks. ▪ Cases no longer infectious after 3 days of antibiotic treatment.	
3	**Mode of Transmission:** ▪ Humans are the only known reservoir. ▪ Transmitted through aerosolized secretions from patients with pharyngeal/respiratory disease; direct contact with skin ulcers can spread infection. ▪ *C. ulcerans* can be spread by infected animals or unpasteurized dairy products.	
4	**Confirmation (diagnosis):** Clinical ▪ Symptoms not diagnostic; toxigenicity vital (laboratory confirmation). Laboratory ▪ Diagnosis based both on culturing organism and demonstrating toxin production; culture takes 48 hours; a variety of molecular techniques can identify organisms and test for toxin-producing capability. Initial isolation carried out in local microbiology department; confirmation by reference laboratory.	
5	**Action:** Early Detection; Treatment; Isolation and Infection Control: ▪ Confirmed or probable case(s) should be isolated in hospital. ▪ Implement appropriate precautions for droplet-borne infection or direct contact. ▪ Non-hospitalized patient should restrict contact with others until 3 days course of antibiotics. Prophylaxis (Vaccination/immunoglobulin/Antibiotics/Antivirals): ▪ Five doses needed: vaccine given at 2, 3, 4 months of age, pre-school and school-leaving booster. ▪ Following completion, >99% develop protective antibodies expected to last many years, if not life-long.	
6	**Report/Communication:** ▪ Diphtheria is notifiable; if toxigenic inform Director of Public Health, relevant local professionals including Infectious Disease physicians; inform national centres.	
7	**Disease Trends, clusters and significant situations:** ▪ National and local disease activity surveillance via NOIDS for trends. Any incident (toxigenic case) should managed by an incident management team.	

A1.1.9 *E.coli* O157 SIMCARD

(Not notifiable in the UK)
But notifiable as a cause of infectious bloody diarrhoea or Haemolytic Uraemic Syndrome (HUS).
Gastrointestinal infection caused by bacteria: *Escherichia. coli* O157, Gram-negative bacterium and the most serious illness is that caused by VTEC (verocytotoxic *E. coli*).

		Yes/No
1	**Signs & Symptoms:** ■ *Symptoms:* from mild diarrhoea to bloody diarrhoea, abdominal pain, vomiting, with or without fever. ■ *Signs:* pallor, rash, reduced urine output, haemolytic uraemic syndrome (HUS).	
2	**Incubation Period & Infectivity:** ■ Incubation 2–10 days. ■ Infective during excretion of pathogen [up to one week (adults); 3 weeks (children)].	
3	**Mode of Transmission:** ■ Transmission is faecal-oral: ingested via food, water, or directly following contact with a contaminated person, environment or various animals.	
4	**Confirmation (diagnosis):** Clinical ■ Abdominal pain (cramps); haemorrhagic colitis with bloody diarrhoea often without fever. ■ HUS with renal failure, anaemia and thrombocytopenia. Laboratory ■ Presumptive case (typical colony morphology on appropriate medium or positive *E.coli* O157 by slide agglutination or latex tests). ■ Confirmed case (confirmation of *E.coli* O157 with genes for vero cytotoxin; serology for *E.coli* O157).	
5	**Action:** Early Detection; Treatment; Isolation and Infection Control: ■ Assess need for hospital admission. ■ Seek specialist advice following single episode of acute bloody diarrhoea in a child. Children, elderly, immunosuppressed patients should have full blood count, urea, electrolytes, lactate dehydrogenase tested to detect possible onset of HUS. ■ Do not administer antibiotics. ■ Notification of case to the local health protection team with the relevant details: name, address, contact details, date of birth, NHS Number, GP, admission date, brief clinical details, date of disease onset; overseas travel, animal or farm contact, nursery or school attended, details of household contacts and their occupation. Public Health Risk Assessment ■ Determine if sporadic case or linked to previously reported case(s), including cases of HUS. ■ Identify potential sources, e.g. foreign travel, farm visit, animal contact, food premises, and social activity. ■ Identify suspect cases within the household or other groups/settings. ■ Decide, in liaison with environmental health and consultant microbiologist, whether there is an ongoing risk to public health. Public Health Advice ■ If case is in gastrointestinal risk group A—D, advise exclusion until microbiological clearance (2 negative faecal specimens 24 hours apart). Group A: those who cannot maintain personal hygiene; Group B: 5 year olds or under attending educational or other settings; Group C: those who prepare or serve food; and Group D: clinical, social care or nursery staff (for further details see Chapter 5). ■ Identify contacts, provide hygiene advice and exclude those in risk groups A—D from work/nursery/school pending microbiological clearance 2 -ve faecal specimen results, i.e., taken at intervals of not less than 24 hours. ■ Visit any suspect source that could pose outbreak risk, e.g. visitor farm, food premises; take immediate action if risk of cross-infection not well controlled. Prophylaxis (Vaccination/immunoglobulin/Antibiotics/Antivirals): ■ Not applicable.	
6	**Report/Communication:** ■ Alert relevant NHS & environmental health colleagues for case finding and identification of source(s). ■ Discuss risk assessment for young children in school as required with head teacher.	
7	**Disease Trends, Clusters, and Significant Situations:** ■ Surveillance by health protection to detect local clusters/outbreaks. ■ Convene an Outbreak Control Team to investigate any clusters/outbreaks.	

A1.1.10 **Fever in the returning traveller SIMCARD**

(Not notifiable in the UK)
But infections such as malaria and VHF that may cause fever in returning travellers are notifiable.

		Yes/No
1	**Signs & Symptoms:** Essential: obtain detailed timeline of travel history, including countries visited, duration of stay, whether urban or rural location, whether malaria prophylaxis taken and appropriate immunizations taken.

Signs—Symptoms	Possible infections*	Geographical areas
Undifferentiated fever	Malaria[1], dengue[2], chikungunya[3], amoebic abscess[1], brucellosis[4]	1. Most tropics 2. S/SE Asia, S America. 3. Sub Saharan Africa, S/SE Asia, Indian ocean, Caribbean, 4. Middle east/N.Africa, 5. Particularly southern Africa. 6. See VHF SIMCARD Appendix 1.1
Fever, rash	Rickettsiae[5], Typhoid,[1] HIV seroconversion[1], (VHF[6])	
Fever, diarrhoea	Typhoid[1], shigella[1], HIV[1], amoebic dysentery[1]	

* Common infectious diseases, but not definitive list; expert clinical infectious disease advice should be sought. | |
2	**Incubation Period & Infectivity:** ■ Determine the time since the patient returned from the tropics, and length of time there to estimate incubation period range, based on date of onset of symptoms and contact with potential source of infection.	
3	**Mode of Transmission:** ■ Vector borne diseases not further transmitted (other than rare blood transfusion incidents) in UK. ■ For suspected typhoid and others with diarrhoea symptoms, faecal-oral is the common mode of transmission.	
4	**Confirmation (diagnosis):** Laboratory Minimum samples to be taken: ■ Blood for malaria film (3 negative films necessary to exclude malaria). ■ Full blood count, full blood sample, serum sample for reference PCR and antibody tests, blood culture. ■ Virology for HIV if appropriate. ■ Stool sample if suspected typhoid or if diarrhoea symptoms.	
5	**Action:** Early Detection; Treatment; Isolation and Infection Control: ■ Most important action for individual patient is to exclude malaria, and arrange appropriate treatment if malaria confirmed. ■ For any confirmed diagnosis of an imported fever, or for patient significantly unwell with an undiagnosed imported fever, contact the regional infectious diseases unit for advice. ***Prophylaxis (Vaccination/immunoglobulin/Antibiotics/Antivirals):*** ■ Depends on the infection, seek specialist advice.	
6	**Report/Communication:** ■ Several imported fevers are notifiable in UK (See appendix 4 for a list of notifiable diseases).	
7	**Disease Trends, Clusters, and Significant Situations:** ■ National collation of imported disease reports may indicate travel areas where there are specific disease risks. ■ World Health Organization (WHO), Centers for Disease Control and Prevention (CDC) Atlanta, Public Health England (PHE) plus other national and international organizations and websites such as NaTHNaC (National Travel Health Network and Centre) contain up to date information about geographical areas with specific disease risks.	

A1.1.11 *Haemophilus influenzae* type b (Hib) invasive disease SIMCARD

(Not notifiable in the UK)
But notifiable as a cause of acute meningitis.
Invasive disease (meningitis and/or septicaemia) caused by bacteria: *Haemophilus influenzae* type b (Hib).

		Yes/No
1	**Signs & Symptoms:** ■ Symptoms: meningism, vomiting, cellulitis, intermittent fever, osteomyelitis, septic arthritis ■ Signs: epiglottitis.	
2	**Incubation Period & Infectivity:** ■ Incubation: exact period unknown but probably between 2–4 days. ■ Infectivity: while organisms present and individuals can carry the bacteria in their nose and throat without showing symptoms.	
3	**Mode of Transmission:** ■ Caused by particular encapsulated serotype of *H. influenzae*. ■ Humans only reservoir; spread through direct contact with respiratory and throat secretions.	
4	**Confirmation (diagnosis):** Clinical ■ Possible case: Isolation of *Haemophilus influenzae* from normally sterile site in case without signs of epiglottitis. ■ Probable: Epiglottitis, *Haemophilus influenzae* isolated from normally sterile site. ■ Confirmed: Clinical diagnosis; *H. influenzae* type b (Hib) isolated from normally sterile site. NB: Hib conjunctivitis is not considered invasive disease. Laboratory ■ A positive culture from blood, cerebrospinal fluid, sterile site aspirate (e.g. joint, pleural, pericardial, peritoneal fluid). ■ Alternatively, *H. influenzae* type b (Hib) antigen detection by latex testing or PCR. ■ Check for alternative diagnoses, e.g. PCR: meningococcal, pneumococcal; viral culture: nasopharyngeal swabs, stool.	
5	**Action:** Early Detection; Treatment; Isolation and Infection Control: ■ Assess for signs of Hib disease, e.g. epiglottitis, and notify health protection team if meningitis suspected or *Haemophilus influenzae* isolated from CSF. ■ Case confidence: Action required if probable or confirmed, not for possible. ■ Hib immunization history should be obtained as soon as possible. ■ Identify vulnerable household individuals: any child <10 years; or, immunosuppressed or asplenic individual of any age. ■ Identify close contacts (household in previous 7 days; boyfriends/girlfriends; sharing dormitory, flat or hospital ward with index case). ■ Attendance at nursery, child-minder, school playgroup, etc. Prophylaxis (Vaccination/immunoglobulin/Antibiotics/Antivirals): ■ Chemoprophylaxis: Rifampicin is antibiotic of choice. ■ Index cases <10 years: chemoprophylaxis should be given before discharge. ■ All household contacts and index cases of any age: chemoprophylaxis if household has vulnerable individual. ■ Vaccination: Consider appropriate *Hib* vaccination, serological testing of index cases <10 years, or cases and contacts with immunosuppression, asplenia, or splenic dysfunction.	
6	**Report/Communication:** ■ Microbiology laboratories should report *Haemophilus influenzae* in blood, or normally sterile site. ■ Inform communications departments of any cases with poor prognosis or death. ■ Prepare press holding statements for clusters.	
7	**Disease Trends, Clusters, and Significant Situations:** ■ Surveillance monitoring for clusters/outbreaks; instigate public health measures as indicated. ■ Two or more cases of invasive disease among nursery or pre-school contacts (staff, children) within 120 days deemed outbreak.	

A1.1.12 **Hepatitis A (HAV) SIMCARD**

(Notifiable in the UK as acute infectious hepatitis)
Viral infection of liver caused by virus: Hepatitis A virus (HAV).

		Yes/No
1	**Signs & Symptoms:** ■ Children: acute onset with non-specific features, including fever, malaise, appetite loss, abdominal discomfort, vomiting, diarrhoea; 30% develop jaundice. ■ Adults: frequently symptomatic; ~70% develop jaundice. ■ Illness duration usually a few weeks; may last 6 months; longer duration in older people. ■ Acute liver failure in 1%, with overall case fatality rate about 0.3%; may be >1% in those aged ≥65.	

2	**Incubation Period & Infectivity:**
	■ Incubation about 28 days (range 15–50 days).
	■ Infectivity:
	  • Maximum from latter half of incubation period (approximately 2 weeks before symptom onset) to 7 days after jaundice onset; and
	  • Asymptomatic patients: during first few days when liver enzymes maximally elevated.
	■ Uncommon viral excretion beyond about 7 days (i.e. after onset of jaundice); may occur in infants and young children up to about 6 months.
	■ No chronic viral excretion.	

3	**Mode of Transmission:** ■ Spread mainly through faecal-oral route; through blood transfusion; and may be transmitted sexually. ■ Humans usual reservoir; occurs in some non-human primates.	
4	**Confirmation (diagnosis):** Clinical and laboratory ■ Appearance of IgM in a patient with compatible illness confirms the diagnosis; IgM appears at the onset of symptoms, lasting about 6 months. ■ IgG appears during convalescent phase, lasting many years; may be lifelong.	
5	**Action:** Early Detection; Treatment; Isolation and Infection Control: ■ Advise index case about good hygiene practices, exclude from work, school or nursery for 7 days after jaundice onset; seek source of infection. Prophylaxis (Vaccination/immunoglobulin/Antibiotics/Antivirals): ■ Offer vaccine to household and sexual contacts seen within 14 days of exposure to index case. ■ Offer Human Normal Immunoglobulin (HNIG) to contacts aged ≥50 years and to those with chronic liver disease. If such household and sexual contacts seen after 14 days but before 8 weeks and multiple exposures have occurred, offer vaccine. ■ Offer HAV vaccine and HNIG to contacts with chronic liver disease seen within 28 days. ■ Advice about food handler and non-household contacts (including where index case in school) should be sought from relevant local public health team. ■ Whole virus, inactivated vaccine available; given as a prime booster, 2-dose schedule with the primary dose given 1–18 months after the first dose; gap depends on vaccine. ■ Efficacy following 2 doses >99%; modelling suggesting antibodies will last at least 25 years in > 99% of vaccine recipients.	
6	**Report/Communication:** ■ Hepatitis A (as acute infectious hepatitis) is notifiable.	
7	**Disease Trends, Clusters, and Significant Situations:** ■ Monitoring of national and local disease activity and trends through surveillance information. Any possible clusters/outbreaks should be managed through establishing OCT.	

A1.1.13 **Hepatitis B disease SIMCARD**

(Notifiable in the UK as acute infectious hepatitis)
Viral infection of liver caused by virus: Hepatitis B virus (HBV).

		Yes/No

1	**Signs & Symptoms:**
	■ Acute infection (none, some or all may be present):
	  • Nausea, vomiting, diarrhoea, abdominal pain, fever, jaundice, abnormal liver enzymes.
	■ Chronic infection:
	  • Symptoms: Liver cirrhosis, hepatocellular carcinoma (may be absent).
	  • History: past blood tests, previous acute symptoms, exposure in high endemnicity country.	

2	**Incubation Period & Infectivity:** ■ Incubation period of 40–160 days, with an average of 60–90 days. ■ Infectivity: the patient is infectious until infection resolves, i.e. HBsAg disappears from the serum.	
3	**Mode of Transmission:** ■ Blood, and other high risk body fluids (semen, vaginal secretions). ■ Sexual, perinatal, household transmission common; other potential blood exposures: tattoos, dialysis, medical procedures.	

4	**Confirmation (diagnosis):**
	Clinical
	■ Acute or chronic:
	  • Suspected case: suggestive history; blood tests – none available other than HBsAg marker.
	  • Confirmed case: full hepatitis B markers available, with symptoms/past history.
	Laboratory
	■ Serology results should be interpreted in conjunction with: the clinical presentation, past medical history, past blood tests, country of origin, travel history and other risk factors.
	■ Acute: HBsAg positive; anti-HBc positive; IgM anti-HBc positive; and anti-HBc negative.
	■ Chronic: HBsAg positive; anti-HepBc positive; IgM anti-HBc negative and anti-HBs negative.	

5	**Action:** Early Detection; Treatment; Isolation and Infection Control: ■ Ensure case informed of diagnosis by responsible clinician. ■ Ensure public health advice given to prevent spread. ■ Obtain full history, request case referred to specialist physician for management, and testing. ■ Test case for other blood-borne viruses, possible referral to sexual health clinic. ■ Ensure case receives written information on condition, and opportunity for personalised advice on preventing spread. ■ Identify, investigate potential sources, e.g. dental practice, tattoo parlour. ■ For newly diagnosed chronic cases: in liaison with responsible clinician contacts need to be followed up like acute case. The case should also be provided with written immunization advice to protect against: pneumococcal disease, hepatitis A, and influenza. Prophylaxis (Vaccination/immunoglobulin/Antibiotics/Antivirals): ■ Identify contacts with high risk exposure in last 7 days (unprotected sex): urgently (within 48hrs of exposure) arrange immunoglobulin (HBIG), vaccine, baseline blood test. Give HBIG up to 7 days after exposure, vaccine any time; delays reduce effectiveness of both. ■ Identify other contacts: arrange vaccine, baseline blood test as soon as possible. ■ If case pregnant, arrange for baby to be vaccinated (and HBIG if indicated) at birth; further vaccines and blood tests as per national guidance.	
6	**Report/Communication:** ■ If common source suspected, notify appropriate authorities to undertake further investigation. ■ Any potential cluster/outbreak inform Director of Public Health and communication team.	
7	**Disease Trends, Clusters, and Significant Situations:** ■ Investigate further, monitor for clusters and outbreaks and convene outbreak control team promptly and implement required measures as appropriate.	

A1.1.14 **Hepatitis C SIMCARD**

(Notifiable in the UK as acute infectious hepatitis)
Viral infection of liver caused by virus: Hepatitis C virus (HCV) genotypes 1–7.
HCV genotype 1 is commonest in Europe and North America.

		Yes/No
1	**Signs & Symptoms:** ■ Most (possibly 75%) acute infections thought to be asymptomatic: in remainder, flu-like symptoms, fatigue, jaundice, dark urine and pale stools, with loss of appetite, nausea, vomiting, abdominal pain and arthralgia are usual. ■ Where symptomatic, duration of illness generally 2–12 weeks.	
2	**Incubation Period & Infectivity:** ■ Incubation usually 6–8 weeks (range 2 weeks to 6 months). ■ Infectivity believed to be higher in last 3 weeks of first 6 months of infection, when exponential doubling of viral replication occurs.	
3	**Mode of Transmission:** ■ Blood borne virus: transmission occurs in unsafe injecting practices, inadequate sterilization of medical equipment, contaminated blood and blood products. Can be spread sexually and vertically from infected mother to child. ■ UK: injecting drug use most important risk factor for transmission. ■ Believed to be human-only pathogen.	
4	**Confirmation (diagnosis):** Clinical and Laboratory ■ Diagnosis of acute infection often not possible because of asymptomatic nature of most infections and overlap between acute and chronic infection. ■ Diagnosis of acute infection more likely when: • Known risk factors for disease present, • Positive HCV antibody and HCV-RNA tests, • Negative anti HAV-IgM and anti-HBc IgM tests, and • Elevated alanine aminotransferase (ALT) levels and blood tests in the previous 12 months showing negative HCV antibody and HCV-RNA tests and normal ALT levels. ■ Diagnosis of chronic HCV infection based on demonstrating persistently positive HCV antibody and HCV-RNA tests for longer than 6 months.	
5	**Action:** Early Detection; Treatment; Isolation and Infection Control: ■ The case should be provided with information to prevent onward transmission, i.e., as per transmission routes. ■ The case should be referred for specialist assessment and treatment. Prophylaxis (Vaccination/immunoglobulin/Antibiotics/Antivirals): ■ No vaccine available against HCV.	
6	**Report/Communication:** ■ Hepatitis C (as acute infectious hepatitis) is notifiable.	
7	**Disease Trends, Clusters, and Significant Situations:** ■ Monitoring national and local disease activity and trends through surveillance. ■ Any incident should be managed by incident management team.	

A1.1.15 **Hepatitis E SIMCARD**

(Notifiable in the UK as acute infectious hepatitis)
Viral infection of liver caused by virus: Hepatitis E virus (HEV) genotypes 1–4.
HEV genotype 4 is commonest in Europe.

		Yes/No
1	**Signs & Symptoms:** ■ Presents with fatigue, loss of appetite, nausea, vomiting, abdominal pain, jaundice, arthralgia, pruritus, dark/brown urine, pale stools. ■ Features vary with genotype; clinical disease increases in frequency and severity with age. ■ Generally mild, self-limiting; can lead to fulminant infection with acute liver failure causing death; women in last trimester of pregnancy and older individuals have higher case fatality rates. ■ Co-infection of young children with Hepatitis A causes more severe disease, with increased incidence of acute liver failure. Immunosuppressed individuals can develop persistent infection, with failure to clear virus and chronic liver disease. ■ Asymptomatic infection relatively common; possibly more frequent than symptomatic disease.	
2	**Incubation Period & Infectivity:** ■ Incubation around 40 days (range 15–60). ■ Infectivity period unknown.	
3	**Mode of Transmission:** ■ Several transmission routes; epidemiological importance varies between industrialized and non-industrialized countries: may relate to infecting genotype or environmental conditions (poor sanitation) or both. ■ In less-industrialized countries (including UK travellers), transmitted by human faecal contamination of food, water; extensive drinking water associated outbreaks commonly reported; outbreaks from consumption of raw/undercooked shellfish. ■ In industrialized countries: sporadic disease common; probably dietary: consumption of undercooked contaminated animal products: pig, raw pork, game meat, shellfish. ■ Person-to-person spread within families in industrialized countries uncommon. ■ Also transmitted from infected mother by perinatal route. ■ Documented parenteral spread: blood transfusions, solid organ transplants..	

4	**Confirmation (diagnosis):**
	Clinical
	■ Symptoms non-specific (fatigue, malaise, loss of appetite, nausea, vomiting, abdominal pain).
	■ Difficult to differentiate from Hepatitis A or B.
	Laboratory
	■ IgM and IgG detection plus HEV RNA testing on plasma or serum.
	■ HEV RNA detection on stool samples.
	■ IgM alone not diagnostic; additional IgG antibody and HEV RNA testing needed to confirm.
	■ Acute HEV infection confirmed by one of:
	  • HEV IgM and IgG positive.
	  • HEV RNA positive (with or without detectable HEV antibodies).
	■ Chronic HEV infection confirmed by:
	  • HEV RNA persisting for at least 3 months (with or without detectable HEV antibodies).	

5	**Action:** Early Detection; Treatment; Isolation and Infection Control: ■ Supportive treatment; in most cases, clears uneventfully. ■ Individuals with persistent infection may require intervention. ■ Although person-to-person spread is thought low in UK, improving personal hygiene is important. ■ Advise index case about good hygiene; exclude from work, school or nursery for 7 days after jaundice onset; seek source of infection. ■ Use enhanced surveillance questionnaire to collect key information from clinician or patient. ■ Advise on enteric precautions, including good personal hygiene. Prophylaxis (Vaccination/immunoglobulin/Antibiotics/Antivirals): ■ No vaccine available against HEV.	
6	**Report/Communication:** ■ Acute infectious Hepatitis is notifiable.	
7	**Disease Trends, Clusters, and Significant Situations:** ■ Monitor national and local disease activity and trends through surveillance.	

A1.1.16 Invasive Group A streptococcal (iGAS) infection SIMCARD

(Notifiable in the UK)
Invasive disease caused by bacteria: Group A streptococcal infection *(Streptococcus pyogenes)*.

		Yes/No
1	**Signs & Symptoms:** ■ Symptoms: toxic shock syndrome, necrotizing fasciitis, bacteraemia, peritonitis, puerperal sepsis, osteomyelitis, septic arthritis, myostitis, surgical site infection. ■ Signs: localized pain, localized inflammation, fever, shock.	
2	**Incubation Period & Infectivity:** ■ Incubation period: 1–3 days (up to 7 days). ■ Infectivity: 2–3 weeks for untreated sore throat. Treatment with penicillin reduces infectivity within 48 hours.	
3	**Mode of Transmission:** ■ Direct contact: blood, body fluids, infected tissues. ■ Droplet exposure: respiratory secretions, splashes with blood, body fluids.	
4	**Confirmation (diagnosis):** Clinical and Laboratory ■ *Group A Streptococci* (also known: *Streptococcus pyogenes)* isolated from sterile site, or from non-sterile site along with severe clinical presentation. ■ Possible sites indicating iGAS: blood, tissues, wound swabs, aspirates, exudate, or pus positive for *Group A Streptococci.* ■ All samples consistent with iGAS should be sent to reference lab for further typing. ■ It is best practice to store all *Group A Streptococci* samples (in-patients, perinatal patients, neonates, immediately post-discharge) for 6 months for retrospective outbreak investigation.	

5	**Action:**
	Early Detection; Treatment; Isolation and Infection Control:
	■ Check lab result, clinical presentation consistent with iGAS.
	■ Check patient receiving appropriate antibiotics.
	■ Check patient isolated (minimum: 24 hours after commencing antibiotics). Isolate high risk cases until microbiological clearance obtained.
	■ Ensure staff access to appropriate infection prevention and control guidance.
	Identify contacts:
	■ Anyone with prolonged close contact with case in household-type setting: 7 days before onset; includes: living and/or sleeping in same household; pupils in same dormitory; boy/girlfriends; and students sharing kitchen in hall of residence.
	■ Healthcare workers (and others) with direct exposure to eyes, nose, mouth or non-intact skin by respiratory droplets, wound exudate, blood, body fluids potentially infected with *Group A Streptococci.*
	■ High risk exposures include: resuscitation, post mortem, abscess drainage, tissue debridement without wearing personal protective equipment (including facial protection); inoculation injuries; caring for person with necrotizing fasciitis.
	Action for Contacts
	■ Give written information; advise to seek medical advice if any symptoms in next 30 days.
	■ Any contact suspected of iGAS: urgent hospital referral.
	■ Assess if case is healthcare associated or part of outbreak.
	Prophylaxis (Vaccination/immunoglobulin/Antibiotics/Antivirals):
	■ Recommend antibiotics to:
	  • Mother and baby if either develops iGAS in first 28 days of life.
	  • Close contacts with symptoms (sore throat, fever, superficial skin infection).
	  • Entire household if two or more cases within 30 days.
	  • Healthcare workers with high risk exposure: risk assess in liaison with occupational health, microbiologist, or infectious diseases physician to consider indication for prophylactic antibiotics.	

6	**Report/Communication:** ■ iGAS is a notifiable disease and if cluster/outbreak suspected, follow local outbreak plan.	
7	**Disease Trends, Clusters, and Significant Situations:** ■ Cases >48hrs after hospital admission or within 7 days post-discharge: consider healthcare associated. ■ Same timescale for cases in residential/institutional settings. ■ If outbreak suspected, investigate thoroughly; consider mass screening and/or prophylaxis.	

A1.1.17 **Influenza (seasonal) SIMCARD**

(Not notifiable in the UK)
Upper respiratory tract infection caused by virus: influenza types A, B, and C.

		Yes/No
1	**Signs & Symptoms:** ■ Starts abruptly: fever, myalgia, headache, malaise; frequently sore throat, non-productive cough, nasal discharge. ■ Spectrum from asymptomatic illness (1/3 infections), through afebrile coryza, to severe, systemic illness. ■ Complications include: secondary bacterial pneumonia; more rarely: myositis with rhabdomyolysis, aseptic meningitis, encephalitis, encephalopathy, transverse myelitis, Guillain Barré syndrome. Cardiac disease, including myocardial infarctions, thought to be associated with influenza. ■ Complications more likely with existing co-morbidity, including chronic lung, heart, kidney, liver, neurological diseases, diabetes, immunosuppression, asplenia or hyposplenia, pregnancy.	
2	**Incubation Period & Infectivity:** ■ Incubation usually about 2 days (range 1–4). ■ Infectivity: from about 24 hours prior to symptom onset, to 3–5 days after onset (children and immunocompromised: up to 7 days); transmission greater during active disease.	
3	**Mode of Transmission:** ■ Largely respiratory—coughing, sneezing, talking generate viral-laden particles; <5 microns diameter remain in air, inhaled into terminal bronchioles, alveoli: larger particles directly impact conjunctiva, oropharynx. ■ Larger particles may contaminate environmental surfaces; can be transferred on hands, causing infection. ■ Influenza viruses widely disseminated through animals, birds; pigs important in generating pandemic strains when co-infected with human and bird strains.	
4	**Confirmation (diagnosis):** Clinical ■ Generally clinical diagnosis: accuracy variable, seek laboratory confirmation. Laboratory ■ Confirmation from combined nose/throat swab. Sensitivity improved if specimens taken from cases with most recent onset. ■ May be appropriate to consider paired sera; plain clotted sample during acute illness; convalescent specimen minimum 14 days later. If single convalescent sample, take 28 days post onset or post exposure.	
5	**Action:** Early Detection; Treatment; Isolation and Infection Control: ■ Cases should be excluded from school/work/other relevant settings until recovered. ■ Advice on individual patient management includes isolation of patient and implementation of enhanced infection control measures (there is a need for infection control specialist input). Prophylaxis (Vaccination/immunoglobulin/Antibiotics/Antivirals): ■ Control is key public health function and may include use of antiviral drugs plus vaccination of close contacts and at-risk individuals to stop spread. ■ UK: influenza programme with selective and universal components. ■ Selective programme: protection for individuals at higher risk (sub-unit influenza vaccine): 6 months to 64 years with possible co-existing morbidity (above). Healthcare workers, registered carers also offered immunization. ■ Universal programme: live attenuated quadrivalent vaccine (Fluenz tetra nasal spray suspension): infants, children aged 2, 3, 4 years; expected extension of programme to 17 years. All individuals aged 65 years and older (sub-unit influenza vaccine).	
6	**Report/Communication:** ■ Not notifiable in UK; if identified by laboratory, reported to local public health authorities.	
7	**Disease Trends, Clusters, and Significant Situations:** ■ Monitoring national and local disease activity and trends through surveillance. ■ During influenza season, clusters/outbreaks of influenza are common in healthcare and community settings such as care homes and prompt implementation of control measure including antivirals for treatment and prophylaxis (when indicated) is essential.	

A1.1.18 Influenza (pandemic) SIMCARD

(Not notifiable in the UK)
Upper respiratory tract infection caused by virus: influenza types A or B.

		Yes/No
1	**Signs & Symptoms:** ■ Pandemic and seasonal influenza may be caused either by type A or B influenza viruses. ■ Pandemic influenza, as with seasonal influenza, typically starts with an abrupt onset of fever associated with myalgia, headache, and malaise: these features are frequently accompanied by a sore throat, non-productive cough and a nasal discharge. ■ Disease attack rates are substantially higher with pandemic viruses because few people, if any, in the population have existing immunity to the new strain. ■ Pandemic disease is due to the infrequent, periodic emergence of a novel viral variant (antigenic shift), which exhibits such major differences with existing circulating strains, and population antibody immunity is non-existent or extremely limited, and thus the novel virus causes widespread infection.	
2	**Incubation Period & Infectivity:** ■ Incubation period for pandemic influenza is the same as seasonal influenza, usually about 2 days with a range of 1–4 days. ■ Infectivity: pandemic influenza virus is transmissible from about 24 hours prior to the onset of clinical symptoms through to about 3–5 days after disease onset.	
3	**Mode of Transmission:** ■ These features are the same for both pandemic and seasonal influenza viruses. ■ Transmission of pandemic influenza is largely through the respiratory route. Coughing, sneezing and even talking generate viral laden mucous particles of varying sizes leading to respiratory infection or contamination of environmental surfaces where they can be transferred to mucosal surfaces on hands and cause infection.	
4	**Confirmation (diagnosis):** Clinical ■ Influenza is generally a clinical diagnosis but the accuracy is variable and laboratory confirmation should be sought. Laboratory ■ All of the following specimens should be considered: 　• Combined nose/throat swab in virus transport medium. Sensitivity is improved if specimens are taken from cases with the most recent onset of symptoms. 　• In certain circumstances it may also be also be appropriate to consider paired sera—if undertaken, a plain clotted sample should be taken during the acute illness, followed by a convalescent specimen a minimum of 14 days later. If only a single convalescent serum is taken this should be taken 28 days post onset or post exposure.	
5	**Action:** Early Detection; Treatment; Isolation and Infection Control: ■ Pandemic influenza disease is a global and national emergency—appropriate infection control is a key public health function involving a combination of respiratory isolation, use of antiviral drugs and vaccination to control disease spread. Prophylaxis (Vaccination/immunoglobulin/Antibiotics/Antivirals): ■ Pandemic vaccines can only be prepared once the emergent pandemic strain has been identified—hence the importance of ongoing global surveillance. 'Pre-pandemic' vaccines may be prepared based on expert assessment of the likely strain (s) that will appear in the future. ■ Vaccination involves mass programmes using a vaccine against the pandemic strain only since this is the one strain that usually circulates during a pandemic. Because there is little population immunity 2 doses of vaccine may be required for full protection. ■ When indicated antivirals should be used promptly for both treatment and prophylaxis.	
6	**Report/Communication:** ■ Neither pandemic nor seasonal influenza are notifiable diseases, but if identified by laboratory testing, then this should be notified to local public health authorities.	
7	**Disease Trends, Clusters, and Significant Situations:** ■ Public health and health protection authorities monitor local and national disease activity and trends through established surveillance systems.	

A1.1.19 **Legionnaires' disease SIMCARD**

(Notifiable in the UK)
Respiratory infection (pneumonia) or a milder febrile illness (Pontaic fever) caused by bacter a:
Legionella pneumophila. There are 16 serogroups, and serogroup 1 is the commonest cause of Legionnaires' disease.

		Yes/No
1	**Signs & Symptoms:** ■ Most early features are non-specific, including: influenza-like illness, fever, non-productive dry cough, lethargy, muscle and joint aches, diarrhoea. ■ Late features may include: pneumonia, confusion, shortness of breath, renal failure, multisystem illness and sepsis.	
2	**Incubation Period & Infectivity:** ■ Incubation period usually 2–10 days, with a median of 6–7 days, but the range can extend to 19–21 days. ■ Legionnaires' disease is not spread from person-to-person.	
3	**Mode of Transmission:** ■ Transmission of Legionnaires' disease is by the inhalation of droplets or aerosols of water containing Legionella bacteria, although *L. longbeachae* is found in soil and compost. ■ Any situation where contaminated water can be aerosolized has the potential to transmit Legionella and cause outbreaks.	
4	**Confirmation (diagnosis):** Clinical ■ Community-acquired pneumonia, but need to be confirmed by the laboratory. Laboratory ■ A clinical or radiological diagnosis of pneumonia with laboratory evidence of one or more of the following: • Isolation (culture) of *legionella* species from clinical specimens. • The presence of *L. pneumophila* urinary antigen determined using validated reagents/kits. • Detection of *Legionella* spp. nucleic acid (e.g. by PCR) in a clinical specimen. • A positive direct fluorescence (DFA) on a clinical specimen using validated *L. pneumophila* monoclonal antibodies (also referred to as a positive result by direct immunofluorescence (DIF).	
5	**Action:** Early Detection; Treatment; Isolation and Infection Control: ■ Details of the case's activities in the 2 weeks prior to onset of symptoms must be collected as soon as possible. If the case is too ill to provide details, a close family member or a friend can be interviewed. ■ Identify all environmental risk factors and potential sources of infection that the patients may have been exposed to in the 14 days prior to onset. For example, a cooling tower up to 6 kilometres from the patient's home or workplace. ■ Assess which possible sources pose the greatest risk to the public, for example a cooling tower known to have had a prohibition order in its recent history. Arrange for local environmental health officers (EHO's) to follow up on any sites highlighted. Prophylaxis (Vaccination/immunoglobulin/Antibiotics/Antivirals): ■ There is no vaccine against Legionnaires' disease.	
6	**Report/Communication:** ■ Legionnaires' disease is a notifiable disease in the UK and relevant local public health/health protection professionals should be informed and public health investigation initiated. ■ Enhanced surveillance form should be completed and sent to the national surveillance centre.	
7	**Disease Trends, Clusters, and Significant Situations:** ■ Possible sources identified in the 14 day patient history are reviewed to determine the most likely source of infection, and should provide a framework to guide the investigation. ■ Cases of Legionnaires' disease are usually sporadic but outbreaks are associated with contaminated evaporative cooling systems (cooling towers), hot and cold water systems and spa pools.	

A1.1.20 **Listeriosis SIMCARD**

(Not notifiable in the UK)
But notifiable if food poisoning (definition includes water) is suspected.
Systemic infection caused by bacteria: *Listeria monocytogenes*, Gram-positive bacterium.

		Yes/No
1	**Signs & Symptoms:** ■ Non-specific flu-like symptoms. More serious cases can develop septicaemia (tachycardia, hypotension, oliguria, collapse) or meningo-encephalitis. ■ Causes miscarriage in early pregnancy. An infected infant presents with poor feeding, lethargy, respiratory distress. ■ Elderly, immunosuppressed individuals, pregnant women, neonates at greater risk.	
2	**Incubation Period & Infectivity:** ■ Incubation 1–70 days (median 3 weeks). ■ Infectivity: person-to-person transmission (excluding vertical) recognized but rare. ■ Can be transmitted mother to child during pregnancy and childbirth.	
3	**Mode of Transmission:** ■ Ingestion of contaminated ready-to-eat foods: commonly soft cheeses, pate, cooked sliced meats, pre packed sandwiches. ■ Direct transmission from animals or an environmental source.	
4	**Confirmation (diagnosis):** Laboratory ■ Aspirate from sterile sites (blood, CSF, joint pleural, pericardial fluid). ■ PCR (blood or CSF). ■ Surface swabs (skin, ears, eyes, umbilicus) in early neonates. ■ NB: Stool cultures and serological testing unreliable.	
5	**Action:** Early Detection; Treatment; Isolation and Infection Control: ■ If suspected in patients showing signs of sepsis or meningo-encephalitis, arrange urgent admission. ■ No exclusion required (enteric precautions advised for in-hospital patients). ■ Check if case is sporadic or possibly linked to other cases. ■ Review local information on exposure settings plus local and national surveillance. ■ Environmental Health Officer (EHO) needs to visit patient, complete *Listeria monocytogenes* Trawling Questionnaire. May be more appropriate for Infection Prevention & Control Nurse (IPCN) to complete questionnaire if patient is hospitalized. ■ EHO needs to collect any suspect food samples from case's home; for cases possibly acquiring infection in hospital, IPCN should determine foods eaten in hospital, investigate kitchens/food storage, in liaison with EHO. ■ Send completed questionnaire to local health protection and national reference centre. Prophylaxis (Vaccination/immunoglobulin/Antibiotics/Antivirals): ■ Not applicable.	
6	**Report/Communication:** ■ Listeriosis not notifiable in UK. Notification should be made by responsible medical practitioner if food poisoning is suspected.	
7	**Disease Trends, Clusters, and Significant Situations:** ■ Case(s) to be discussed with local microbiologist for further serotyping and phagetyping. ■ Consider incident meeting if preliminary investigations reveal potential source and further exposure of at-risk individuals. ■ Incidents/clusters need to be managed by incident management/outbreak control group with relevant local public health professionals' involvement.	

A1.1.21 Measles SIMCARD

(Notifiable in the UK)
A systemic viral infection caused by: Measles (RNA) virus, genus *Morbillivirus*, family *Paramyxoviridae*.

		Yes/No
1	**Signs & Symptoms:** ■ Infection starts with high fever, runny nose, cough, red watery eyes, sore throat: Koplik spots (small red spots, bluish-white centres) seen in 1/3 patients on buccal mucosa opposite molar teeth. ■ Several days later: rash, first on face, upper neck, spreading over body, reaching hands, feet. Rash lasts 5–6 days, disappears in order it started. Rash appears about 14 days after first exposure. ■ Complications include otitis media, primary viral or secondary bacterial pneumonia, encephalitis, exacerbation of tuberculosis, diarrhoea, keratitis, hepatitis, pancreatitis, myocarditis, subacute sclerosing panencephalitis. ■ May be worse in susceptible infants, pregnant women, and immunocompromised individuals.	
2	**Incubation Period & Infectivity:** ■ The incubation period: 7–14 days (average 10–12 days). ■ Infectivity from about 4 days before to about 4 days after onset of rash.	
3	**Mode of Transmission:** ■ Fifteen minutes of face to face contact sufficient for transmission. Human-only pathogen. ■ Highly infectious; 90% susceptible close contacts develop disease following exposure. ■ Coughing, sneezing, talking generate viral-laden particles; particles <5 microns diameter remain suspended, enter body through terminal bronchioles and alveolar mucosa: larger particles initiate infection through direct contact with oropharyngeal mucosa or conjunctiva.	
4	**Confirmation (diagnosis):** Clinical ■ Frequently clinical; generally unreliable in non-outbreak/non-epidemic situations. ■ In liaison with the reporting clinician, experienced health protection professional will classify case as likely (probable), unlikely (possible) based on clinical assessment plus epidemiological information. ■ Assessment plus case's occupation, location (primary or secondary care), household contacts, local measles epidemiology (other cases) determines actions: https://www.gov.uk/government/uploads/system/uploads/attachment_data/file/322932/National_Measles_Guidelines.pdf Laboratory ■ Laboratory confirmation on oral fluid or serum for IgM, IgG antibodies, +/- measles RNA. ■ Take diagnostic laboratory samples at earliest opportunity; send oral fluid samples by post to national viral reference department (for surveillance).	
5	**Action:** Early Detection; Treatment; Isolation and Infection Control: ■ Confirmed or likely case prompts immediate public health action, for patient and community. ■ Cases should be excluded from school/workplace for 4 days from onset of rash. Prophylaxis (Vaccination/immunoglobulin/Antibiotics/Antivirals): ■ Individual: assess immune status, as MMR vaccination or immunoglobulin may be recommended. Detailed advice on post exposure prophylaxis with immunoglobulin: http://webarchive.nationalarchives.gov.uk/20140714084352/; http://hpa.org.uk/webc/hpawebfile/hpaweb_c/1238565307587 ■ MMR (live attenuated vaccine) can be given to susceptible contacts up to 5 days after exposure to modify/prevent disease. ■ First dose of MMR is normally given at one year of age, second dose age 3–5 years. Second dose overcomes primary vaccine failure (for measles component of MMR, there is 5% primary vaccine failure).	
6	**Report/Communication:** ■ Measles is notifiable in the UK. Detailed information can be found in PHE document - *Measles: guidance, data and analysis*: https://www.gov.uk/government/collections/measles-guidance-data-and-analysis.	
7	**Disease Trends, Clusters, and Significant Situations:** ■ National and local disease activity and trends surveillance. If cluster/outbreak, convene OCT.	

A1.1.22 Meningococcal disease SIMCARD

(Notifiable in the UK)
Invasive meningococcal disease (meningitis, septicaemia or a combination) caused by bacteria:
Neisseria meningitidis, Gram-negative bacterium.

		Yes/No
1	**Signs & Symptoms:** • *Symptoms:* meningism, nausea & vomiting, rash, (symptoms maybe non-specific in infants) • *Signs:* petechial non-blanching rash and/or Kernig's sign.	
2	**Incubation Period & Infectivity:** • Incubation period is 2–5 days. • Infectivity: while organism present in nasopharynx.	
3	**Mode of Transmission:** • Invasive disease caused by Gram-negative bacterium (meningococcus) spreads through exchange of respiratory and throat secretions.	
4	**Confirmation (diagnosis):** Clinical • Possible case: other diagnosis at least as likely. • Probable: most likely diagnosis. • Confirmed: by laboratory tests. Laboratory • Blood: culture, PCR. • Serum on admission, and 2–6 weeks later. • CSF and aspirate from any suspect sterile site: microscopy, culture and sensitivity, PCR. • Nasopharyngeal swab (normally through mouth): bacterial culture. • Where appropriate, check for alternative diagnoses, e.g. test nasopharyngeal swabs, stool for viral culture.	
5	**Action:** Early Detection; Treatment; Isolation and Infection Control: • Arrange urgent admission if petechial non-blanching rash +/- Kernig's sign. • Immediate parenteral antibiotics (iv/im benzylpenicillin: aged ≥10 years: 1.2g; 1–9y 600mg; <1y 300mg); do not delay transfer to complete. • Notify case to local health protection team with relevant details: name, address, contact details (parents/guardian), date of birth, NHS Number, GP, admission date, ward, consultant, brief clinical details (date of onset; nursery/School/College and contact details); names, dates of birth, addresses of overnight contacts (overnight stay in previous 7 days); vaccination history, current antibiotic treatment. Prophylaxis (Vaccination/immunoglobulin/Antibiotics/Antivirals): • Chemoprophylaxis: Ciprofloxacin is antibiotic of choice. • Identify close contacts (household, shared dormitory or kitchen, boy/girlfriend; staff involved in resuscitation without appropriate face protection for droplets); arrange chemoprophylaxis as soon as possible (ideally within 24 hours); can be given up to 4 weeks after onset if reporting delayed. • Arrange prophylaxis for index case if not treated with ceftriaxone. • Consider, arrange appropriate meningococcal vaccinations for cases and contacts (see Chapter 11 for details).	
6	**Report/Communication:** • Inform heads of educational intuitions about cases attending their institutions: send letters to staff, students. • Inform public health communications departments for individual cases with poor prognosis or death with poor prognosis or death. • Prepare press holding statements for clusters/outbreaks.	
7	**Disease Trends, Clusters, and Significant Situations:** • National and local disease activity and trends surveillance. If cluster/outbreaks, convene OCT. • Clusters/Outbreaks may require mass prophylaxis/vaccination for contacts.	

A1.1.23 Middle East Respiratory Syndrome (MERS) SIMCARD

(Not notifiable in the UK)
But as new and emerging infection any suspected case should be notified as soon as possible.
Respiratory infection caused by virus: Coronavirus [Middle East Respiratory
Syndrome (MERS-CoV infection)].

		Yes/No
1	**Signs & Symptoms:** Elicit symptoms and signs consistent with MERS-CoV ■ Upper respiratory tract symptoms. ■ Severe, acute respiratory illness, including: • Breathlessness • Cough • Rapidly progressive pneumonitis • Respiratory failure ■ Shock ■ Multi-organ failure, leading to death (30% of cases)	
2	**Incubation Period & infectivity:** ■ Incubation: 2–13 days (median 5 days). ■ Infectivity: probably while virus in respiratory tract and increases when patient is symptomatic.	
3	**Mode of Transmission:** ■ Animal reservoir young camel (particularly <2years age). ■ Routes of person-to-person transmission are not fully understood, close contact, and healthcare exposure are strongly associated with risk of transmission from infected cases.	
4	**Confirmation (diagnosis):** Clinical ■ Possible case: compatible with clinical description; and with travel to an affected area in the 10 days prior to onset of illness, or prolonged face-to-face contact with someone symptomatic with MERS-CoV infection. ■ Probable: Meeting possible case criteria and negative for seasonal respiratory virus screen. ■ Confirmed: laboratory confirmed. Laboratory ■ Seasonal respiratory virus screen. ■ Respiratory, blood, or stool sample for PCR testing for MERS-CoV.	
5	**Action:** Early Detection; Treatment; Isolation and Infection Control: ■ Consult national guidelines: https://www.gov.uk/government/collections/middle-east-respiratory-syndrome-coronavirus-mers-cov-clinical-management-and-guidance ■ No specific treatment available. ■ Supportive therapy as required. ■ Consult national algorithm and guidelines: https://www.gov.uk/government/publications/mers-cov-public-health-investigation-and-management-of-possible-cases ■ Ensure use of standard barrier, droplet and respiratory precautions are implemented. ■ Establish travel and exposure history (animal contacts, healthcare attendance, contact with confirmed or probable cases) to aid identification of source of infection and mode of transmission. Prophylaxis (Vaccination/immunoglobulin/Antibiotics/Antivirals): ■ At present not applicable, but seek expert advice.	
6	**Report/Communication:** ■ Reporting to national and international surveillance systems. ■ Probable media interest warrants preparation of proactive media statements with advice for public about risk of transmission.	
7	**Disease Trends, Clusters, and Significant Situations:** ■ Since 2012, cases of MERS-CoV have been reported from countries in the Middle East including Jordan, Kuwait, Oman, Qatar, Saudi Arabia, United Arab Emirates and Yemen. Travel-related cases have also been reported in Europe, North Africa, South East Asia, China, North America. Health-care associated outbreak in Republic of (South) Korea in 2015. ■ (For epidemiological update, see http://www.who.int/csr/disease/coronavirus_infections/en/) ■ Clusters and outbreaks of infection (including among health workers and hospital contacts) have occurred in hospitals in Saudi Arabia, United Arab Emirates and South Korea.	

A1.1.24 MRSA (Methicillin-resistant *Staphylococcus aureus*) SIMCARD

(Not notifiable in the UK)

Invasive disease (bacteraemia, pneumonia, joint infection) or minor localized infection (skin, venous ulcer, pressure sores) caused by bacteria: methicillin-resistant *Staphylococcus aureus*.

		Yes/No
1	**Signs & Symptoms:** ▪ Patients colonized with MRSA show no signs or symptoms. ▪ Patients with clinical infections have signs and symptoms according to infected site. ▪ Infections can include bacteraemia, pneumonia, surgical wounds, venous ulcers, pressure sores, bone and joint infections. ▪ Colonization occurs in nose, throat, axilla, perineum, in eczema, and on medical devices, e.g. intravenous lines.	
2	**Incubation Period & Infectivity:** ▪ For many patients, MRSA infection arises from endogenous colonization. ▪ Incubation period: for non-colonized patients, acquisition may occur within 48 hours of exposure to carrier or case. ▪ Infectivity: transmission may occur from any colonized patient, particularly nasal carriers, and those with eczema and discharging wounds.	
3	**Mode of Transmission:** ▪ Major route of transmission from a colonized/infected patient to others via staff hands. This has been one of the main drivers for improved hand hygiene in healthcare settings. ▪ With skin carriers or discharging wounds, MRSA may contaminate the ward environment, leading to a high risk of transmission to other patients.	
4	**Confirmation (diagnosis):** Laboratory ▪ Appropriate specimens should be taken from patients with suspected infections. The laboratory will be able to report a presumptive MRSA result in 24–48 hours. ▪ Rapid screening tests able to provide a result in 2–4 hours are becoming increasingly available. ▪ Patients may be screened for MRSA carriage on admission to hospital, or to high risk units, such as surgery, ITU, and oncology. The nose and perineum are the principal screening sites, but this will depend on local guidelines.	
5	**Action:** Early Detection; Treatment; Isolation and Infection Control: ▪ In hospitals, colonized patients should be decolonized, generally with mupirocin nasal ointment and body washes. ▪ Clinical infections should be treated with appropriate antibiotics, with microbiology advice. Ideally colonized patients should be placed in single rooms with infection control precautions (hand hygiene, aprons etc.). ▪ Where isolation facilities are limited, high shedders such as those with eczema or open wounds should be prioritized. ▪ In the community, decolonization is rarely required, but infections such as pressure sores and venous ulcers should be treated to reduce the risk of bacteraemia. Prophylaxis (Vaccination/immunoglobulin/Antibiotics/Antivirals): ▪ Not applicable.	
6	**Report/Communication:** ▪ MRSA infection is not a notifiable disease, but in UK there is a mandatory reporting system for bacteraemias, in hospitals and the community.	
7	**Disease Trends, Clusters, and Significant Situations:** ▪ Any incident should be managed through convening an incident management team.	

A1.1.25 **Needle Stick (Inoculation Injury) SIMCARD**

(Not notifiable in the UK)
But any suspected blood borne viruses, e.g. acute hepatitis B should be notified
as soon as possible.

		Yes/No
1	**Signs & Symptoms** ▪ Injury with needle, human teeth or sharp object of known or unknown origin; may be contaminated with blood or body fluids. In healthcare settings, handling sharp-containing waste is a major issue. ▪ Risk mainly infection by Blood Borne Viruses: Hepatitis B, Hepatitis C, Human Immunodeficiency Virus (HIV) from infected blood, cerebrospinal fluid, pleural fluid, breast milk, amniotic fluid, vaginal secretions, peritoneal fluids, pericardial fluids, semen, wound exudate, unfixed human tissues, saliva in association with dentistry, other fluids that contain blood. ▪ Other body fluids with minimal risk of transmission include urine, faeces, sputum, tears, sweat, and vomit.	
2	**Incubation Period & infectivity:** ▪ Incubation: Hepatitis B, Hepatitis C, HIV, 2 weeks- 6 months. ▪ Risk from exposure, if source person infected, estimated: Hepatitis B: seroconversion rate of 30%; Hepatitis C: seroconversion rate of 0.5–1.8%; and HIV: seroconversion rate of 0.3%.	
3	**Mode of Transmission:** ▪ Nose, eyes, mouth, non-intact skin contaminated with blood or body fluids; sexual exposure possible. ▪ Indirect contact through contaminated objects, e.g. discarded, used needle. ▪ Direct exposure to blood or body fluids of another person, e.g. blood splashed into eye.	
4	**Confirmation (diagnosis):** Clinical and laboratory ▪ Assess if inoculation injury has occurred. ▪ Injury: skin broken? Mucous membranes, non-intact skin contaminated? ▪ Contaminant: injury site contaminated with blood or body fluids? ▪ Consider known risk factors of (suspected) source. ▪ If known, someone other than recipient should ask their permission for testing for blood borne viruses. However, it is best practice to seek expert advice or incident management team agreement before proceeding with this action.	

5	**Action:**
	Early Detection; Treatment; Isolation and Infection Control:
	▪ Wash injury site; gently encourage injury site to bleed (if appropriate); advise injury recipient not to suck or rub; cover with dressing.
	▪ Ensure any sharp objects are disposed of safely and promptly.
	▪ Assess likely risk from injury; consider injury type, object involved (hollow bore needle holds fluid).
	▪ Consider Hepatitis B immunization status of recipient.
	▪ Refer promptly: Occupational Health, GP, Accident and Emergency.
	▪ Collect baseline bloods for storage.
	▪ Offer follow-up blood tests over next 6 months to ascertain if acquired blood borne virus.
	Prophylaxis (Vaccination/immunoglobulin/Antibiotics/Antivirals):
	▪ Depending on initial risk assessment, may require:
	  • Hepatitis B vaccine booster dose, Hepatitis B vaccine accelerated course.
	  • Hepatitis B immunoglobulin.
	  • HIV antiviral prophylaxis. When indicated, antiretroviral should be initiated promptly within 72 hours for the best chance of success. Further guidance on HIV post-exposure prophylaxis can be found at: https:// www.gov.uk/government/news/hiv-post-exposure-prophylaxisguidance-from-the-uk-chief-medical-officers-expert-advisory-group-on-aids.	

6	**Report/Communication:** ▪ If in workplace, record injury. ▪ Inform Occupational Health/GP to ensure follow up of recipient and donor. ▪ Inform appropriate authorities to prevent reoccurrence (may include: Infection Prevention and Control, Environmental Health, Health and Safety Executive). ▪ Consider safeguarding issues (if appropriate).	
7	**Disease Trends, Clusters, and Significant Situations:** ▪ Rare; can occur if equipment inappropriately re-used, not decontaminated effectively between patients (blood glucose meters/lancets). Healthcare associated incidents and trends need to be monitored regularly and reported to relevant national surveillance scheme. ▪ Be vigilant for similar injuries; if cluster suspected, seek advice promptly from senior colleague.	

A1.1.26 **Norovirus SIMCARD**

(Not notifiable in the UK)
But notifiable if food poisoning (definition includes water) is suspected.
Gastrointestinal infection caused by virus: Norovirus
[Also called as small round structured viruses (SRSV) or Norwalk-like viruses].

		Yes/No
1	**Signs & Symptoms:** ■ *Signs:* forceful vomiting, diarrhoea (usually without blood, or mucous), fever. ■ *Symptoms:* may include headache, nausea, abdominal pain, aching body. ■ In UK, norovirus infection also known as: winter vomiting disease, gastric flu, viral gastroenteritis.	
2	**Incubation Period & Infectivity:** ■ Incubation: 12–48 hours. ■ Infectivity: until full recovery and symptom-free for at least 48hrs; longer excretion possible.	

3	**Mode of Transmission:**
	■ Highly contagious
	  • Direct contact: with faeces or vomit from infected person.
	  • Indirect contact: with surfaces contaminated by faeces or vomit of infected person.
	  • Droplets: dispersed from vomit or faeces of infectious person, those within <1metre radius of person vomiting/having diarrhoea most at risk.
	  • Food: naturally contaminated (e.g. shell fish); contaminated by infectious food handlers.
	  • Water: swimming in or drinking contaminated water.	

4	**Confirmation (diagnosis):** Clinical ■ Sudden onset of vomiting not attributable to another cause (with or without diarrhoea). Laboratory ■ Test faeces or vomit (not all laboratories test vomit). Virus detected by antigen test, PCR; electron microscopy. ■ Laboratory confirmation not always necessary; for uncomplicated cases, clinical diagnosis sufficient.	
5	**Action:** Early Detection; Treatment; Isolation and Infection Control: ■ Maintain good fluid intake and avoiding dehydration is the most important clinical measure. ■ Self-limiting illness, usually resolves within 48–72 hours. ■ All cases should be advised not to return to school/workplace until 48 hours from last episode of diarrhoea or vomiting. Clearance samples not required. ■ Avoid preparing food for others during the infectious period. ■ Provide hygiene advice to individual or family about preventing spread within household: hand hygiene (soap, water), separate hand towels, cleaning of toilet areas and spills. ■ Assess if case part of wider outbreak. Prophylaxis (Vaccination/immunoglobulin/Antibiotics/Antivirals): ■ Not applicable.	
6	**Report/Communication:** ■ Offer information on norovirus, and enteric precautions including hand hygiene. ■ If outbreak suspected, inform infection prevention and control team. If food premises involved, involve environmental health officers. Inform local laboratory. ■ Norovirus outbreak with significant impact on public health, convene OCT and inform: Director of Public Health, media/communications team, microbiologist, reference laboratory.	
7	**Disease Trends, Clusters, and Significant Situations:** ■ Outbreaks common (schools, nurseries, hospitals, hotels, cruise ships, restaurants). Virus has many strains, survives well in environment, transmits readily; host immunity short term, low infective dose can cause illness. ■ It is important to ascertain if transmission is person-to-person, or from food or water source, in order to instigate effective control measures. ■ It is also important to exclude other causes for outbreak, such as bacterial infection or chemical poisoning. Further guidance on managing norovirus outbreaks can be found at: https://www.gov.uk/government/uploads/system/uploads/attachment_data/file/322943/Guidance_for_managing_norovirus_outbreaks_in_healthcare_settings.pdf	

A1.1.27 **PVL: Panton Valentine Leucocidin-producing** *S. aureus* **SIMCARD**

(Not notifiable in the UK)
Severe soft tissue infections caused by a toxin-producing bacteria [can occur in both methicillin sensitive (MSSA) and methicillin resistant S. aureus (MRSA)].

		Yes/No
1	**Signs & Symptoms:** ▪ PVL MSSA and MRSA can cause severe skin and soft tissue infections (SSTIs), abscesses, necrotizing pneumonia, wound infections, osteomyelitis and bacteraemia. ▪ SSTIs may be more painful and severe than the clinical signs might otherwise suggest. Necrotizing pneumonia, which may occur in young adults in the community, is a particularly severe infection with a high mortality.	
2	**Incubation Period & Infectivity:** ▪ Incubation period in cross infection is commonly 2–3 days. ▪ Infectivity: any exposed lesions can be infectious. ▪ Patients may be colonized with PVL MSSA/MRSA (mostly nasal or skin colonization) before infection, or infection may be transmitted from a colonized or clinical case.	
3	**Mode of Transmission:** ▪ Transmission by direct physical contact, or sharing of towels or other household items. Patients with uncovered skin lesions or pneumonia may transmit infection. ▪ In the community transmission occurs in close community settings such as households, sports teams, gyms and military training camps.	
4	**Confirmation (diagnosis):** Clinical ▪ Symptoms not diagnostic. Laboratory ▪ Clinical samples (from abscesses, boils, sputum) and screening samples (anterior nares) should be sent for microscopy and culture with a specific request for PVL detection. ▪ Most laboratories can detect PVL rapidly by molecular methods if S.aureus is cultured. For screening, some laboratories can detect PVL directly from nasal samples.	
5	**Action:** Early Detection; Treatment; Isolation and Infection Control: ▪ Household contacts of a case should be screened, if any are positive, decolonization should be offered to the whole family. ▪ In schools, care homes and other institutions where PVL infections have occurred, decisions on screening and decolonization should be decided locally, preferably by incident control team. ▪ Hospital cases should follow the hospital MRSA policy, with a heightened priority for isolation. Prophylaxis (Vaccination/immunoglobulin/Antibiotics/Antivirals): ▪ No applicable.	
6	**Report/Communication:** ▪ PVL is not a notifiable disease in UK, but laboratories must report all positive isolates to local health protection teams, so case follow-up is undertaken.	
7	**Disease Trends, Clusters, and Significant Situations:** ▪ Incidents/outbreaks need to be managed by incident management/outbreak control team.	

A1.1.28 **Parvovirus B19 SIMCARD**

(Not notifiable in the UK)
A viral infection caused by Parvovirus B19 *(the commonest parvovirus found in humans), also known as erythema infectiosum, fifth disease, or slapped cheek syndrome.*

		Yes/No
1	**Signs & Symptoms:** ■ About 25% asymptomatic. ■ Five clinical syndromes, determined by the patient's age, haematological and immunological status: I. Erythema Infectiosum (fifth disease): mild febrile illness and a later appearing rash ('slapped cheek syndrome') in children. II. An acute and symmetrical arthralgia/arthritis more common in adults, especially females, with or without a rash. III. Failure of red blood cell production (aplastic anaemia) in people with existing blood disorders (e.g. iron deficiency anaemia). IV. Foetal infection may cause a severe anaemia leading to miscarriage, intra-uterine death or non-immune foetal hydrops. V. A temporary interference of erythropoiesis, in immunosuppressed individuals. May result in severe anaemia and death.	
2	**Incubation Period & Infectivity:** ■ Incubation period: usually 4 to 14 days (range: 3 to 20 days). ■ Infectivity for: • Fifth disease, infectivity is thought to be during the acute febrile illness. • Temporary aplastic crises: for about a week after onset. Transmission from chronically infected immunosuppressed individuals may occur over months or years.	
3	**Mode of Transmission:** ■ Inhalation of infectious respiratory droplets, direct contact with infected droplets or saliva, and contaminated fomites; ■ During pregnancy from mother to foetus across the placenta (risk greatest in the first 20 weeks); and ■ Through blood products if these are donated during the (unrecognized) viraemic phase of an acute illness.	
4	**Confirmation (diagnosis):** Clinical ■ Clinical diagnosis unreliable. Laboratory ■ Serology for Parvovirus B19 specific IgM. ■ The absence of IgM excludes acute infection in the 4 weeks prior to the date of testing: however, infection cannot be excluded if testing is undertaken more than 4 weeks after onset. ■ In the first 20 weeks of pregnancy, confirmation of positive serology requires alternative assays—seek expert advice. ■ If a pregnant woman is in contact with a (presumed) Parvovirus B19 infection, the demonstration of specific IgG in her serum without IgM is evidence of existing immunity—seek expert advice.	
5	**Action:** Early Detection; Treatment; Isolation and Infection Control: ■ Widely distributed in community, therefore emphasis on prompt identification and management of vulnerable individuals. ■ For individual cases, exclusion from school or workplace is not advised. Prophylaxis (Vaccination/immunoglobulin/Antibiotics/Antivirals): ■ Not applicable.	
6	**Report/Communication:** ■ Not a notifiable disease.	
7	**Disease Trends, Clusters, and Significant Situations:** ■ Public health and health protection authorities monitor local and national disease activity and trends through established surveillance systems.	

A1.1.29 **Pertussis (whooping cough) SIMCARD**

(Notifiable in the UK)
A respiratory infection caused by bacteria (Bordetella pertussis and parapertussis).

		Yes/No
1	**Signs & Symptoms:** Disease has 3 stages: ■ Stage 1 (catarrhal phase, 1–2 weeks) presents as any common upper respiratory infection with low-grade fever, sneezing, nasal congestion, rhinorrhoea and conjunctival irritation. Towards the end of this stage the individual usually develops an intermittent nocturnal cough. ■ Stage 2 (paroxysmal phase, 1–6 weeks) usually presents as bouts of forceful coughing lasting several minutes—these episodes are more common at night and have a characteristic inspiratory whoop; following paroxysms, the child may vomit. ■ Stage 3 (the convalescent phase, 1 week—3 months) presents with a non paroxysmal chronic cough. ■ Severe complications, including pneumonia, seizures, encephalitis and an increased risk of death.	
2	**Incubation Period & Infectivity:** ■ Incubation period: usually between 7 and 10 days (range: 4 to 21 days, and occasionally as long as 42 days). ■ Infectivity: highly transmissible during the catarrhal phase, and for 3 weeks after the onset of cough.	
3	**Mode of Transmission:** ■ Virus-laden mucous participles generated through coughing, sneezing and talking.	
4	**Confirmation (diagnosis):** Clinical and Laboratory ■ Typical clinical symptoms may provide a probable diagnosis, especially in young children. ■ Diagnosis of whooping cough is based on PCR (nasopharyngeal swabs or aspirates or pernasal swabs), serology or culture. ■ Patients treated with antibiotics are likely to generate false negative results.	
5	**Action:** Early Detection; Treatment; Isolation and Infection Control: ■ Cases should be excluded from school/workplace/other relevant settings for 5 days from starting antibiotics or 21 days from onset of illness if no antibiotic treatment is initiated. Prophylaxis (Vaccination/immunoglobulin/Antibiotics/Antivirals): ■ Early recognition of case(s) in a setting where there is a vulnerable individual (particularly those under 3 months of age), should lead to the prompt implementation of chemoprophylaxis and vaccination to limit further spread i.e., regardless of their immunisation status. ■ Pregnant women and healthcare workers who are more likely to transmit the infection, should also be considered for post-exposure prophylaxis. ■ The primary schedule consists of 3 doses at monthly intervals with a pre-school booster given at 3 years 4 months of age or soon thereafter. ■ In the UK, pregnant women are offered vaccine in every pregnancy between 16–32 gestational weeks (vaccination is probably best offered on or after the foetal anomaly scan at around 20 weeks, and expectant women may still be immunised after 32 weeks, but this may not offer as high a level of passive protection to the baby). ■ Protection following vaccination fades with time.	
6	**Report/Communication:** ■ Notifiable disease.	
7	**Disease Trends, Clusters, and Significant Situations:** ■ Outbreaks may occur among vulnerable individual groups and require outbreak control team management to interrupt transmission.	

A1.1.30 *Pseudomonas* SIMCARD

(Not notifiable in the UK)

Invasive infection occasionally (septicaemia) caused by Gram-negative bacteria, *Pseudomonas spp.* These are widely distributed in the environment. Most infections are caused by *Pseudomonas aeruginosa*, referred to below as *Pseudomonas*.

		Yes/No
1	**Signs & Symptoms:** ■ *Pseudomonas* causes urinary tract infections, infections of venous ulcers and pressure sores, respiratory infections, and occasionally bacteraemia and septicaemia. ■ While there are no specific signs, *Pseudomonas* wound infections may have a characteristic 'musty' odour.	
2	**Incubation Period & Infectivity:** ■ Incubation: Usually 24–72 hours, but varies by infection, and most patients are colonized with *Pseudomonas* prior to infection. ■ Infectivity: patients with open skin lesions and respiratory infections may be infectious via respiratory droplet secretions.	
3	**Mode of Transmission:** ■ Pseudomonas is ubiquitous in the hospital/care home environment, including from taps, sinks and vases of flowers. ■ Transmission may be directly from environmental contact by patients, by healthcare staff from patient-to-patient or from environment to patient, or from *Pseudomonas* containing water used to clean equipment or in ancillary equipment, e.g. humidifiers.	
4	**Confirmation (diagnosis):** Clinical ■ Symptoms are not diagnostic. Laboratory ■ Screening for *Pseudomonas* carriage is not currently recommended (e.g. prior to hospital admission). ■ In suspected infection, specimens should be sent for microscopy and culture. ■ In outbreaks, environmental samples may be appropriate, with guidance from microbiology.	
5	**Action:** Early Detection; Treatment; Isolation and Infection Control**:** ■ Individual cases of clinical infection should be treated with antibiotics guided by sensitivity patterns. ■ In the community, resistance to oral antibiotics often creates difficulties for treatment. It is important to distinguish infection from colonization in catheter urine and wound specimens. ■ Promote hygiene and handwashing. ■ While it is not possible to eradicate from the environment, there are specific guidelines (in UK) for reducing pseudomonas in water supply/distribution systems. Prophylaxis (Vaccination/immunoglobulin/Antibiotics/Antivirals): ■ Not applicable.	
6	**Report/Communication:** ■ Pseudomonas infection is not a notifiable infection in the UK. Outbreaks should be notified to the local public health bodies.	
7	**Disease Trends, Clusters, and Significant Situations:** ■ Incidents/outbreaks need to be managed by incident management/outbreak control group with relevant local public health professionals' involvement.	

A1.1.31 **Rabies SIMCARD**

(Notifiable in the UK)
An acute viral encephalitis caused by viruses of the genus Lyssavirus.

		Yes/No
1	**Signs & Symptoms:** ■ Early stages: headache, fever, malaise, progressing to excitability, hydrophobia, delirium and convulsions ('furious rabies'). ■ May also present with limb and respiratory muscle paralysis ('dumb rabies'). ■ Coma and death within 1–2 weeks. ■ Invariably fatal once symptoms begin.	
2	**Incubation Period & Infectivity:** ■ Incubation period: usually 3–8 weeks after the bite from an infected animal, but may be a few days to several years. ■ Infectivity: Infected animals may be infective from 3–7 days before the onset of symptoms.	
3	**Mode of Transmission:** ■ Transmission occurs through a bite or scratch by mammals (dogs, foxes, wolves, racoons, bats) in endemic area. ■ Case reports of person–to-person transmission through solid organ transplant. ■ Insectivorous bats in UK may carry European bat lyssavirus (EBLV 1, 2) and may rarely cause human disease.	
4	**Confirmation (diagnosis):** Clinical ■ Ante-mortem diagnosis is based mainly on history and clinical presentation. Laboratory ■ While PCR/viral antigen may be investigated in saliva, CSF and tissue biopsy, these are often negative. In many cases, confirmation is only post-mortem from brain tissue.	
5	**Action:** Early Detection; Treatment; Isolation and Infection Control: ■ Undertaking comprehensive risk assessment and providing good public health advice for those travellers to high risk areas is essential. ■ Prophylactic vaccination can be offered to workers and travellers in at-risk situations. Prophylaxis (Vaccination/immunoglobulin/Antibiotics/Antivirals): ■ Following exposure, risk assessment and post exposure prophylaxis (PEP) plan must be implemented:	

Rabies risk based on exposure assessment	Prior no or incomplete immunization	Prior fully immunized
No risk	None	None
Low risk	5 doses rabies vaccine	2 doses rabies vaccine
High risk	5 doses vaccine plus Human rabies immunoglobulin	2 doses rabies vaccine

■ Two inactivated rabies vaccines are available in the UK. For pre-exposure prophylaxis three doses (0, 7, 28 days) are required. If there is ongoing risk a booster is given at 12 months, and thereafter at 3–5 year intervals.

		Yes/No
6	**Report/Communication:** ■ Rabies is a notifiable infection in the UK. ■ Appropriate public health department should be contacted for any suspected case or exposure.	
7	**Disease Trends, Clusters, and Significant Situations:** ■ Incidents of rabies need to be managed by incident management team with relevant local public health professionals' and multi-agency partner involvement.	

A1.1.32 Rash in pregnancy, i.e., exposure to viral rash during pregnancy SIMCARD

(Not notifiable in the UK)

But, exposure to a rash in pregnancy that may be caused by viral infections (rubella, chickenpox, parvovirus B19, measles) may pose significant health risks to the pregnant women and foetus, therefore should be reported to local public health/health protection team.

		Yes/No

1	**Signs & Symptoms:**
	▪ Rash can be classified as:
	  • Vesicular rash: a rash with vesicles (blisters): chickenpox/shingles.
	  • Non-vesicular rash: a rash without vesicles (blisters): measles, rubella, parvovirus B19.
	▪ Identify the trimester and gestation of the pregnant women:
	  • Trimester: 1st 0–12 weeks, 2nd 13–28 weeks, 3rd, 28 weeks to delivery.
	▪ Assess the exposure:
	  • Significant exposure: Direct face-to-face exposure. Being in the same room as someone with a rash illness for 15 minutes or more. If the pregnant woman is immunosuppressed shorter exposures should be considered significant.
	▪ Chickenpox/shingles:
	  • Risk of congenital varicella syndrome is highest in the first 20 weeks of gestation. If the mother develops chickenpox 7 days before/after delivery the neonate may develop severe disseminated haemorrhagic neonatal chickenpox. Increased risk of maternal pneumonia and death after 18 weeks gestation.
	  • Susceptibility: 90% of adults raised in the UK are estimated to be immune.
	▪ Measles:
	  • Severe maternal morbidity, foetal loss and preterm delivery.
	  • Susceptibility: 90% of adults raised in the UK are estimated to be immune but susceptibly varies with age.
	▪ Rubella:
	  • Substantial risk (>90%) of major congenital deformities in first 16 weeks of gestation.
	  • Large majority of UK women immune.
	▪ Parvovirus B19
	  • 9% risk of intrauterine death, 3% risk of hydrops fetalis in the first 20 weeks of gestation.
	  • No increased risk to the mother.
	  • Susceptibility: 60% of adults in the UK are estimated to be immune.
	NB: Other possible causes of rash are not covered in this SIMCARD.	

2	**Incubation Period & Infectivity:** ▪ Chickenpox: 14–16 days (range 10–21 days). ▪ Measles: 10–12 days (range 7–18 days). ▪ Rubella: 14–21 days. ▪ Parvovirus B19: 4–14 days (range 3–20 days).	
3	**Mode of Transmission:** ▪ All spread by respiratory droplets. Chickenpox vesicles also infectious by direct contact.	
4	**Confirmation (diagnosis):** Clinical and Laboratory ▪ Establish gestation and timing, nature and duration of exposure to rash and likelihood person with rash was infectious. ▪ Establish pregnant women's immunity to viruses (vaccination status, self-reported e.g. chickenpox, previous serology e.g. pregnancy booking bloods, testing of stored bloods or new blood sample).	
5	**Action:** Early Detection; Treatment; Isolation and Infection Control: ▪ Early confirmation of exposure to a probable or confirmed case is essential for prompt public health action. Prophylaxis (Vaccination/immunoglobulin/Antibiotics/Antivirals): ▪ Immunoglobulin (chicken pox or measles) may be required to attenuate infection and reduce risk of adverse events to foetus. ▪ Ensure outstanding vaccinations are completed.	
6	**Report/Communication:** ▪ Rubella and measles infections are notifiable. Appropriate public health/health protection professionals should be informed of any suspected case or exposure.	
7	**Disease Trends, Clusters, and Significant Situations:** ▪ Incidence of these viral diseases in pregnancy is very low, but consequences are serious, so relevant public health/health protection authorities need to informed in order to provide appropriate advice and intervention.	

A1.1.33 **Rubella (German measles) SIMCARD**

(Notifiable in the UK)
A systemic viral infection caused by: Rubella virus, member of *Togaviridae*.

		Yes/No
1	**Signs & Symptoms:** ■ Infection in childhood is generally mild with a fever, conjunctivitis, nausea and a rash. ■ Rash (50–80% of cases), starts on the face and neck before progressing down the body, lasting between 1 and 3 days. ■ Post auricular lymphadenopathy (swelling behind the ear). ■ Adults (up to 20%) may develop joint pain in hands. ■ The principal concern is that a pregnant female who develops infection during the first 16 weeks of pregnancy has a 90% chance of passing the virus transplacentally and infecting her foetus. This can cause miscarriage, stillbirth, or congenital rubella syndrome (CRS). CRS may present with microcephaly, cataracts, heart defects, hearing loss. ■ Rubella infection between 16 and 20 weeks has a minimal risk of causing high tone deafness only. Infection after 20 weeks conception carries no documented risk.	
2	**Incubation Period & Infectivity:** ■ Incubation period: usually 14 to 21 days. ■ Infectivity: most infectious between one and 5 days after the appearance of rash. (Virus has been isolated from the throat, faeces and urine up to 14 days).	
3	**Mode of Transmission:** ■ Person-to-person transmission via inhalation and direct contact with respiratory droplets.	
4	**Confirmation (diagnosis):** Clinical ■ Clinical symptoms not diagnostic. Laboratory ■ Confirmed by presence of IgM/IgG in oral fluid, serum, or plasma; PCR of oral fluid, throat swabs, nasopharyngeal aspirate, urine, CSF, amniotic fluid, placenta or foetal tissue.	
5	**Action:** Early Detection; Treatment; Isolation and Infection Control: ■ Exclusion of the case from vulnerable individuals, school or workplace for 4 days after onset of their rash. ■ Babies born with CRS may excrete virus for up to a year after birth; care must be taken to prevent transmission to susceptible individuals. Prophylaxis (Vaccination/immunoglobulin/Antibiotics/Antivirals): ■ Readily preventable by vaccination (virtually eliminated in UK since introduction of MMR vaccine). ■ Live attenuated vaccine given as combined MMR at 12–13 months of age and 3 years and 4 months. ■ Although it is not recommended to administer the vaccine during pregnancy, there has never been any evidence of damage to the fetus from vaccinating the mother during pregnancy.	
6	**Report/Communication:** ■ Notifiable disease. Prompt notification of rubella to local public health/health protection team is required to ensure public health action can be taken promptly.	
7	**Disease Trends, Clusters, and Significant Situations:** ■ Outbreaks may occur among groups with low uptake of MMR vaccination. In the UK, infants with suspected congenital rubella infection should be reported to the National Congenital Rubella Surveillance Programme (directly to the Institute of Child Health or via the British Paediatric Surveillance Unit).	

A1.1.34 **Salmonella (non-typhoidal) infection SIMCARD**

(Not notifiable in the UK)
But notifiable if food poisoning (definition includes water) is suspected.
Gastrointestinal infection (diarrhoeal disease) caused by bacteria: *Salmonella species.*

		Yes/No
1	**Signs & Symptoms:** ■ Diarrhoea, stomach cramps, nausea, vomiting and fever usually lasting from 4 to 7 days. ■ Rarely, may spread from the bowel to other areas of the body causing abscesses or may cause septicaemia (blood poisoning), especially among immunocompromised.	
2	**Incubation Period & Infectivity:** ■ Incubation: 6 to 72 hours. ■ Infectious period varies; cases excrete from a few days to a few months with a median of 5 weeks.	
3	**Mode of Transmission:** ■ Faecal-oral route. ■ Transmission can be person-to-person or animal to person. ■ Transmission can be food or waterborne (ingestion of food or water that has been contaminated with human or animal faeces). ■ Salmonella infections are documented following exposure to exotic pets, especially reptiles (up to 90% of reptiles are salmonella carriers).	
4	**Confirmation (diagnosis):** Clinical ■ Symptoms not diagnostic. Laboratory ■ Confirmation by stool culture. ■ Laboratories may use PCR methods for primary diagnosis (requires culture for confirmation). ■ Reference laboratory typing and genetic sequencing of cultured isolates.	
5	**Action:** Early Detection; Treatment; Isolation and Infection Control: ■ Advice on enteric precautions, particularly hand hygiene. ■ Symptomatic patients should be excluded from work/school for 48 hours after symptoms resolved. ■ No microbiological clearance is required. ■ Establish whether travel related, and identify and screen symptomatic close contacts. ■ In outbreak, identify and manage possible sources. Prophylaxis (Vaccination/immunoglobulin/Antibiotics/Antivirals): ■ Not applicable.	
6	**Report/Communication:** ■ Salmonella (non-typhoid) is not a notifiable infection, but should be notified if food poisoning is suspected.	
7	**Disease Trends, Clusters, and Significant Situations:** ■ Outbreaks are common and are frequently related to contaminated foodstuffs, or pets (e.g. reptiles). ■ Epidemiological investigations and establishment of multidisciplinary outbreak team may be required to identify and manage source. May require regional/national/international collaboration (e.g. if linked to food production chains).	

A1.1.35 **Shigella infection SIMCARD**

(Not notifiable in the UK)
But notifiable if food poisoning (definition includes water) is suspected.
Gastrointestinal infection (diarrhoeal disease) caused by bacteria:
Shigella spp. (S. sonnei, S. flexneri, S. boydii, S. dysenteriae) bacteria.

		Yes/No
1	**Signs & Symptoms:** ■ Diarrhoea, abdominal cramps, fever, nausea, vomiting, headache, malaise. ■ 10–50% develop bloody diarrhoea. ■ Haemolytic uraemic syndrome (*Shigella dysenteriae type 1*)	
2	**Incubation Period & Infectivity:** ■ Range 12 hours to 4 days (usually 1–3 days); *Shigella dysenteriae* can be up to 7 days. ■ Infectious period is mainly during diarrhoeal phase of illness. Cases may excrete for 2–4 weeks and maintain a low level of infectivity.	
3	**Mode of Transmission:** ■ Faecal-oral transmission. ■ Direct person-to-person spread or spread via contaminated food, water and environment.	
4	**Confirmation (diagnosis):** Clinical and Laboratory ■ Symptoms not diagnostic. ■ Stool culture. ■ PCR may be used for rapid diagnosis but confirmation should be done by culture. ■ Confirmatory tests and strain typing can be carried by the reference laboratory.	
5	**Action:** Early Detection; Treatment; Isolation and Infection Control: ■ Hygiene advice; inform and advice contacts about the disease.	

Type of Shigella	Case-Exclusion/clearance	Contacts Exclusion/clearance
sonnei	Exclude until 48 hours after symptoms resolve.	Asymptomatic contact: No exclusion Symptomatic contact: Exclude until 48 hours after symptoms resolve.
flexneri and *boydii*	Not in risk group: Exclude until 48 hours after symptoms resolve. Risk group: Exclude until one negative clearance sample (culture) 48 hours after symptom free or completing antibiotics.	Asymptomatic contact: No exclusion Symptomatic contact not in a risk group: Exclude until 48 hours after symptoms resolve. Symptomatic contact in a risk group: Exclude until 48 hours after symptoms resolve and a negative culture result obtained from specimen collected 48 hours after recovery.
dysenteriae	Not in risk group: Exclude until 48 hours after symptoms resolve Risk group: exclude until 2 negative clearance samples 24 hours apart after symptom free. ■ If negative for Shiga Toxin – consider stepping down to measures for boydii/flexneri.	Asymptomatic contact: No exclusion Symptomatic contact not in a risk group: one sample to be tested. If positive treat as case. Symptomatic contact in a risk group: exclude until 2 negative clearance samples 24 hours apart after recovery ■ If negative for Shiga Toxin –consider stepping down to measures for boydii/flexneri.

		Yes/No
5	Prophylaxis (Vaccination/immunoglobulin/Antibiotics/Antivirals): ■ Not applicable.	
6	**Report/Communication:** ■ Shigella is not a notifiable infection unless food poisoning is suspected. In addition, dysentery should be notified as infectious bloody diarrhoea.	
7	**Disease Trends, Clusters, and Significant Situations:** ■ Relevant public health/health protection authorities undertake surveillance to monitor trends, exceedance, clusters/outbreaks and instigate public health measures as indicated.	

A1.1.36 **Tuberculosis (TB) SIMCARD**

(Notifiable in the UK)
nfection of any organ, but predominately lungs, caused by bacteria: *Mycobacterium tuberculosis.*

		Yes/No

1	**Signs & Symptoms:**
	■ Infection: may be asymptomatic, cause primary progressive systemic illness, or reactive months to years later.
	■ Active disease: fever, night sweats, poor appetite, and weight loss.
	  • Pulmonary TB: prolonged cough, sputum (may be blood-stained), chest pain and shortness of breath. May present as acute pneumonia, especially in immunocompromised patients.
	  • Other symptoms of TB depend on affected body part (e.g. bone, brain, gastrointestinal system, urinary system, lymph nodes etc.).	

2	**Incubation Period & Infectivity:** ■ The incubation period (time to tuberculin conversion) is usually 3–8weeks; the latent period (time to development of disease) may be many decades, but is accelerated in immunosuppressed (e.g. HIV infection). ■ The infectious period is for as long as viable organisms persist in the sputum (sputum smear positive most infectious). Most cases of TB are non-infectious after two weeks of treatment.	
3	**Mode of Transmission:** ■ Respiratory droplet transmission requires prolonged, close contact with sputum-smear positive cases.	
4	**Confirmation (diagnosis):** Clinical ■ Symptoms, and indicative Chest X-ray but need to be confirmed by laboratory tests. Laboratory ■ Microscopy of stained sputum (or other clinical) samples indicates presence of mycobacterial organisms. ■ Culture and drug sensitivity testing (liquid culture may require 2–3 weeks before positivity). ■ Rapid molecular testing (e.g. Xpert MTB/RIF) is becoming increasingly available.	
5	**Action:** Early Detection; Treatment; Isolation and Infection Control: ■ Early diagnosis and treatment essential to preventing transmission. ■ Most cases can be treated at home as become rapidly non-infectious with treatment. ■ If admitted to hospital, untreated suspected pulmonary TB, or drug resistant TB, should be nursed in a negative pressure room. Prophylaxis (Vaccination/immunoglobulin/Antibiotics/Antivirals): ■ Close prolonged contacts of a case should be screened for active disease. Those with immunological evidence of TB infection (latent TB infection) may be offered TB preventive therapy (chemoprophylaxis). ■ UK national programmes promote pre-entry and GP-based screening for latent and active TB for migrants from high TB incidence countries. ■ BCG vaccination of neonates in the UK is offered to babies born in families at higher risk for TB.	
6	**Report/Communication:** ■ Notifiable disease. ■ Occupational health departments of work places and heads of educational institutions should be informed about potentially infectious cases who attend their institutions.	
7	**Disease Trends, Clusters, and Significant Situations:** ■ Clusters may occur in at-risk groups (e.g. homeless) or in congregate settings (e.g. prisons/hostels) and can be investigated using classical and genomic epidemiology. Often challenging to manage and require multidisciplinary input.	

A1.1.37 **Tetanus SIMCARD**

(Notifiable in the UK)
Paralytic and spasmic disease of central nervous system caused by bacterial toxin from:
Clostridium tetani.

		Yes/No

1	**Signs & Symptoms:**
	■ Characterized by muscle rigidity and painful muscle spasms.
	  • Often begin in the jaw muscles ('lock jaw') and/or neck, shoulder and abdomina muscles.
	  • Spasms are triggered by stimuli such as touch, loud noises and bright lights.
	■ As the disease progresses, generalized seizure-like spasms develop.
	■ Autonomic dysfunction (alteration of blood pressure and heart rate).
	■ Death usually from respiratory muscle failure.	

2	**Incubation Period & Infectivity:** ■ Usually 3–21days (range one day to several months). ■ The shorter the incubation period, the more heavily contaminated the wound has been and the worse the prognosis. ■ Not transmitted from person-to-person.	
3	**Mode of Transmission:** ■ Tetanus spores (excreted by animals in faeces) enter the body usually through a penetrating wound and release toxin. ■ Associated with contaminated injecting drug use paraphernalia. ■ (Neonatal tetanus in some developing countries associated with cultural practices of spreading dung on healing umbilicus stump).	
4	**Confirmation (diagnosis):** Clinical ■ Diagnosis made from clinical signs and symptoms, and history of penetrating injury (may not always be apparent). Laboratory ■ Only occasionally possible to isolate bacteria from wound.	
5	**Action:** Early Detection; Treatment; Isolation and Infection Control: ■ Thorough cleaning of wound is essential. Prophylaxis (Vaccination/immunoglobulin/Antibiotics/Antivirals): ■ For tetanus-prone wound (wounds/burns that require surgical intervention but delayed for >6hrs; wounds/burns with a significant degree of devitalized tissue; wounds containing foreign bodies; compound fractures; wounds or burns in patients who have systemic sepsis), human tetanus immunoglobulin should be given for immediate protection, irrespective of the tetanus immunization history of the patient. ■ Tetanus vaccine is not considered adequate for treating a tetanus-prone wound, but it is an opportunity to ensure the individual is protected for future exposure. ■ Tetanus vaccination is provided as part of UK national immunization schedule [5 doses (at 2,3 and 4 months, 4 years, between 13 and 18 years)] are required for full protection. ■ Booster may be required for fully vaccinated adults at ongoing risk of exposure (e.g. travel to area with limited medical facilities). ■ Patients who are immunosuppressed may not be adequately protected, despite having been fully immunized. Therefore, they should be managed as if they were incompletely immunized.	
6	**Report/Communication:** ■ Notifiable disease.	
7	**Disease Trends, Clusters, and Significant Situations:** ■ Large majority of global cases reported from developing countries where expanded programme on immunization not fully implemented and/or infection control procedures not strictly followed. ■ Recent large outbreaks among injecting drug users in Europe.	

A1.1.38 **Toxic Food (Marine) Poisoning SIMCARD**

(Notifiable in the UK)

Toxic poisoning caused by ingestions of fish and shellfish.

	Signs & Symptoms:	Incubation Period & Infectivity:	Mode of Transmission:	Confirmation (diagnosis):
Ciguatera	Flushing, headache, nausea, vomiting, urticaria. Paraesthesia of arms, legs, tongue. Rarely cardiac arrhythmia.	1–4 hours	Consuming fish that have eaten and concentrated toxins produced by dinoflagellates (e.g. Barracuda, snapper, sea bass, moray eel).	History of eating fish known to carry ciguatera toxin. Testing of fish is unreliable.
Scromboid	Skin flushing, pruritus, throbbing headache, dizziness, nausea, vomiting, abdominal cramps, diarrhoea.	10–60 minutes	Ingestion of fish that has been inadequately refrigerated allowing bacteria to multiply and produce high levels of histamine (e.g. tuna, mackerel, herring, sardines, anchovy, mahi-mahi).	Clinical presentation. Histamine level of fish can be tested.
Pufferfish	Perioral paraesthesia, dizziness, nausea. Generalized paraesthesia can develop with numbness, ataxia and ascending paralysis, headache nausea and diarrhoea. In severe cases respiratory paralysis can be fatal.	Within minutes	Ingestion of fish that has concentrated Tetradoxin (concentrated in the viscera of puffer fish, porcupine fish and ocean sunfish).	Clinical presentation and history of eating Pufferfish Toxins in fish can be measured in a specialist laboratory.
Paralytic shellfish poisoning	Parathesia of face, lips and tongue, headache nausea, vomiting and diarrhoea. In severe cases ataxia, decreased mental status, flaccid paralysis and respiratory failure.	30–60 minutes	Consuming shell fish that have eaten and concentrated toxins (Saxitoxin) produced by algae (e.g. Bivalve shellfish or mussels).	Clinical Presentation. Toxins in fish can be measured in a specialist laboratory.

Action:

Early Detection; Treatment; Isolation and Infection Control:

- Suspected cases should be investigated in liaison with the local Environmental Health officers to identify and control the source in order to reduce the chance of other cases.

Prophylaxis (Vaccination/immunoglobulin/Antibiotics/Antivirals):

- Not applicable.

Disease Trends, Clusters, and Significant Situations:

- Public health/health protection authorities should follow up and ascertain if there are other cases and instigate public health measures as indicated.

A1.1.39 Typhoid/Paratyphoid fever (enteric fever) SIMCARD

(Notifiable in the UK)

Potentially fatal systemic febrile illness with diarrhea and rash caused by bacteria
[*Salmonella enterica serovar Typhi* (typhoid) or *S. paratyphi A, B and C* (paratyphoid)].

		Yes/No

1	**Signs & Symptoms:**
	■ Symptoms and signs vary considerably and are determined by the strain and host factors.
	■ First week:
	  • Myalgia, weakness, diffuse abdominal pain (may be severe), constipation,
	  • Stepwise increase in temperature with peaks (reaching to about 39–40°C) and troughs,
	  • Headache,
	  • Dry cough, and/or
	  • Delirium.
	■ Second week:
	  • Rose red maculopapular rash on trunk.
	■ Third to fourth week:
	  • Encephalitis,
	  • Metastatic abscesses,
	  • Reduction of fever by end of third week, and/or
	  • Deterioration with intestinal haemorrhage and bowel perforation, leading to death.	

2	**Incubation Period & Infectivity:** ■ Usually 8–14 days (range: 3 days–1 month) related to infecting dose. ■ Infectious from first week to convalescence (or rarely longer). ■ Up to 10% of untreated patients with typhoid excrete *S typhi* in the faeces for up to 3 months. ■ Between 1% and 4% of cases become chronic *S typhi* carriers (persistence in urine or faeces for >1 year).	
3	**Mode of Transmission:** ■ Faecal-oral transmission: acquired by ingesting food and water contaminated with excreta from acutely ill cases and typhoid carriers.	
4	**Confirmation (diagnosis):** Clinical and Laboratory ■ Symptoms not diagnostic. ■ Culture of faeces, urine, blood, bone marrow, other sterile sites (repeated cultures may be required). ■ Widal test may be unreliable, culture is the mainstay of the diagnosis of typhoid.	

5	**Action:**
	Early Detection; Treatment; Isolation and Infection Control:
	■ Provide hygiene and sanitation advice.
	■ Determine whether travel-related (if not, identify possible source of infection).
	■ Identify and screen (stool samples) symptomatic co-travellers or close contacts.
	■ Provide written advice to other non-symptomatic contacts.
	■ Exclude for 48 hours after resolution of symptoms. If in a risk group (A–D), will require microbiological clearance of stool samples before return to duties (2 negative clearance samples 24 hours apart, 5 days after completion of antibiotics).
	Prophylaxis (Vaccination/immunoglobulin/Antibiotics/Antivirals):
	■ Vaccination should be considered for at-risk travellers to endemic areas.
	■ Two vaccines available:
	  • Oral live attenuated whole bacterial (booster every 5 years).
	  • Injectable subunit polysaccharide vaccine (booster every 2 years).	

6	**Report/Communication:** ■ Notifiable diseases.	
7	**Disease Trends, Clusters, and Significant Situations:** ■ Endemic in many tropical and subtropical countries. ■ Clusters related to acutely ill cases or chronic excreters may be challenging to manage and OCT should be established promptly.	

A1.1.40 *Varicella* (chickenpox) SIMCARD

(Not notifiable in the UK)
A systemic infection caused by bacteria: *Varicella-zoster (VZV) virus.*

		Yes/No
1	**Signs & Symptoms:** ■ Primary infection: chickenpox; reactivation or secondary infection causes zoster (shingles). ■ Chickenpox normally starts with fever, headache, tiredness, loss of appetite. 1–2 days later, characteristic three stage rash appears: • stage one: itchy, red, generalized maculopapular lesions, over several days; • stage two: small fluid-filled blisters (vesicles) develop from papules over day or two; and • stage three: blisters leak, form scabs and crusts, healing over 7–10 days. ■ All three stages can be present together. ■ Disease more severe in adults (especially pregnant women) and immunocompromised; • Complications: secondary bacterial skin infection, primary or secondary pneumonia, encephalitis, septicaemia, toxic shock syndrome.	
2	**Incubation Period & Infectivity:** ■ Usually 14–16 days (range 10–21). ■ Infectivity: from approximately 48 hours before vesicles, to 4–5 days (until all vesicles crusted). ■ Highly infectious: affects most unvaccinated people by adulthood.	
3	**Mode of Transmission:** ■ Respiratory droplets (coughing, sneezing), or direct contact with skin lesions before crusted. ■ Intimate contact: mother, new-born; face-to-face conversation; same room for 15 minutes or more; continuous home contact.	
4	**Confirmation (diagnosis):** Clinical ■ Diagnosis usually clinical: characteristic rash with all three stages present. ■ Breakthrough varicella (chickenpox in immunized individual) usually milder, afebrile, fewer lesions (<50), may remain papular. Laboratory: ■ Laboratory tests available: • PCR identifying VZV in vesicles most sensitive. • IgM ELISA suggests primary infection; not as sensitive as PCR (does not exclude re-activation or reinfection). • Single positive IgG test indicates existing immunity in most, but not all, cases.	
5	**Action** Early Detection; Treatment; Isolation and Infection Control: ■ Immunocompetent adolescent (≥14 years), or adult with severe chickenpox, or at risk of severe chickenpox (e.g. a smoker or on corticosteroids), presenting within 24 hours of rash: consider acyclovir; no evidence acyclovir benefits immunocompetent child. ■ Development of pneumonia, encephalitis, bacterial superinfection of skin lesions: seek specialist advice. ■ Ascertain risk in exposed individual: • If has had chickenpox, or known immune, and/or not had significant exposure, reassure as unlikely to develop chickenpox. • If no history of prior chickenpox, and significant exposure, and immunocompetent, advise may develop chickenpox. If developed chickenpox, should be advised to stay away from school or workplace until all vesicles have crusted over (7–10 days). Prophylaxis (Vaccination/immunoglobulin/Antibiotics/Antivirals): ■ If pregnant, check serological status, refer for immediate specialist advice as may need passive protection with Varicella Zoster Immunoglobulin (VZIG). ■ If healthcare worker, check serological status, refer for immediate occupational health advice. Cases should be excluded from work until all vesicles have crusted over. ■ If neonate, seek immediate specialist paediatric advice. If serology result not available within 48 hours seek specialist advice.	
6	Report/Communication: ■ Chickenpox is not notifiable in the UK.	
7	**Disease Trends, Clusters, and Significant Situations:** ■ Manage as single case; cluster/outbreaks in community or institution—follow local outbreak control plan.	

A1.1.41 *Varicella* (shingles) SIMCARD

(Not notifiable in the UK)

Shingles is a reactivation of a dormant varicella *Varicella-zoster virus (VZV)* that causes chickenpox.

		Yes/No
1	**Signs & Symptoms:** ■ Once chickenpox resolves then the virus (VZV) spreads along sensory nerves to dorsal root ganglia where it remains dormant. What causes VZV reactivation is not known but associated with declining adaptive immunity, which may occur as a result of advancing age, malignancy, drugs or immunosuppressive disease as may occur with HIV infection. Re-exposure to VZV has also been postulated as a cause of shingles. ■ Shingles describes the characteristic, red, painful unilateral rash that occurs along the distribution of a spinal sensory nerve. The rash starts as erythematous papules, which rapidly become vesicular (i.e. blisters) and then pustular: within 7–10 days they crust, by this stage they are usually regarded as non-infectious.	
2	**Incubation Period & Infectivity:** ■ Incubation period: 15- 18 days (range 7–21days), i.e., time between direct contact with shingles skin lesions before they crust and a VZV naïve individual developing chickenpox. ■ Infectivity: direct contact between an exposed skin lesion, i.e. before it crusts over (7–10 days) and a susceptible individual can spread VZV.	
3	**Mode of Transmission:** ■ Shingles is infectious by direct contact, but less so than chickenpox.	
4	**Confirmation (diagnosis):** Clinical and Laboratory ■ Shingles diagnosis is generally based on the history and clinical findings, specifically the appearance and distribution of the rash and associated pain (intense). ■ Laboratory confirmation of VZV infection using PCR is not generally undertaken but may be used in an outbreak situation.	
5	**Action:** Early Detection; Treatment; Isolation and Infection Control: ■ Pustular skin lesions should be covered appropriately, and infection control precaution implemented if these skin lesions are in exposed parts of the body. ■ Recommend exclusion from school/workplace if rash is weeping and cannot be covered, i e., until rash crusts over. Prophylaxis (Vaccination/immunoglobulin/Antibiotics/Antivirals): ■ In October 2013, vaccination with live attenuated Oka/Merck strain varicella zoster vaccine, Zostavax®, was introduced for all 70 year olds, with a catch-up programme for those aged 78 and 79 years of age in the UK. ■ In those aged 70 years and above, vaccine efficacy for reducing shingles occurrence is estimated to be ~ 38% and ~ 67% for reducing post-herpetic neuralgia (PHN). ■ Because shingles vaccine can lead to transmission of vaccine virus, individuals at high risk of complications from VZV exposure should be considered for passive protection with chickenpox immunoglobulin.	
6	**Report/Communication:** ■ Shingles is not a notifiable disease—neither is chickenpox—but relevant public health advice should be sought from local public health/health protection professionals.	
7	**Disease Trends, Clusters, and Significant Situations:** ■ Public health/health protection authorities monitor national and local disease activity and trends through established surveillance systems.	

A1.1.42 **Viral haemorrhagic fevers (VHF) SIMCARD**

(Notifiable in the UK)

Haemorrhagic fever caused by Ebola virus, Marburg virus, Lassa virus, Crimean-Congo haemorrhagic fever virus (CCHF).

		Yes/No

1	**Signs & Symptoms:**
	■ Suspect in any patient returning from endemic areas with fever.
	  • Ebola: Central and west Africa.
	  • Lassa: West Africa.
	  • Marburg: central/southern Africa.
	  • CCHF: rural areas of central Asia, sub Saharan Africa.
	■ Fever, malaise, headache, abdominal pain. Bleeding (haemorrhage) may be uncommon in early stages.	

2	**Incubation Period & Infectivity:** ■ Ebola: 2–21 days. ■ Lassa, Marburg: 6–21 days. ■ CCHF: 1–12 days. ■ Infectivity: while the patient is symptomatic (from the onset of fever until the patient is symptom free).	

3	**Mode of Transmission:**
	■ Reservoirs:
	  • Ebola: Primates (likely exposure through infected bush meat).
	  • Marburg: Bats.
	  • Lassa: Rodents.
	  • CCHF: Domestic animals (vector—ticks).
	■ Person-to-person transmission: Body fluids (blood, saliva, sweat, possibly urine) infectious in symptomatic cases.
	■ No aerosol transmission reported.
	■ High risk of hospital (requires full PPE) and laboratory-associated transmission (requires Category 4 facilities)	

4	**Confirmation (diagnosis):** *The remainder of this section is specifically related to Ebola virus disease.* Clinical and Laboratory ■ In a suspected case (clinically), no samples should be taken except a blood sample to exclude malaria. The sample must be processed in the Category 3 cabinet of the hospital microbiology laboratory (rapid malaria test). ■ In UK, PHE Imported Fever Service should be contacted for advice on further specimens and advice on case management.	
5	**Action:** Early Detection; Treatment; Isolation and Infection Control: ■ Essential to follow the current national protocol for infection control and public health management of suspected VHF cases. ■ Febrile patients, who have returned from a current Ebola outbreak area within 21 days, are regarded as High Risk and the Imported Fever Service or equivalent expert department and local public health department should be contacted for directions on further action including isolation and infection prevention and control procedures. Prophylaxis (Vaccination/immunoglobulin/Antibiotics/Antivirals): ■ Seek expert advice on prophylaxis, but at present no vaccine available.	
6	**Report/Communication:** ■ VHF's are notifiable diseases in the UK, once relevant local public health department is contacted follow up action relating to notification, prevention, investigation, control (including contact tracing) and public health management will proceed.	
7	**Disease Trends, Clusters, and Significant Situations:** ■ The 2014–15 Ebola outbreak in West Africa has demonstrated the global impact of VHF's, and the need for all countries, including those outside endemic zones, to have robust plans for assessment and management.	

Abridged SIMCARDs providing information on less common infections with potential public health significance in the UK

A1.2.1 **Anthrax (bacterial infection, *Bacillus anthracis*)**

(Notifiable in the UK)

Anthrax is a zoonosis, the reservoir being cattle and other domestic and wildlife herbivores in endemic areas. Disease may be cutaneous, inhalational, or gastrointestinal. Transmission is by contact with infected animals or their products, or, in IV drug users, contamination of heroin with anthrax spores. Anthrax is a potential agent for bioterrorism. Incubation period 1–7 days, person-to-person transmission is very rare. Laboratory confirmation requires culture from a cutaneous lesion and/or blood culture. Reference laboratory advice should be obtained. The local public health department should be notified of a suspected case and an epidemiological assessment undertaken to determine the possible source.

A1.2.2 **Botulism (bacterial toxin infection, *Clostridium botulinum*)**

(Notifiable in the UK)

Botulism is an acute, neurotoxin-mediated illness, often presenting with difficulty in swallowing and impaired vision, progressing to bilateral descending paralysis. The incubation period is dependent on the toxin dose, in most cases 12 hours to three days. Transmission may be from toxin-contaminated foodstuffs, including inadequately preserved fruits or vegetables and fermented fish, and also from wounds contaminated with *C. botulinum*. Diagnosis is based on clinical suspicion from the typical signs, and laboratory confirmation of botulinum toxin in serum. In individual cases rapid administration of anti-toxin is essential. Public health action involves food history and rapid recall of implicated foodstuffs.

A1.2.3 **Chikungunya (mosquito-borne flavivirus)**

(Not notifiable in the UK)

Chikungunya infection occurs in much of Africa, Asia, and Indian and Pacific Ocean islands. It may be suspected in febrile returning travellers from endemic areas. Symptoms include fever, polyarthralgia, conjunctivitis, and a maculopapular rash. The incubation period is 1–12 days. Transmission is mosquito-borne (*Aedes aegypti* and others) from an infected individual. Laboratory confirmation requires a blood sample for PCR or serology. Transmission was reported in Italy in 2007, and surveillance for possible European infections must be considered.

A1.2.4 **Cholera (bacterial infection: *Vibrio cholerae*)**

(Notifiable in the UK)

Cholera is a water-borne bacterial infection, caused by *Vibrio cholerae*, and transmitted by the faecal-oral route. It presents with acute profuse diarrhoea and vomiting, and severe dehydration if not treated rapidly. The incubation period is 6–48 hours, and cases are infective while symptomatic and for seven days after symptoms subside. Diagnosis is by stool microscopy and culture. Imported cases are rare, and should be excluded from school/work as for other enteric infections.

A1.2.5 **Dengue and dengue haemorrhagic fever (DHF) (mosquito-borne flavivirus)**

(Not notifiable in the UK)

Dengue is widely distributed in tropical areas, and should be considered in any returning traveller with fever. It is an acute-onset febrile illness, with headache, myalgia, and often a maculopapular rash. DHF is a severe disease, associated with haemorrhage and shock, with high mortality. The incubation period for both forms is 3–14 days. Transmission is mosquito-borne (*Aedes aegypti* mosquito) from an infected individual. Diagnosis is by serology or PCR for dengue virus usually in a specialist laboratory. Travellers to endemic areas should be given advice on preventing mosquito exposure.

A1.2.6 **Enterovirus D-68**

(Not notifiable in the UK)

Enterovirus D-68 (EV-D68) is a non-polio enterovirus causing mild to severe respiratory illness, and in some cases polio-like neurological symptoms including paralysis and meningo-encephalitis. An increasing number of cases have occurred in North America and Europe since 2014. Both children and adults are affected. Many asymptomatic infections may occur. Incubation period and infectivity are considered to be similar to other respiratory viruses, 1–5 days incubation, and infectivity for five days after symptoms begin. Humans are the only reservoir. EV-D68 would not normally be included in laboratory respiratory screens, and reference laboratory advice should be sought in suspected cases.

A1.2.7 **Extended spectrum beta lactamases (ESBLs)**

(Not notifiable in the UK)

ESBLs are enzymes produced by coliform bacteria (*E.coli, Klebsiella*) that cause resistance to commonly used antimicrobial agents (penicillins, cephalosporins). ESBL-producing bacteria may be carried in the gastrointestinal tract of hospitalized or community patients, leading to endogenous infection, or may be transferred between patients by healthcare staff, by commonly used equipment, and in toilet areas. Hospital laboratories routinely test coliform bacteria for ESBL production. Screening for ESBL carriage is not indicated unless there is a cluster of infections in units such as neonatal or intensive care. Strict hand hygiene is essential to reduce transmission.

A1.2.8 *Giardiasis* (protozoon parasite, *Giardia lamblia*)

(Not notifiable in the UK)

Giardiasis is a protozoal infection, causing diarrhoea, abdominal cramps, nausea, and anorexia, that typically lasts 2–3 weeks. The incubation period is 5–16 days, and infectivity may last for several weeks. Up to 30% of infections may be asymptomatic. Transmission may be through faecal contamination of recreational or drinking water and direct person-to-person, particularly in nurseries. Laboratory diagnosis is by demonstrating the presence of Giardia cysts by stool microscopy. Cases should not attend school or work until symptoms are resolved. Epidemiological investigations in relation to recreational water exposure, nursery attendance, etc. should be undertaken when clusters occur.

A1.2.9 **Gonorrhea (bacterial infection, *Neisseria gonorrhoeae*)**

(Not notifiable in the UK)

Gonorrhea is a sexually transmitted infection (STI), presenting with urethritis and epididymitis in males, and urethritis, cervicitis, and later pelvic inflammatory disease in females. The incubation period is 1–14 days. Infectivity may persist for months in untreated cases, but treated cases are non-infectious within days. Transmission is by sexual contact. Mother-to-child transmission can occur at birth leading to severe neonatal conjunctivitis. Laboratory diagnosis is by culture or molecular testing of urethral or cervical discharge. Assessment of cases for other STIs, contact tracing, and advice on safe sex are necessary follow up actions.

A1.2.10 **HIV/AIDS (human immunodeficiency virus and opportunistic infections)**

(Not notifiable in the UK)

Infection with HIV has several phases if untreated. The initial acute retroviral syndrome has symptoms of fever, malaise, lymphadenopathy, followed by a variable period of months or years with limited symptoms. Acquired immunodeficiency syndrome (AIDS) is associated with opportunistic infections, neoplasms, and other organ dysfunction (e.g. renal failure). Transmission is from infected blood, by sexual contact, and mother to child. Incubation period from exposure to HIV positivity is 1–4 weeks. Laboratory diagnosis is by serology and molecular blood tests, requiring experienced interpretation. Anti-retroviral therapy has a major impact on disease progression and transmission. Local policies should be followed regarding pre- and post-exposure prophylaxis.

A1.2.11 **Lyme disease (*Borrelia burgdoferi*)**

(Not notifiable in the UK)

A systemic infection following the bite of an infected tick. The initial manifestation is an itchy, red area at the site of the bite, *erythema migrans*. Systemic symptoms include fever, myalgia, and lymphadenopathy. Neurological or cardiac complications develop months or years later in a small number of patients. The incubation period is 3–30 days. Infection reservoirs include deer and rodents. Laboratory diagnosis is serological, available at reference laboratories. Early treatment is important to reduce the risk of long-term complications. Public health action includes education to avoid tick bites for outdoor activities in endemic areas.

A1.2.12 **Lymphogranuloma venereum (LGV) (*Chlamydia trachomatis* types L1, L2, L3)**

(Not notifiable in the UK)

A sexually transmitted infection presenting with a painless penile/urethral or cervical lesion, followed by regional lymphadenopathy, which may undergo suppuration with pelvic involvement and proctitis. LGV is endemic in tropical areas, but is increasing among Europe in men who have sex with men (MSM), particularly those HIV positive. Incubation period 3–30 days; infectivity remains throughout the period of active lesions. LGV transmission is through sexual contact. Laboratory diagnosis is by immunofluorescence or PCR of lesion exudates.

A1.2.13 **Malaria (*Plasmodium species*)**

(Notifiable in the UK)

Despite advice on prophylaxis, the possibility of malaria remains a serious risk in travellers from tropical areas. Patients may present with fever, rigors, headache, or diarrhoea. *P. falciparum* infection, if not treated early, can lead to cerebral malaria with significant mortality. Incubation period 9–14 days for *P. falciparum*, 12–18 days for *P. vivax* and *P. ovale*, longer for *P. malariae*. Transmission is mosquito-borne (anopheles mosquitoes) from an infected individual. Laboratory diagnosis is by blood film microscopy or a rapid antigen test for *P. falciparum*. Urgent treatment, with specialist infectious disease advice, is essential. Confirmed cases should be reported to national surveillance programmes.

A1.2.14 **Mumps (Paramyxovirus)**

(Notifiable in the UK)

Mumps is a systemic infection, with or without parotid and other salivary gland involvement, up to 30% of infections are asymptomatic. Complications can include orchitis and meningitis or encephalitis. Complications may occur more frequently in adults. Incubation period 16–18 days (range 12–25 days). Maximum infectivity is two days before onset of symptoms to four days after onset of symptoms. Asymptomatic cases may be infectious. Transmission is primarily by respiratory droplet spread. Laboratory confirmation is by PCR of throat swabs or nasopharyngeal aspirates or by serology. Detection of specific IgM in oral fluid (saliva) samples, ideally between one and six weeks after the onset of parotid swelling, has also been shown to be highly sensitive and specific for confirmation of mumps. Cases should be excluded from school for five days from the onset of symptoms.

A1.2.15 **Plague (*Yersinia pestis*)**

(Notifiable in the UK)

Plague is a bacterial infection caused by *Yersinia pestis*. There are three clinical types, bubonic, septicaemic, and pneumonic. Transmission is by a flea bite from an infected rodent, but person-to-person transmission can occur in pneumonic plague. The incubation period is 1–6 days. Confirmation of diagnosis is by culture of bubo exudate, blood, or sputum. Advice from a reference laboratory should be obtained. Public health action should include confirmation of travel history, identification of individuals with shared exposure, and of contacts of a case of pneumonic plague.

A1.2.16 **Pneumococcal disease (*Streptococcus pneumoniae*)**

(Not notifiable in the UK)

Pneumococcal infections include respiratory diseases (pneumonia, otitis media, etc.), bacterae-mia, and meningitis. There are many serotypes of *S. pneumoniae*. Humans are the reservoir, and symptoms develop within a few days of exposure, though much of the population will be col-onized. Laboratory diagnosis includes microscopy, culture, and molecular tests of appropriate specimens. Polyvalent pneumococcal vaccines are offered to risk groups (age ≥65 years, chronic disease, immunosuppression), and Pneumococcal Conjugate Vaccine (PCV) is included in child-hood vaccination in most developed countries including the UK. Clusters may occur in closed settings including long-term healthcare, military camps, and children's day centres.

A1.2.17 **Poliomyelitis (polio virus types 1, 2, 3)**

(Acute poliomyelitis is notifiable in the UK)

Polio is an acute virus infection of the nervous system which can lead to permanent paralysis, though most infections are asymptomatic. It continues to be endemic in a small number of coun-tries. Symptomatic cases may present with acute flaccid paralysis, which is usually asymmetric. Incubation period in paralytic cases is 7–14 days. Transmission is by the faecal-oral route; humans are the only reservoir. Live vaccine-derived virus may result in cases. Laboratory diagnosis is by viral culture from stool specimens. Urgent notification to the public health department is neces-sary for suspected cases. Most European countries now use inactivated vaccine (see Chapter 19).

A1.2.18 **Psittacosis (*Chlamydophila psittaci*)**

(Not notifiable in the UK)

Psittacosis presents as an 'atypical' pneumonia, with fever and headache. Occasionally cases develop myocarditis or encephalitis, and in untreated cases mortality may be 20%. Incubation period is 1–28 days. The reservoirs are psittacine birds (parrots, parakeets, etc.) and other birds including pigeons and poultry. Transmission is by inhalation of dust from droppings, nasal secre-tions, or feathers of infected birds. Laboratory diagnosis is by serology or PCR. A suspected case should be investigated for risk exposure, and potential sources investigated with veterinary colleagues.

A1.2.19 **Q fever (*Coxiella burnetii*)**

(Not notifiable in the UK)

Q fever is a zoonosis, transmitted to humans through contact with infected cattle, goats, and sheep. It presents as an acute febrile illness, with headache, malaise, and cough. Chronic Q fever endocarditis occurs in 1–2% of cases up to two years after initial infection. The incubation period is 2–3 weeks. Transmission is by aerosol transmission from dust and fomites from animal excreta, and the products of parturition. There is no person-to-person transmission. Laboratory diagnosis is serological. Public health input includes collaboration with veterinary colleagues for improved hygiene practices in animal management and premises. There is a whole-cell killed-inactivated vaccine produced and licensed in Australia. The vaccine is used for defined risk groups in Australia but is not licensed or used in any other country, and no vaccine for Q fever is available in the UK.

A1.2.20 **Rotavirus**

(Not notifiable in the UK, unless food poisoning is suspected)

Infection occurs primarily in young children, and presents with sudden onset of fever, vomiting, and diarrhoea, with the risk of severe dehydration. Incubation period is 1–3 days. Transmission is faecal-oral; there is also possible direct contact or respiratory spread. Infectivity is during the symptomatic stage, and for several days after. Most transmission will occur via adults caring for children, hence strict hygiene measures are essential. Clusters may occur in nurseries, and isolation of hospital cases is essential to prevent hospital transmission. Laboratory diagnosis is by the detection of rotavirus in stool specimens by PCR. Oral vaccine is now included in childhood immunization in some countries including the UK (see Chapter 19).

A1.2.21 **SARS: Severe Acute Respiratory Syndrome (Coronavirus, SARS Co-V)**

(Notifiable in the UK)

First described in China in 2002, leading to a pandemic affecting 26 countries. The last reported case was in China in 2004. Typical cases presented with fever, cough, and shortness of breath. Severe cases develop rapidly progressing respiratory distress. Incubation period 2–10 days, infectivity period may be up to 21 days after the start of symptoms. Transmission is through airborne droplets (respiratory). Diagnosis is by virus detection in respiratory samples; special laboratory facilities are required. There are strict case definitions and protocols based on WHO guidance for suspected cases should SARS reoccur.

A1.2.22 **Scarlet fever (group A *Streptococcus*)**

(Notifiable in the UK)

Early symptoms may include sore throat, fever, and headache, with the characteristic red, pinhead rash developing after 12–48 hours. Complications include ear infection or throat abscess, and rarely glomerulonephritis or rheumatic fever. The incubation period is 1–5 days. Transmission is by respiratory secretions and contact with contaminated utensils. Laboratory confirmation is by culture of group A *Streptococci* from a throat swab. Cases should be excluded from school until they have received 24 hours of appropriate antibiotics. In suspected outbreaks in schools or nurseries the local health protection team should be informed, and enhanced infection control strategies implemented.

A1.2.23 **Smallpox**

(Notifiable in the UK)

The last naturally acquired case of smallpox occurred in Somalia in 1977. Smallpox presents with an initial high fever and malaise for 2–4 days, with the classic vesicular and pustular rash subsequently developing. Incubation period is 7–19 days. Infectivity is from the first appearance of the rash to the disappearance of all scabs, about three weeks. Humans are the only reservoir. Transmission is by airborne droplets (respiratory). Smallpox is considered as a possible agent for deliberate release. Laboratory diagnosis, in designated laboratories, by PCR of vesicular fluid. In a suspected case/possible deliberate release incident, immediate contact must be made with the health protection team.

A1.2.24 **Syphilis (Spirochaete, *Trepenoma pallidum*)**

(Not notifiable in the UK)

A sexually (rarely congenital) transmitted infection with defined stages; primary: a painless sore on mucocutaneous membranes with regional lymphadenopathy; secondary: a maculopapular rash, fever, malaise; tertiary: a wide range of systemic involvement, including cardiac, and neurological and destructive infiltrates. Congenital syphilis may result in stillbirth, hepatosplenomegaly, and neurological abnormalities. Incubation period for primary 3–90 days; secondary may develop from two weeks to six months after primary infection; and tertiary, in untreated cases, many years after initial infection. Laboratory diagnosis may be by dark-field microscopy/PCR of lesion exudates, or appropriate serology. Cases should be managed with advice from GUM clinics.

A1.2.25 **Tickborne encephalitis (TBE) (flavivirus)**

(Not notifiable in the UK)

TBE occurs in forested areas of central and Eastern Europe, and Scandinavia (and related Louping ill in Scotland). It presents as a biphasic illness, with a week of influenza-like symptoms and then encephalitis in one-third of cases. Incubation period is 7–14 days. Woodland ticks are the principal reservoir, but also tick-infected woodland mammals and, in some areas, goats and sheep. Transmission is by tick bite, but some cases arise from unpasteurised goat's milk. Laboratory diagnosis in specialized laboratories is by serology and PCR. Travellers to infected areas should be advised regarding tick exposure. Vaccination is available for travellers intending to visit rural areas in endemic countries in late spring and summer months. Full details are available at the NaTHNaC website: (http://www.nathnac.org/yf_centres/yfvcinitiative.htm), but there is no specific treatment.

A1.2.26 **Typhus fever (epidemic louse-borne typhus, *Rickettsia prowazekii*)**

(Notifiable in the UK)

A febrile illness occurring in many low-and middle-income countries. Recent epidemics have occurred among refugees and displaced communities in Ethiopia and Rwanda. Presents with a sudden onset of fever, headache, and myalgia, with a macular rash. Symptoms subside after about two weeks. The case fatality rate in untreated cases ranges from 10–40%. Incubation is 1–2 weeks. Transmission is human to human by body lice, in crowded and unhygienic conditions. Patients are infective for lice during the febrile period. Laboratory diagnosis is by serology or PCR. Imported cases have occurred in aid workers working in endemic refugee areas.

A1.2.27 **VRE: vancomycin (glycopeptide)-resistant *Enterococci* (*Enterococcus faecium/faecalis*)**

(Not notifiable in the UK)

VRE are Gram-positive bacteria that are resistant to vancomycin and similar antimicrobials. VRE infections include urinary tract infections, wound infections, bacteraemia, and endocarditis. Infections may be endogenous from intestinal carriage, or transmitted from colonised or infected patients by healthcare workers or by contaminated shared equipment. VRE are detected by standard laboratory methods. In clusters of infection isolates may be sent to a reference laboratory for strain typing. Individual carriers or cases must be managed with strict hygiene, even if isolation is not possible.

A1.2.28 **West Nile Virus (West Nile Fever) (mosquito-borne flavivirus)**

(Not notifiable in the UK)

Symptoms include fever, rash, gastrointestinal symptoms, malaise, and conjunctivitis, lasting for 7–10 days. A proportion of patients (more common in the elderly) develop encephalitis. Incubation period 2–14 days. West Nile Virus (WNV) occurs in North America, Africa, Asia, and parts of southern Europe. Wild birds are the reservoir of WNV, and transmission to humans is by mosquitoes. There is no person-to-person transmission. Laboratory confirmation is by serology or PCR. Veterinary departments will provide advice on the potential risks of WNV.

A1.2.29 **Yellow fever (mosquito-borne flavivirus)**

(Notifiable in the UK)

Present in sub-Saharan Africa, South America, and parts of the Caribbean. Many cases are asymptomatic, or have only a febrile illness with headache and myalgia, lasting 4–5 days. 15–20% of symptomatic cases progress to severe disease with haemorrhage and jaundice. Incubation period is 3–6 days. No direct person-to-person transmission. Transmission is by mosquitoes, human to human in the urban cycle, and from non-human primates via mosquitoes in the forest cycle. Laboratory diagnosis is by blood PCR and serology. A suspected imported case should be managed by the regional infectious diseases unit. The live attenuated 17-D yellow fever vaccine gives protection for ten years.

A1.2.30 **Zika (mosquito-borne flavivirus)**

(Not notifiable in UK)

Zika infection had previously ocurred sporadically in Africa, SE Asia, and Oceania, but in 2015 a widespread epidemic began in south and central America. The incubation period is 3–12 days. Symptoms include fever, myalgia, exanthem and conjunctivitis, lasting 2–7 days. Most cases (around 80%) are asymptomatic. There are reports that infection has been associated with Guillain-Barré syndrome (GBS) and, if infection occurs during pregnancy, higher than expected incidence of foetal microcephaly. Transmission is primarily by Aedes mosquitoes (predominantly day-biters often found in urban environments), but mother to foetus infection and sexual transmission have been described. Diagnosis is by PCR for the virus in a patient's blood during the acute disease, and so only cases with active or very recent symptoms can be reliably tested. In the absence of a vaccine, protection is by mosquito control and prevention of mosquito bites. Travel advice suggests if possible pregnant women should not visit Zika infected areas. However, if travel to these areas is unavoidable, pregnant women should implement insect bite avoidance measures both during daytime and night-time hours. Women who are planning to become pregnant should discuss their travel plans with their healthcare provider to assess the risk of infection.

Brief SIMCARDs providing basic information on relatively rare infections with low public health significance in the UK

Acinetobacter

Actinomycosis

Ameobiasis

Roundworm

Aspergillosis

Babesiosis

Bartonella

Blastomycosis

Brucellosis

Burkholderia

Candidiasis

Genital chlamydia

Chlamydial pneumonia

Chromoblastomycosis

Clostridium perfringens

Coccidioidomycosis

Coxsakievirus

Cryptococcosis

Cyclosporiasis

Cytomegalovirus

Dracunculiasis

Encephalitis

Epstein–Barr Virus

Exanthema subitum/Roseola infantum

Lymphatic filariasis

Genital herpes

Genital warts

Hantaviral diseases

Head lice

Helicobacter pylori

Hepatitis delta

Herpes simplex

Histoplasmosis

Hookworm

Hydatid disease

Japanese encephalitis

Kawasaki disease/syndrome

Klebsiella species

Leishmaniasis

Leprosy

Leptospirosis

Loa loa

Molluscum contagiosum

Mycetoma

Mycoplasma pneumoniae

Onchocerciasis

Orf

Pasteurellosis

Rat-bite fever

Tick-borne relapsing fever and louse-borne relapsing fever

Respiratory syncytial virus

Ringworm

Scabies

Schistosomiasis

Strongyloidosis

Tapeworms

Threadworms

Toxocariosis

Toxoplasmosis

Trematodes

Trichinosis

Whipworm

African Trypanosomiasis

American Trypanosomiasis

Tularaemia

Vibrio parahaemolyticus

Virus: Arenaviridae

Virus: Bunyaviridae

Virus: Flaviviridae

Virus: Paramyxoviridae

Virus: Poxviridae

Warts

Yersiniosis

Infectious disease	Signs and symptoms	Incubation	Infectivity (person to person)	Mode of transmission	Confirmation	Action (public health)	Report/ communication	Disease trend, cluster
Acinetobacter spp.	Systemic infections in immunosuppressed, including pneumonia, septicaemia. Can colonize open wounds	May be endogenous	While colonized or infected	Usually nosocomial, especially in ITU	Culture from appropriate specimens	Hospital outbreaks may require intervention	Laboratory reporting to national laboratory may be indicated	Increasing antimicrobial resistant strains
Actinomycosis (*Actinomyces spp.*)	Localized chronic abscesses (jaw, thorax abdomen)	Years after colonization	Unknown	Unknown, case studies show instances of transmission by human bite	Culture	Promotion of dental hygiene	Not applicable	Not applicable
Ameobiasis (*Entamoeba histolytica*)	90% asymptomatic. Diarrhoea, abdominal pain. Occasionally dysentery. Liver (and other organ) abscesses	1–4 weeks	Infectious whilst cysts are passed in stool (may be years)	Faecal-oral transmission of cysts. Via contaminated food or water	Microscopy for cysts or trophozoites	Reinforce hygiene. Exclude for 48h after symptom resolution. Stool clearance required if in risk group. Screen close contacts	Notifiable if food poisoning is suspected	Identify possible outbreak sources
Roundworm (*Ascaris lumbricoides*)	Asymptomatic. Nutritional deficiencies. Rarely passage of live worms, pneumonitis, intestinal obstruction	4–8 weeks	Humans infectious while worms living in intestines (up to 24 months)	Ingestion of eggs in soil or food contaminated with human faeces	Microscopy	Promote improved hygiene and sanitation. Identify and screen contacts	Not applicable	Not applicable
Aspergillosis (*Aspergillus spp.*)	Asthma-like symptoms. Pulmonary fibrosis, bronchiectasis	2 days to 3 months	Not applicable	Inhalation of environmental spores	Microscopy and culture	Investigate for linked cases	Not applicable	Outbreaks may occur in healthcare settings
Babesiosis (*Babesia genus parasites*)	Asymptomatic. Fever, flu-like symptoms. Haemolytic anaemia	Usually: 1–3 weeks. Up to 1 year	Not applicable	Bite of infected hard ticks from deer reservoir. Rarely blood transfusion	Microscopy, serology	Investigate for linked cases with common exposures	Not applicable	Recognized increased geographical distribution

(continued)

Infectious disease	Signs and symptoms	Incubation	Infectivity (person to person)	Mode of transmission	Confirmation	Action (public health)	Report/ communication	Disease trend, cluster
Bartonella (*Bartonella spp.*)	Spectrum of illness related to species. Most common is cat-scratch disease with red papule at injury site, with lymphadenopathy and occasionally encephalopathy	3–14 days (cat-scratch disease)	Not applicable	Bite, lick or scratch of infected cats. Other species may be transmitted by sand flies	Immunodetection and histology of lesion	Not required	Not required	Not applicable
Blastomycosis (*Blastomyces dermatitidis*)	Fever, cough, infiltrated lung fields on x-ray. Cutaneous papules (may crust or ulcerate). Disseminated granulomatous disease	Unclear: likely weeks to months	No person-to-person transmission	Inhalation of environmental spores	Microscopy and culture	Not required	Not required	Sporadic cases only
Brucellosis (*Brucella abortus*)	Acute influenza-like illness. Chronic systemic illness with myalgia, fever, weight loss and neuropsychiatric symptoms	Variable: 1–2 months usual	Person-to-person transmission rare	Consumption of meat or unpasteurized milk from infected ungulates. Direct transfer through broken skin/mucous membranes (e.g. hunters/lab workers). Sexual/ breastfeeding (rare)	Culture. Agglutinating antibody response	Identify source. Investigate for linked cases	Notifiable. Potentially inform Health and Safety Executive & DEFRA	IMT need to be established. Slaughter of infected herds may be required
Burkholderia spp.	*B. pseudomallei* causes meliododis (SE Asia) Fever, localized abscesses, pneumonia. (*B.cepacia* respiratory infections in cystic fibrosis)	Meliodosis: 1–21 days, but may be years before symptoms appear	Meliodosis: person-to-person transmission rare	Meliodosis: contact with infected soil/ water, e.g. rice farmers. Tourists after 2004 tsunami	Culture from appropriate specimens or serology	Consider deliberate release	Not required	Extreme/ adventure tourist groups clusters could occur

Disease (organism)	Clinical features	Incubation period	Infectious period	Transmission	Laboratory diagnosis			
Candidiasis (*Candida spp.*)	Superficial mycotic rash on skin or mucous membranes. Can cause disseminated infection in immuno-compromised	2–5 days	Cases infectious whilst lesions present	Direct contact with secretions	Microscopy and culture	Not required	Not required	Outbreaks may occur in healthcare settings (e.g. healthworker-associated transmission, or contaminated intravenous solutions)
Genital chlamydia (*Chlamydia trachomatis*)	Asymptomatic. Urethritis, with or without discharge. Women: cervicitis. Opthalmia neonatorium in baby	7–14 days	Unknown	Sexual, interpartum (mother-to-child)	Nucleic acid amplification (urine)	Not required	Not required	Outbreaks in defined populations may require case-finding and prevention activities
Chlamydial pneumonia (*Chlamydia psittaci* *Chlamydophila pneumoniae*)	Pneumonia and bronchitis. Prolonged cough, laryngitis. Fever, malaise	*C. psittaci:* 4 days to 4 weeks. *C. pneumoniae:* 10–30 days	*C. psittaci* (Not applicable) *Chlamydophila pneumoniae* (post-infection carriage can occur up to 8 weeks)	*C. psittaci:* inhalation of infected bird (psitticine) droppings. *C. pneumoniae:* presumed person-to-person via droplets	Serological	Identify source (*C. psittaci*)	Not notifiable but may need to liaise with veterinarians to identify infected birds (*C. psittaci*)	Clusters occur and may require outbreak investigation
Chromo-blastomycosis (Various soil fungal pathogens)	Spreading fungal infection of skin, commencing as a papule but may become massive and cauliflower-like. May be locally destructive	Months	Not transmitted person-to-person	Fungi usually introduced via penetrating wound (e.g. wood splinter)	Microscopy	Not required	Not required	Not applicable

(continued)

Infectious disease	Signs and symptoms	Incubation	Infectivity (person to person)	Mode of transmission	Confirmation	Action (public health)	Report/communication	Disease trend, cluster
Clostridium perfringens	Diarrhoea, abdominal pain. Vomiting, fever, necrotizing enteritis (rarely)	6–24 hours	Not applicable	Ingestion of food contaminated with spores. Frequently associated with suboptimal storage/refrigeration	Detection of toxin in stool. Culture, serotyping	Exclude for 48 hours after symptoms resolved. Identify source	Notifiable if food poisoning is suspected	Identify and remove common source in outbreaks
Coccidioidomycosis (*C. immitis, C. posadasii*)	Acute influenza-like illness. <1% lead to disseminated infection	1–4 weeks	Not transmitted person-to-person. Immuno-suppressed (e.g. HIV-positive) at increased susceptibility	Inhalation of fungi from soil and dust (esp. desert conditions)	Microscopy and serology	Not required	Not required	Outbreaks may require dust control interventions
Coxsackievirus	Wide variety of disease including: pharyngitis, conjunctivitis, 'hand, foot, and mouth disease', uveitis, meningitis, carditis, epidemic myalgia	3–5 days	Several weeks	Direct or faecal-oral	Clinical	Promotion of hand washing	Not required	Outbreaks can occur, often in congregate settings (schools, nurseries)
Cryptococcosis (*Cryptococcus spp.*)	Immunocompetent: pneumonia. Immuno-compromised (e.g. HIV): meningitis, disseminated infection	Unknown (may be as long as months or years)	No person-to-person transmission	Inhalation of fungal spores from environment	Microscopy. Antigen test	Not required	Not required	Not applicable
Cyclosporiasis (*Cyclospora cayetanensis*)	Diarrhoea, abdominal pain, which may persist. Endemic in developing countries	1 week	Up to a month	Faecal-oral transmission of oocytes via contaminated food or water	Microscopy	Hand washing, washing of contaminated foodstuffs and water purification required	Not required	Outbreaks have been associated with imported fruit and vegetables

Organism	Clinical features	Incubation period	Period of infectivity	Transmission	Diagnosis	Infection control	Notification	Comments
Cytomegalovirus	Mild febrile illness (may be severe and disseminated, with multiple system sequelae in immunosuppressed individuals and in-utero)	3–12 weeks	Neonates who were congenitally infected and <3% of adults may be chronic (up to 5–6 years) sporadic viral shedders	Through direct exposure to infected bodily secretions	Virus isolation or PCR from urine. Viral antigen detection. Serology	Reinforce hygiene	Not required	Not applicable
Dracunculiasis (*Drancunculus medinensis*, "Guinea worm").	Generalized urticaria. Itchy blister on lower limb, from which long worm emerges	1 year	No person-to-person transmission	Nematodes shed larvae into water (e.g. ponds) that are ingested by crustacean copepods, and subsequently drunk by humans	Visual inspection of worm. Microscopy of larvae	Filter drinking water in areas where cases occur	Report to international surveillance systems	Only 4 countries endemic in 2014, with 126 cases reported from Chad, Mali, Ethiopia and South Sudan (reduced 99% from ~3.5 million cases in 1986)
Encephalitis (acute)	Fever, headaches, altered consciousness, seizures, focal neurological signs including cranial nerve defects	Wide range of causative organisms, commonest herpes simplex virus	Dependent on causative organism	Dependent on causative organism	Clinical, CT/MRI brain, examination of CSF (microscopy, biochemistry and PCR for organisms)	Not required	Notifiable	Action dependant on causative organism and epidemiological links
Epstein–Barr Virus (Infectious mononucleosis/ Glandular fever/ Human herpesvirus 4 (HHV-4))	Mild febrile illness (young children). Tonsillitis, lymph node swelling, hepato-splenomegally	4–6 weeks	Several months	Direct contact with infectious saliva (e.g. kissing), fomites	Clinical, atypical mononuclear cells in blood. Monospot test. Serology	Personal advice on infection control measures	Not required	Not applicable

(continued)

Infectious disease	Signs and symptoms	Incubation	Infectivity (person to person)	Mode of transmission	Confirmation	Action (public health)	Report/ communication	Disease trend, cluster
Exanthema subitum/Roseola infantum (Human herpesvirus 6)	Acute febrile illness (lasting 3–5 days) with maculopapular rash first on trunk and spreading peripherally	10 days (range 5–15)	Unknown	Likely salivary contact	Clinical, serology.	None	Not required	Not applicable
Lymphatic filariasis (*Wuchereria bancrofti, Brugia malayi, Brugia timori*)	Lymphatic damage resulting in swelling and oedema (may result in elephantiasis and hydrocele), with secondary bacterial infection. Tropical pulmonary eosinophilic syndrome	Between 3 and 12 months (depending on species)	Not directly transmitted from person-to-person	Bite of mosquitoes (various species) with infective larvae	Microscopy	Not required	Not required	Endemic in many tropical countries. Outbreaks unlikely to occur
Genital herpes (Predominantly Human herpesvirus 2)	Painful, recurrent ulceration on cervix, vagina, perineal skin, buttocks, anus, penis (may be extensive and destructive in immunosuppressed)	2–12 days	Up to 7 weeks in primary genital ulcers	Sexual	Clinical. Viral isolation from swabs	Not required	Not required	Not applicable
Genital warts (human papillomavirus, HPV)	Small fleshy growths, found on genital/anal areas	2 weeks to 8 months	Sexually transmitted infection, from skin to skin contact	Sexual	Clinical, can be confirmed with biopsy	Barrier contraception and HPV vaccine available	Not required	Some HPV types associated with neoplastic changes
Hantaviral diseases (*Hantaviruses spp*)	Symptoms related to strain. Flu-like illness. Haemorrhagic fever with renal syndrome. Acute respiratory distress syndrome	Up to 2 months	Person-to-person transmission rare	Inhalation of aerosolized rodent faeces.	Acute and convalescent stage serology. Viral RNA sequencing	Advise nurse in isolation with respiratory precautions. Ascertain travel and exposure history	Report to international surveillance systems. Possible media interest	UK outbreaks linked to breeding of rats

Organism/disease	Clinical features	Incubation period	Period of infectivity/epidemiology	Transmission	Laboratory diagnosis	Control measures	Exclusion/notification	Comments
Head lice (pediculosis). *Pediculus humanus capitis*	Asymptomatic. Itching of scalp after 4–6 weeks. Bacterial infection of scratches	Life cycle of adult louse about 1 month	Lice cannot jump or fly, and survive for only 48h off of scalp. Children aged 3–12 most commonly infested	Direct contact	Wet combing with visual inspection for live lice (empty eggshells do not confirm infestation)	Not necessary to exclude children from nursery or school. Inspection of contacts (e.g. siblings, fellow pupils) for lice	Not required	Clusters frequently reported from schools and other congregate settings. Multidisciplinary approach (e.g. teachers, parents, infection control nurses, GP, pharmacist) required
Helicobacter pylori	Most asymptomatic. Gastritis, gastric and duodenal ulceration	Unknown	Unclear. Prevalence high (20–50%) in developed countries and increases with age and deprivation	Unknown	13C urea breath test (may be false negative if using protein pump inhibitors, in an acute bleed, or if taking antibiotics). Serological	Not required	Not required	Not applicable
Hepatitis delta	Always associated with coexistent hepatitis B virus infection. Acute hepatitis (new coinfection with hepatitis B virus), or acute-on-chronic hepatitis 'flare' (new superinfection of pre-existing hepatitis B virus infection)	2–8 weeks	Infectious during active phase of hepatitis delta infection	Same as for hepatitis B virus: Bloodborne, sexual. Intrafamily	Detection of antibodies to hepatitis delta (IgM indicates on-going replication) PCR	Prevention as for hepatitis B infection	Notifiable as acute infectious hepatitis	Highest prevalence occurs where hepatitis B virus infection is endemic (Africa, Asia, Eastern Europe)

(*continued*)

Infectious disease	Signs and symptoms	Incubation	Infectivity (person to person)	Mode of transmission	Confirmation	Action (public health)	Report/ communication	Disease trend, cluster
Herpes simplex (*Herpes simplex virus 1 and 2*) (Both can be implicated in genital transmission. Also maternal–neonate transmission of HSV2. HSV1 can cause acute encephalitis)	Classically, primary HSV–1 results in painful mouth and gum ulceration and HSV–2 results in painful genital ulceration, see genital herpes above	2–20 days	Primary gingivostomatitis: 2 weeks. Primary genital ulceration: up to 7 weeks. Virus shed from mucosal site intermittently for years in chronic infection	Direct contact with oral secretions (e.g. kissing). Sexual transmission	Clinical. PCR	Advice to minimize transmission to others. Personal protective equipment (gloves) for HCWs at risk of infection	Not required	Increased prevalence of infection in individuals with multiple sexual partners emphasizes importance of prevention messaging
Histoplasmosis (*Histoplasma capsulatum*)	Most infections asymptomatic. Acute influenza-like respiratory illness (may have scattered lung/spleen/ liver calcification). Acute disseminated infection (diarrhoea, fever, bone marrow suppression, lymphadenopathy, death, esp. in children and immunosuppressed). Chronic disseminated infection with wasting, fever, haematological abnormalities, death after about 1 year). Chronic pulmonary form, mimicking tuberculosis	3–17 days	Not transmitted person-to-person	Inhalation of airborne fungus from soil or bird droppings	Microscopy and culture of sputum or blood. Serology	Investigate, identify and control environmental source of infection	Not required	Rare in Europe. Outbreaks may occur in workers exposed to soil or bird droppings

Disease	Clinical features	Incubation period	Person-to-person transmission	Transmission/Reservoir	Diagnosis	Control	Immunization	Distribution
Hookworm (*Ancylostoma spp.*)	Iron deficiency anaemia. Neurodevelopmental delay in children. Delayed physical development. Rarely acute respiratory/ GI reaction (Loeffler's syndrome)	From a few weeks to many months	Not directly transmitted person-to-person	Eggs passed in human stool. Infective larvae in soil penetrate skin	Microscopy of stool for ova.	Improved hygiene, sanitation and footwear	Not required	Endemic in tropical and subtropical countries. May be imported to UK
Hydatid disease (*Echinococcus spp.*)	Slow growing fluid-filled cysts in liver, lungs and other organs. May be asymptomatic or have symptoms relating to local pressure. Cysts may rupture causing anaphylaxis-like reaction	Usually >1 year	Not directly transmitted from person-to-person	Dogs are infected by eating raw infected animal (e.g. sheep) viscera. Humans infected directly (ingestion of tapeworm ova from dog faeces) or indirectly from contaminated food, soil or water	Ultrasound, CT, serology. Microscopy of surgical specimens	Investigate close household contacts for presence of infection	In endemic areas work with animal health officers to improve livestock inspection, reduce feeding of raw viscera to dogs, offer periodic mass drug treatment to dogs, and improve hygiene and sanitation	Endemic in many tropical countries. May be imported into UK
Japanese encephalitis (*Japanese encephalitis virus*)	>99% asymptomatic/ febrile illness. <1% encephalitis	5–15 days	Not applicable	Vector is *Culex spp.* mosquitoes. Reservoirs are pigs and wild birds (esp. herons)	Acute and convalescent stage serology.	Vaccination available for at-risk travellers	Not required	Japanese encephalitis does not occur in the UK but can be imported
Kawasaki disease/ syndrome	Acute, febrile childhood illness (fever >5 days) with irritability, lymphadenitis, vasculitis, red lips, strawberry tongue, rash, oedema, conjunctivitis. May be long convalescent period	Unknown	Unknown	Unknown	Clinical diagnostic criteria	Not required	Not required	Occurs worldwide

(continued)

Infectious disease	Signs and symptoms	Incubation	Infectivity (person to person)	Mode of transmission	Confirmation	Action (public health)	Report/ communication	Disease trend, cluster
Klebsiella species	Hospital and community infections including urinary tract, wounds/ diabetic ulcers, bacteraemia and neonatal meningitis	Endogenous, or a few days after colonization	While colonized or infected	If not endogenous, via healthcare workers if hand hygiene not adequate	Culture of appropriate specimens	Hospital outbreaks may require intervention	Laboratory reporting of multiply resistant strains	Highly resistant strains of Klebsiella are increasingly prevalent
Leishmaniasis (*Leishmanania spp.*)	i) Cutaneous and mucosal form: indolent ulceration (primary lesion) which may result in chronic, destructive granulomatous lesion on nasopharynx. ii) Visceral form (kala-azar): fever, hepato-splenoemgally, lymphadenopathy, blood dyscrasias, wasting	2- 6 months	Not usually directly transmitted from person-to-person (cases of transmission between injecting drug users have been reported)	Through the bite of infected sandflies	Microscopic identification of parasites in sample from lesion (cutaneous form) or in blood in visceral form	Not required	Not required	Endemic in many tropical and subtropical countries. May be imported into the UK
Leprosy (*Mycobacterium leprae*)	Hypopigmented skin lesions; peripheral nerve thickness with loss of sensation/function. Spectrum of clinical apperaranceappearance dependent on the degree of cell mediated immune reaction	9 months to 20 years	Cases rapidly become non-infectious after commencing drug treatment	Nasal secretions	Clinical. Microscopy of stained skin smears for acid-alcohol fast bacilli	Early detection and treatment of cases key to prevention. BCG vaccination	Notifiable	Global incidence declining and WHO targeted for elimination. Because of long duration of infection, cases may be diagnosed in UK

Organism	Clinical features	Incubation period	Person-to-person transmission	Transmission	Laboratory diagnosis	Control advice	Exclusion	Epidemiology
Leptospirosis (*Leptospira spp.*)	Flu-like illness, jaundice, renal failure, haemorrhage, myocarditis, meningoencephalitis	Usually 5–14 days. Range: 2–30 days	Person-to-person transmission rare	Contact (broken skin, mucous membrane) with water or soil contaminated with urine of infected animals (e.g. rats)	Microscopy of blood, CSF, urine. Acute and convalescent stage serology	Identify source. Investigate for linked cases	Not required	Identify sources of outbreak, e.g. rivers, lakes, swimming pool
Loa loa	Transient swellings on any body part with pain and itching. Migration of adult worm under conjunctiva causing pain and oedema	4 months to several years	Adult worms may live in humans and shed microfilariae for decades	Transmitted between humans during feeding of infected *Chrysop. spp* flies	Microscopy to identify microfilariae in stained blood samples (blood drawn during daylight hours)	Not required	Not required	Endemic in rainforest areas of Africa countries, especially in Central and West Africa. May be imported into the UK
Molluscum contagiosum	Smooth, umbilicated papules on face and trunk (children) or genitalia and thighs and abdomen (adults). May be extensive in HIV-positive individuals	7 days to 6 months	Unknown	Direct contact. Sexual	Clinical. Microscopy of core of lesion. Histology	Advise avoid direct contact to reduce risk of transmission	Not required	Incidence peaks in childhood. No requirement for exclusion of children from school or activities
Mycetoma (chronic bacterial infection, *Nocardia brasiliensis*, *Actinomadura madurae* and others)	Subcutaneous swelling and ulceration, with formation of sinus tracts	Months	Not transmitted from person-to-person	From soil through penetrating wounds	Histology or culture	In endemic areas, encourage foot protection/care.	Not applicable	Endemic in Central America, parts of tropical Africa and Asia

(continued)

Infectious disease	Signs and symptoms	Incubation	Infectivity (person to person)	Mode of transmission	Confirmation	Action (public health)	Report/ communication	Disease trend, cluster
Mycoplasma pneumoniae	Community-acquired pneumonia (estimated 40% of community acquired pneumonia is attributable to *M. pneumoniae*), upper respiratory tract infection, erythema multiforme	1–4 weeks	Unknown	Respiratory droplets	Culture of sputum. Serology. Quantitative PCR	Increase hand and respiratory hygiene/cough etiquette in outbreak situation	Not required	Outbreaks may occur in congregate settings (e.g. university halls, barracks, homeless shelters)
Onchocerciasis (*Onchocerca volvulus*)	Chronic infection with skin changes including nodulation, loss of elasticity and depigmentation. Visual impairment (river blindness)	Microfilariae found in skin for 1 year after infected blackfly bite	Not directly transmitted person-to-person	Via the bite of infected blackflies, which breed near fast-flowing rivers	Clinical, including eye signs. Microscopy of skin biopsy for microfilariae, or of excised nodule for adult worm	Mass periodic drug administration (with ivermectin) in endemic communities	Not required	>99% of cases occur in sub-Saharan Africa. May be imported to the UK
Orf (*orf virus*)	Red pustules on hands, arm and face that may form weeping pustules	3–6 days	Unknown	Direct contact with infected ungulates (esp. sheep, goats) e.g. during milking	Clinical, serology.	Improved hygiene and hand washing in farm environments	Not required	Infection ubiquitous in farm workers
Pasteurellosis: (*Pasteurella spp.*)	Rapidly progressive soft tissue infection (may be locally destructive) following animal bite (e.g. dogs, cats). Disseminated infection, including: endocarditis, meningitis	24 hours	Not directly transmitted from person-to-person	*Pasteurella spp.* are oral commensals of many animals. Infection occurs following animal bite	Microscopy and culture	Not required	May need to report dog bites to vets and police	Not applicable

Disease (organism)	Clinical features	Incubation period	Person-to-person	Route of transmission	Diagnosis	Prevention/control	Public health action	Epidemiology
Rat-bite fever (Spirillum minus, Streptobacillus moniliformis)	Slow healing wound with prolonged fever following rodent exposure (spirillosis, 'Sodoku'). Acute febrile illness with polyarthralgia and macular widespread rash (Streptobacillosis 'Haverhill fever')	Spirillosis: 2–4 weeks. Streptobacillosis: 2–10 days	Not directly transmitted from person-to-person	Exposure to rodent urine or mucous secretions (e.g. bite)	Microscopy	Rodent control. Reduce risk of laboratory injury	May need to communicate with municipal/LA rodent control departments	Spirillosis predominately reported from Japan. Streptobacillosis reported widely. Associations with rodent pet ownership and (putatively) laboratory animal handlers
Tick-borne relapsing fever & louse-borne relapsing fever (Borrelia spp.)	Intermittent fever lasting about 3 days and separated by about 7 days, malaise, headache, nausea, vomiting, cough, light sensitivity, confusion, spontaneous 'crisis' with delirium, hyperpyrexia, hypotension. Tick-borne relapsing fever tends to be milder than louse-borne	7 days	Not directly transmitted from person-to-person	Bite of infected soft ticks (Ornithodoros) or lice (Pediculus humanus)	Microscopy of peripheral blood smears	Identification and insecticide spraying of tick habitats (e.g. infested cabins, rural houses)	Not required	Tick-borne relapsing fever outbreaks have been associated with rural cabins. Louse-borne relapsing fever outbreaks associated with war, famine, homelessness and poverty
Respiratory syncytial virus	Lower respiratory tract infections, bronchiolitis	4–5 days	Can be transmitted from person-to-person	Droplet spread	PCR or viral culture	Not required	Not required	Very common virus. Almost all children are infected with RSV by the time they are 2 years old

(continued)

Infectious disease	Signs and symptoms	Incubation	Infectivity (person to person)	Mode of transmission	Confirmation	Action (public health)	Report/ communication	Disease trend, cluster
Ringworm (*Trichophyton spp.*, *Microsporum spp.*)	Fungal infection, silvery/ red rash on skin	1–3 weeks	Can be transmitted from person-to-person	Direct skin contact and contact with towels/clothes. Transmission from animals	Clinical	Good hand hygiene	Not required	10–20% of people will have ringworm in their lifetime, more common in children
Scabies (*Sarcoptes scabiei var. hominis*)	Itchy papules and linear burrows around finger webs, wrists, elbows, genitalia. May have bacterial superinfection from scratching	2–6 weeks	Until treatment successfully removes mites and eggs	Direct contact	Clinical	Exclude cases until after first application of treatment. Identify and treat all household, close and sexual contacts, regardless of whether symptomatic	Not required	Clusters may occur in schools, residential homes and healthcare settings and often require a multidisciplinary response
Schistosomiasis (*S. haemotobium*, *S. mansoni*, *S. japonicum*)	Related to egg load and location. Acute: systemic Katayama fever. Urinary (*S. haemotobium*): haematuria, frequency, obstruction, cancer. Abdominal (*S. japonicum*, *S. mansoni*): diarrhoea, abdominal pain, hepatosplenomegaly, liver fibrosis, portal hypertension, cancer. Rarely, local CNS, lung symptoms	2–6 weeks to acute symptoms	Not directly transmitted person-to-person	Cercariae develop in fresh-water snails before penetrating swimmer's skin. Cercariae mature in liver and adult schistosomes migrate to mesenteric or pelvic veins. Eggs are excreted into water, before hatching and infecting snails	Microscopy of urine and stool. Histology of affected tissues. Serology	Education and improved sanitation to reduce water-borne transmission. Mass periodic drug administration in affected communities	Not required	Endemic in many countries in Asia, Africa and the Middle East, especially in communities that live and work near fresh water sources

Organism	Symptoms	Incubation period	Infectious period	Transmission	Diagnosis	Prevention	Exclusion	Epidemiology
Strongyloidosis (*S. stercoralis*, *S. fulleborni*)	Asymptomatic, skin rash at worm entry point, cough, pneumonitis, abdominal pain, diarrhoea. Wasting may be profound in immunocompromised	2–4 weeks	As long as worms are in intestine	Adult female worms shed eggs into the intestine, which develop into larvae and are excreted into soil. Larvae penetrate human skin	Microscopy for larvae in stool	Promote improved hygiene and sanitation	Not required	Endemic in tropical and subtropical countries. May be imported to UK
Tapeworms (cestodes)	Commonly asymptomatic, abdominal pain, diarrhoea and vomiting	Variable, can be years	Low risk of person-to-person transmission e.g. food preparation by infected person	Faecal-oral route, or eating raw or contaminated beef, pork or fish	Microscopy for larvae in stool	Good hand hygiene and avoid eating contaminated raw beef, pork or fish	Not required	Commonly seen in developing countries and are rare in the UK
Threadworms (*Enterobius vermicularis*)	Intense itching around the anus or vagina, particularly at night; disturbed sleep; lack of appetite	2 to 6 weeks	High risk of person-to-person transmission	Faecal-oral route	Clinical diagnosis	Good hand hygiene	Not required	Most common type of worm infection in the UK, and they are particularly common in young children under the age of 10
Toxocariosis (*T. canis*)	Asymptomatic generally, or mild flu like symptoms. Rarely infects organs such as the liver, lungs, eyes or brain and causes severe symptoms	10–21 days	Not directly transmitted person-to-person	Faecal-oral route, from contaminated animal faeces (cats, dogs)	Microscopy for larvae via biopsy	Good hand hygiene, deworming pets	Not required	Rare in UK, cases seen around the world

(continued)

Infectious disease	Signs and symptoms	Incubation	Infectivity (person to person)	Mode of transmission	Confirmation	Action (public health)	Report/ communication	Disease trend, cluster
Toxoplasmosis (*T.gondii*)	Asymptomatic in healthy. In-utero infection: miscarriage, stillbirth, congenital abnormalities. In immunosuppressed: fever, confusion, cerebral lesions leading to focal neurological signs	5–23 days	Not directly transmitted person-to-person	Ingestion of undercooked meat containing cysts or handling cat faeces. Intrauterine	Microscopy of clinical specimens (e.g. CSF). Serology. PCR for parasite DNA in amniotic fluid	Identify possible sources of infection	Not required	Not applicable
Trematodes (flukes)	Depending on the type of trematodes, can affect blood, lung, liver, intestine	Few days to months	Not directly transmitted person-to-person	Parasitic infections acquired through ingestion of food contaminated with the larval stage of the parasite	Microscopy	Improved food hygiene and sanitation	Not required	Prevalent in east and south-east Asia, and in central and south America
Trichinosis (*Trichinella spiralis*)	Early symptoms— Diarrhoea, abdominal pain, fatigue, nausea and vomiting; late symptoms—fever, muscle pain and tenderness, facial swelling, weakness, headache	1–2 days (enteral phase) to 2 to 8 weeks (parenteral phase)	not transmitted person-to-person	Ingestion of larvae of trichina worm, usually through undercooked pork or game	Clinical, confirmation with identification of *Trichinella* larvae in biopsy	No	Not required	Infects humans throughout North America, parts of South America, central America, parts of Africa, Asia, New Zealand, and Tasmania. The parasite is highly prevalent in Europe, Asia, and Southeast Asia and is endemic in Japan and China

Disease	Clinical features	Incubation	Infectivity	Transmission	Diagnosis	Prevention	Treatment	Distribution
Whipworm (*Trichuris trichiura*)	Asymptomatic. Diarrhoea (may be bloody), rectal prolapse. Developmental delay in children	indefinite	Years	Ingestion of vegetables or soil containing ova	Microscopy of stool	Improved hygiene, hand washing and sanitation	Not required	Endemic in many tropical and subtropical countries. May be imported into the UK
African Trypanosomiasis (*Trypanosoma brucei rhodesensia*, *Trypanosoma brucei gambiense*)	'Sleeping sickness'. Starts as painful chancre at bite site. Fever and systemic illness. Progressive neurological decline, including disruption of sleep cycle, eventually leading to death. May be acute (*T. brucei rhodesensia*) or chronic (*T. brucei gambiense*)	*T. brucei rhodesensia*: 3 days to several weeks. *T. brucei gambiense*: several months	Not directly transmitted person-to-person. Infectious to tsetse flies whilst parasitaemic	Ungulates (esp. bushbuck and cattle) are reservoir for *T. brucei rhodesensia*. Humans only reservoir for *T. brucei gambiense*. Human infection occurs via the bite of infected tsetse flies	Microscopy of blood and CSF for trypanosomes	Not applicable	Not required	Endemic in Central and west Africa. May be imported to UK
American Trypanosomiasis (*Trypanosma cruzi*) (Chagas disease)	Acute: fever, lymphadenopathy, hepatosplenomegally. Chronic (Chagas disease): cardiac involvement resulting dilatation and arrhythmias. Occasionally, oesophageal and intestinal dilatation (megaviscera)	1 to 3 weeks	Not directly transmitted person-to-person. Infectious to Reduviidae (kissing bugs) whilst parasitaemic	Wide range of wild and domestic animal reservoirs. Transmitted to humans by Reduviidae rubbing their faeces into a blood-feed wound, often located in dwellings. Occasional transmission by blood transfusion	Microscopy of blood for trypanosomes	Not applicable	Not applicable	Endemic in South and Central America. May be imported to the UK

(continued)

Infectious disease	Signs and symptoms	Incubation	Infectivity (person to person)	Mode of transmission	Confirmation	Action (public health)	Report/communication	Disease trend, cluster
Tularaemia (*Francisella tularensis*)	Indolent skin ulcer. Acute influenza-like illness. Painful lymphadenopathy. Pneumonia. If swallowed: pharyngitis. If inhaled: pneumonia and septicaemia	1–14 days	Not directly transmitted person-to-person	Zoonotic, with reservoir in rabbits, hares, beavers, muskrats, voles. Transmitted to humans by bite of infected ticks	Clinical, serology, PCR	Investigate possible sources of infection	Not required	Consider possible laboratory exposure or deliberate aerosol release if epidemiologically-linked cases with no identified source of infection
Vibrio parahaemolyticus	Explosive, watery diarrhoea, fever. Can cause infections of eyes, skins, ears and wounds	24 hours	No person-to-person transmission	Faecal-oral route through uncooked seafood; contact with contaminated water	Stool culture	No	Not required	Most common in Asia, central and South America
Virus: *Arenaviridae* (e.g. VHF)	Argentine, Bolivian, Brazilian, Chapare, and Venezualan haemorrhagic fevers; and old world (Lassa and Lujo haemorrhagic fevers and Lymphocytic choriomeningitis). Similar symptoms of fever, myalgia, malaise, headache, abdominal pain, haemorrhage	Usually 7–14 days	Rarely transmitted from person-to-person	Inhalation of rodent excreta particles. Rarely person-to-person transmission among healthcare workers and household contact. Laboratory associated transmission reported	Serology. Viral PCR or isolation in cell culture	Support physicians and microbiologists in making risk assessment, accessing reference laboratory testing services and in implementing infection control for cases in community and health facilities	Notifiable as cause of VHF	Geographical distribution related to rodent host range and incidental human contact

Virus	Clinical features	Incubation	Person-to-person	Transmission/Exposure	Diagnosis		Notifiable	Geographical distribution
Virus: *Bunyaviridae* (e.g. Rift valley)	Over 300 viruses in 5 genera. Most important: Rift valley fever, Crimean-Congo Haemorrhagic fever and Hantavirus (see above). May be asymptomatic, or present with fever, headache, backache, encephalitis, haemorrhage (<1%, with up to 50% case fatality).	RVF: 2–6 days, CCHF: 1–9 days (usually 1–3 days)	Not usually transmitted directly person-to-person	RVF: Exposure to blood/viscera of RVF infected animals (e.g. sheep). Bite of infected mosquitoes. CCHF: Bite of infected hard ticks	Serology. Viral PCR or isolation in cell culture	As above	Notifiable as cause of VHF	Usually restricted to geographical area inhabited by animal reservoirs. Potential laboratory-associated outbreaks from aerosolized material. RVF: Outbreaks have occurred in South Africa (2010), Kenya, Tanzania, and Somalia (2010), and Saudi Arabia and Yemen (2000)
Virus: *Flaviviridae* (e.g. yellow fever, dengue, WNV)	Important flaviviruses include: Alkhuma virus (Saudi Arabia), Dengue virus, Kyasanur Forest virus (India, Karnataka State), Omsk virus (Siberia), yellow fever virus, Japanese Encephalitis, West Nile Virus, Tick-borne encephalitis. Symptoms and signs related to virus	Variable, dependent on virus, but rarely longer than 21 days	Not usually transmitted directly person-to-person	Transmission via mosquito and tick vectors	Serology. Viral PCR or isolation in cell culture	As *Arenaviridae*	Yellow fever is notifiable	Usually restricted to geographical area inhabited by animal reservoirs. Dengue virus distribution increasing globally

(continued)

Infectious disease	Signs and symptoms	Incubation	Infectivity (person to person)	Mode of transmission	Confirmation	Action (public health)	Report/communication	Disease trend, cluster
Virus: *Paramyxoviridae* (e.g. Nipah; Hendra)	Encephalitis, fever, headaches.	Nipah: 5–14 days. Hendra: 9–16 days	Unknown	Nipah: Usually via bat secretions and close contact with infected pigs. Person-to-person transmission among caregivers reported in India and Bangladesh. Hendra: Exposure to secretions of infected horses (flying fox reservoir)	Serology. Viral isolation in cell culture	As *Arenaviridae*	Not required	Nipah: Outbreaks reported from Asia. Henrda: small number of cases reported from Eastern Australia
Virus: *Poxviridae* (e.g. cowpox)	Painful vesicles and pustules on hands and face that may become disseminated. Develop into black eschar before falling off. May resemble smallpox	9–10 days	Not transmitted person-to-person	Direct contact with infected animals (cow's udders, cats, rodents, exotic animals)	Electron microscopy of swab from vesicle. Viral cell culture	Support physicians and microbiologists in making risk assessment to differentiate from smallpox, and in accessing laboratory testing services	Not required	Clusters associated with animal owners
Warts (non-genital) (HPV, many types)	Various morphlogies of skin warts.	weeks to months	Rarely transmitted from person-to-person	Direct skin to skin contact, indirect contact e.g. at swimming pool	Clinical diagnosis	Caution when feet are wet (e.g. at swimming pool)	Not required	Not applicable
Yersiniosis (*Yersinia paratuberculosis, Yersinia enterocolitica*)	Acute diarrhoea, fever, abdominal pain (may mimic acute appendicitis). Post infectious arthropathy, erthyema nodosum	3–7 days	Untreated may excrete bacteria for 2–3 months, but person-to-person transmission is rare	Faeco-oral via contaminated food or water (esp. raw or undercooked meat, milk)	Stool culture	Hygiene and hand washing advice. Exclude case and symptomatic contacts if in risk group for 48 hours after first normal stool. No stool microbiological clearance required	Notifiable if food poisoning is suspected	Outbreaks require investigation for possible food sources

Books and on-line resources for the SIMCARDs and other infections

(For an exhaustive list of infectious diseases and detailed information on clinical, epidemiological, microbiological, and public health actions, readers are referred to the following reference books and websites.)

Books

Bennett J, R Dolin, JB Martin. 2015. *Principles and Practice of Infectious Diseases*. 8th edition. 2 vols. Oxford: Elsevier. http://www.elsevierhealth.co.uk/infectious-disease/mandell-douglas-and-bennett-principles-and-practice-of-infectious-diseases-expert-consult/9781455748013/

Farrer J, P Hotez, T Junhanss, et al. 2015. *Manson's Tropical Diseases*. 23rd edition Oxford: Elsevier.

Hawker J, N Begg, I Blair, et al. (eds). 2012. *Communicable Disease Control and Health Protection Handbook*. 3rd edition. London: John Wiley & Sons.

Heymann LD (ed.). 2014. *Control of Communicable Diseases Manual*. 20th edition. Washington, DC: American Public Health Association.

Salisbury D, M Ramsay, K Noakes. 2006. *Immunisation against Infectious Disease - The Green Book*. London: Stationery Office. https://www.gov.uk/government/collections/immunisation-against-infectious-disease-the-green-book

Online resources

British Infection Association: Disease Guidelines. http://www.britishinfection.org/guidelines-resources/published-guidelines/

British HIV Association. http://www.bhiva.org/guidelines.aspx

Centers for Disease Control and Prevention (CDC). http://www.cdc.gov/

European Centre for Disease Prevention and Control. Updates and Guidelines available online. http://ecdc.europa.eu/en/Pages/home.aspx

European Society of Clinical Microbiology and Infectious Diseases. Guidelines available on line. https://www.escmid.org/escmid_library/medical_guidelines/escmid_guidelines/

Healthcare Infection Society: Access to a wide range of guidelines on different aspects of healthcare associated infections. http://www.his.org.uk/resources-guidelines/#.VY-JNPlViko

Infectious Diseases Society of America. Disease guidelines available on line. http://www.idsociety.org/IDSA_Practice_Guidelines/

National Travel Health Network and Centre: *Advice for Health Professionals*. http://www.nathnac.org/pro/index.htm

ProMED Mail. International Society for Infectious Diseases. Internet-based reporting system for providing early warning of emergent and re-emergent infections. http://www.promedmail.org/

Public Health England (PHE), Animal and Plant Health Agency (APHA), Department for Environment, Food and Rural Affairs (DEFRA). *Health Protection: Infectious Diseases A to Z*. https://www.gov.uk/topic/health-protection

World Health Organization (WHO). Information on a wide range of infectious diseases. http://www.who.int/topics/infectious_diseases/en/

World Health Organization (WHO). Information on current disease outbreaks. http://www.who.int/csr/don/en/

Appendix 2

SIMCARDs for dealing with emergency situations

A2.1 **Chemical spill/leak of unknown type SIMCARD**

Potentially toxic spillage, often from a storage tank

		Yes/No
1	**Situation:** Report, usually from emergency services, 'something leaking' in a particular place.	
2	**Incubation Period (Lead Time):** Unknown; the spill may be old and only recently uncovered, or recent. Health effects depend on the chemicals.	
3	**Mode of Transmission (Exposure):** Inhalation, ingestion, skin and eye exposure are all possible and not mutually exclusive. Potential risk of explosion with associated trauma.	
4	**Confirmation (Criteria):** Contact emergency services, environmental health, Environment Agency or other relevant body; elucidate as much information as possible: especially time, people exposed, place, source, known history of incident.	
5	**Action** *Immediate:* *Acute situation*: Call local health protection team together for a meeting, assess urgency and size of risk and incident; allocate tasks. Remember your business continuity issues and continue to provide essential services. If the incident is too big, call extra staff in from meetings. If the incident is small, respond within normal structures. *Chronic leak*: less urgency, but need for full information remains. *Public Health:* *Acute situation*: Consider whether a major incident needs to be called, thus mobilizing health protection and other agencies' resources in an organized and coherent manner. Establishing a Strategic Coordinating Group, possibly with Scientific and Technical Advice Cell, takes time; continue to gather information during establishment. *Chronic leak*: need for multi-agency response may still be present, but urgency is less. Assess the capacity needed to respond: time may need to be allocated over the coming weeks (months, years) to respond fully. *Planning:* Lessons identified from hot debriefs (acute incident), or during the ongoing response (chronic incident), should be acted upon, in planning for future events, and/or in current response (particularly chronic incident). Involve appropriate emergency planning staff within public health, the local resilience forum, the local health resilience partnership and relevant others. Develop an exit strategy, with partners if possible: different partners may exit (or enter) the response at different times, depending on their responsibilities.	
6	**Report/Communication:** Initially, with emergency services, the wider public health teams, environmental health, emergency planning colleagues. Support Strategic Coordinating Group media response with health messages. As months and years pass in long-standing incidents, do not forget to communicate; ensure the situation is standing item in appropriate forum.	
7	**Disease Trends, Clusters, and Significant Situations:** Acute responses unlikely to need health studies (consider if risk register needed for longer term surveillance). Long-standing issues may need consideration of health studies, although the numbers may be too small for meaningful investigation.	

Useful information on a variety of chemicals can be found at:

Public Health England (PHE). n.d. *Health Protection: Chemical Hazards*. https://www.gov.uk/health-protection/chemical-hazards (accessed 31 December 2015).

A2.2 **Chemical suicides SIMCARD**

For suspected, confirmed, or attempted chemical suicides

		Yes/No
1	**Situation:** Attending emergency services consider someone within a polluted building, room or vehicle has tried to commit suicide through chemical release, probably partly as gas. Commonly available chemicals are often mixed to release toxic gas, which can be highly concentrated in confined spaces.	
2	**Incubation Period (Lead Time):** Immediate.	
3	**Mode of Transmission (Exposure):** Inhalation of toxic chemical, likely still to be present where casualty lies; occasionally ingestion, with off-gassing (release of gas) from casualty, rendering room unsafe.	
4	**Confirmation (Criteria):** Suspicious circumstances, confined space (car, room), perhaps notice on door: 'Do not enter!' or a suicide note, sealed door or vents, empty containers (cleaning fluid, pesticide, paint), smell (e.g. rotten eggs: hydrogen sulphide; bitter almonds: cyanide), others nearby complaining of symptoms (e.g. breathing problems). Clinical examination by responding emergency services, with casualty showing no signs of trauma.	
5	**Action** *Immediate:* Emergency services should enter in appropriate personal protective equipment, including gas-tight suits if necessary. Remove casualty: if dead, in gas-tight body bag; if alive, to A&E, but do not contaminate A&E: decontaminate first; ventilate room, extinguish any fire or source of chemical release. *Public Health:* Consider neighbouring properties or rooms: has the chemical penetrated? Take history of situation, possible chemical, details of symptoms or casualty, then discuss with regional or national toxicological colleagues. Remember, the site may be a crime scene. Consider liaising with local authority public health and their suicide reduction strategist.	
6	**Report/Communication:** Doctor determining death should inform the coroner. Inform Director of Public Health as there may be media interest. The emergency services will inform police.	
7	**Disease Trends, Clusters, and Significant Situations:** Suicide can come in waves, with copy-cat successes. There are websites that advertise what chemicals are useful for suicide. Chemical suicides are increasing in numbers.	

Further information

Public Health England (PHE). 2014. *Suicide Prevention: Developing a Local Action Plan.* https://www.gov.uk/government/publications/suicide-prevention-developing-a-local-action-plan (accessed 31 December 2015).

A2.3 **Carbon monoxide SIMCARD**

Carbon monoxide (CO) poisoning (accidental, indoor, residential; suicide)

		Yes/No
1	**Situation:** CO: colourless, odourless, tasteless gas, produced by burning any fossil fuel without enough air.	
2	**Incubation Period (Lead Time):** Exposure to high indoor levels quickly fatal; exposure to lower levels can result in symptoms including headache, dizziness, drowsiness, and may resemble, viral infections or food poisoning.	
3	**Mode of Transmission (Exposure):** Exposure to incompletely burnt fuel in boiler or fire (including wood burning stoves) not recently (annually) serviced, particularly where room ventilation is poor. Cooking inside tents, caravans, canal barges, and camping cabins also results in poisoning and fatalities. Barbeques used indoors in inadequately ventilated rooms. Also used to commit suicide or attempt murder. Use of internal combustion engines indoors can be fatal, for instance with pumps after flooding. Can occur in hotels and work premises so consider full situation. Elderly and fetus are most vulnerable to exposure. Note: cigarette smoke contains CO.	
4	**Confirmation (Criteria):** Clinical confirmation difficult, particularly if patient given oxygen by emergency responders. Keep high level of suspicion. Carboxyhaemoglobin (HbCO) levels elevated; in smokers this may be difficult to interpret. Link between carboxyhaemoglobin level and outcome is weak. Use clinical algorithm: https://www.gov.uk/government/publications/carbon-monoxide-co-algorithm-to-diagnose-poisoning. Fire brigades and some ambulance crews can measure CO in indoor air. Do not ignore CO once possibility raised; negative readings in building or patient not conclusive proof of absence of previously raised CO concentrations.	
5	**Action** *Immediate:* Remove everyone within the immediate vicinity inside building. Consider neighbouring flats (above, below, next door): CO crosses walls, floors, ceilings. If there is suspicion of suicide (see Chemical Suicide SIMCARD) the site is a police crime scene. *Public Health:* Ensure the premises safe and possible sources of CO (particularly gas boilers, fires) identified and switched off before being checked by qualified personnel (http://www.gassaferegister.co.uk/). Chimney flues should be swept. *Planning:* Develop coordinated responses with local emergency services, environmental health and other agencies (e.g. housing) to ensure comprehensive, timely emergency response.	
6	**Report/Communication:** With emergency services and environmental health; report plans and developments to Director of Public Health. Consider media campaigns to alert community to risks and need for vigilance in servicing appliances. Encourage use of CO alarms (inexpensive but, unlike smoke detectors, needs replacing every five years as detector wears out).	
7	**Disease Trends, Clusters, and Significant Situations:** Epidemiology of CO poisoning not clear; at least 40 deaths and 4000 A&E attendances each year in England. Rural populations may be at slightly greater risk than urban populations. Chronic exposure associated with neurological effects, including difficulties in concentration. The health risk from low level exposure remains unclear.	

Further information

Public Health England (PHE). 2009. *Carbon monoxide (CO)*. https://www.gov.uk/government/collections/carbon-monoxide-co (accessed 21 April 2016).

A2.4 **Decontamination—chemical SIMCARD**

Responding to possible decontamination need following chemical exposure

		Yes/No
1	**Situation:** Questions about decontamination of people or premises arise from large or small pollution incidents, including A&E if a contaminated person presented there unexpectedly.	
2	**Incubation Period (Lead Time):** Immediate, where the people are already: do not move without decontamination, otherwise second site (car, ambulance, A&E) can be contaminated.	
3	**Mode of Transmission (Exposure):** Surface of clothes/footwear, skin, eyes, hair, and ornaments; inhalation or ingestion from off-gassing/splashes/particles from contaminated persons is also possible.	
4	**Confirmation (Criteria):** Gases do not adhere, so someone exposed to a gas does not need decontamination. Liquids and solids adhere to surfaces and need removal.	
5	**Action** *Immediate:* Removal of a person's clothes reduces subsequent exposure by around 80%. Dry wiping with paper towel now preferred to complete the process. If showering: for chemicals which react with water, use copious amounts of water to dilute pollutant. Dry decontamination can usually be achieved simply. When large numbers need showering, portable decontamination is needed, organized by ambulance and fire services; temporary replacement garments needed. It takes time to organize showering facilities for large numbers; keeping people on site may prove difficult. Safe capture and handling of run-off water and clothing is important to prevent secondary contimantion offsite. Decontamination of buildings is largely outwith the health protection remit, but advice on cleaning affected health premises may be needed. Consult with specialist national environmental and toxicology colleagues. Communication to members of the public, with both health-focused explanations about decontamination and sufficient practical information, is essential for the smooth-running of any decontamination process; failure to communicate effectively is likely to result in public non-compliance and anxiety. *Public Health:* Liaise with emergency services over the need for decontamination and the best method for the particular incident. Seek advice from specialist environmental and toxicological colleagues in health protection. But do not delay decontamination while finding information and decisions are being made. *Planning:* Review and exercise multi-agency plans for decontamination, particularly for large numbers. Feed all learning back into the plans.	
6	**Report/Communication:** Report findings from review and exercise debrief to public health colleagues who may have to deal with such situations. Share with regional and national colleagues as appropriate. Consider whether a report should be published in relevant newsletters or journals.	
7	**Disease Trends, Clusters, and Significant Situations:** With good decontamination, there should be very limited ongoing health risks.	

(*continued on the next page*)

References

Carter H, J Drury, R Amlôt, et al. 2014. Effective responder communication improves efficiency and psychological outcomes in a mass decontamination field experiment: implications for public behaviour in the event of a chemical incident. *PLoS One*, 9(3): e89846.

Further reading

UK Government Decontamination Service. 2015. *Strategic National Guidance: The Decontamination of Buildings, Infrastructure and Open Environment Exposed to Chemical, Biological, Radiological Substances or Nuclear Materials*, 4th edition. https://www.thenbs.com/PublicationIndex/Documents/Details?DocId=309655 (accessed 20 April 2016).

A2.5 **Deliberate release SIMCARD**

To be used when responding to deliberate releases: Chemical, Biological, Radiological, Nuclear

		Yes/No
1	**Situation:** An incident presenting with unusual numbers affected, unusual clinical presentation, known but locally rare disease, known cause but not responding to standard treatment; other unusual situation that 'does not feel right': consider a deliberate act.	
2	**Incubation Period (Lead Time):** Immediate. 'Rising tide' deliberate release scenarios are possible but uncommon, e.g. radiation release.	
3	**Mode of Transmission (Exposure):** Inhalation, ingestion, skin and eye contact, radiation exposure, explosive blast.	
4	**Confirmation (Criteria):** The presenting symptoms of those exposed/injured plus the nature of an acute incident may raise suspicions of deliberate release but delayed identification of the harmful agent may occur when index of suspicion is low.	
5	**Action** *Immediate:* Inform relevant authorities of suspicion of deliberate release. Care for the sick and exposed worried, control the source, determine the extent of the possible incident/exposure (emergency services). Get clinical and environmental samples sent to appropriate laboratories (microbiology, chemical, radiation). *Public Health:* Seek advice on identity of the possible agent from regional or national toxicology or microbiology colleagues. Ensure attendance at the Strategic Coordinating Group and STAC (Scientific and Technical Advice Cell) as well as staffing your own local incident/outbreak response room. Consider business continuity issues for your own staff and resources; this is likely to be a 24/7 response for a while. Priorities are to prevent others being affected, monitor the effectiveness of measures taken, prevent a recurrence, consider the needs of staff and other patients. Identify and support public health leadership for high-pressure media communications. For decontamination support see decontamination SIMCARD *Planning:* Ensure robust local multi-agency plans are up-to-date with the changing face of deliberate actions. Such plans should not differ in concept from standard multi-agency plans for incidents and outbreaks but use tried and tested local approaches. People respond better under stress when taking their usual approach to an incident or outbreak. Try to establish a register of exposed people for follow up.	
6	**Report/Communication:** There will be many pressures for communications. Decide who (upward and horizontal communication) needs to know and who does not; communicate with the former, ignore the latter. Provide regular health updates to the Strategic Coordinating Group and support media communications with health messages.	
7	**Disease Trends, Clusters, and Significant Situations:** Will depend on agent, dose, personal factors (age, health etc). Review exposed.	

Further reading

Health Protection Agency. 2008. *CBRN Incidents: Clinical Management and Health Protection.* https://www.gov.uk/government/publications/chemical-biological-radiological-and-nuclear-incidents-recognise-and-respond (accessed 31 December 2015).

Health Protection Agency. 2010. *Initial Investigation and Management of Outbreaks and Incidents of Unusual Illnesses.* https://www.gov.uk/government/publications/unusual-illness-investigation-and-management-of-outbreaks-and-incidents (accessed 31 December 2015).

Public Health England (PHE). 2013. *Deliberate and Accidental Releases: Investigation and Management.* https://www.gov.uk/government/collections/deliberate-and-accidental-releases-investigation-and-management (accessed 31 December 2015).

A2.6 **Evacuation SIMCARD**

		Yes/No
1	**Situation:** Question of evacuation from affected location(s) during any incident.	
2	**Incubation Period (Lead Time):** Usually urgent decision. May be enough warning (e.g. of adverse weather) to prepare and organize a specific mass evacuation.	
3	**Mode of Transmission (Exposure):** Anxiety or ill health may arise from evacuation due to missing essential medicines, hypothermia or injury, exposure to toxins (e.g. smoke) during the evacuation, loss of home and possessions, and if separated from family, pets, neighbours, carers, support networks and friends.	
4	**Confirmation (Criteria):** Limited number of situations warrant evacuation as a precaution or during incident: bomb threat, some radiation releases, accidental explosion risk, flooding, spread of fire, prolonged chemical release rendering indoor sheltering ineffectual (indoor and outdoor air equilibrate). Some fires, chemical releases and smoke themselves may be reasons for NOT evacuating people and exposing them to further risk, that indoor sheltering might avoid. However, there may be pressures from other agencies to evacuate, with limited understanding of risks.	
5	**Action** *Immediate:* Be very clear that benefits for evacuation overwhelm disbenefits. Local authority arranges mass transport; this takes time, especially for large numbers. Guided evacuation may be best from festivals or public events; public safety comes first. Coordinate activity through Strategic Coordinating Group, factoring in human behaviour; think broadly about public communications. *Public Health:* Be flexible, encourage mutual aid for responsible local authority. Ensure evacuation plans remove people from immediate danger but do not place them in further danger. Few people attend local authority rest centres; most go to friends and family. Consider setting up disease register (e.g. in flooding or other long-term disruption) for follow-up and learning lessons. *Planning:* Support flexible, proportionate, scalable, local multi-agency planning. Exercise and learn: rewrite the plan if necessary. Remember, the responding agencies may be caught and need to evacuate their premises: consider business continuity. In some situations, the military may assist; in many situations, assistance by voluntary organizations (Red Cross) is vital. Remember psychological needs following evacuation; offer support through voluntary and public bodies. Needs of long-term evacuees are different from short-term, including stability, sense of home, coping with loss. Encourage early local public health input to Reception Centres and temporary settlements.	
6	**Report/Communication:** Communicate in multiple ways with the affected community. Police have manpower; although social media reaches many unexpected corners, many do not use electronic communications easily. Communicate clearly with partner agencies and professional colleagues, including the wider public health community, local authority, emergency services.	
7	**Disease Trends, Clusters, and Significant Situations:** Not well understood, but mental health issues recognized, although they may relate to the incident as well as the evacuation.	

Further reading

Health Protection Agency. n.d. *Sheltering or evacuation checklist.* http://www.who.int/ipcs/emergencies/shelter_or_evacuation.pdf (accessed 31 December 2015).

HM Government. 2014. *Evacuation and Shelter Guidance.* London: Cabinet Office. https://www.gov.uk/government/uploads/system/uploads/attachment_data/file/274615/Evacuation_and_Shelter_Guidance_2014.pdf (accessed 31 December 2015).

A2.7 **Explosion SIMCARD**

To be used when responding to explosions or the risk thereof

		Yes/No
1	**Situation:** Explosions can occur during a fire, a chemical release, or due to deliberate act. Emergency services may inform health protection staff of the imminent danger affecting a local population (often due to acetylene or other cylinders in the vicinity of the fire) or of an evacuation already in place due to the magnitude of the risk.	
2	**Incubation Period (Lead Time):** Immediate usually.	
3	**Mode of Transmission (Exposure):** Injury from debris. Inhalation from smoke or acetylene released from cylinder. Possible chemical or radiation contamination, particularly if a deliberate act in a public place.	
4	**Confirmation (Criteria):** Confirm details with emergency services: history of incident, risk of explosion, number of people involved, site and radius of safety zone (standard is 200m but may be more; never less).	
5	**Action** *Immediate:* Ensure community understands what is happening and why, with sufficient practical information. *Public Health:* Support evacuation (see evacuation SIMCARD) and consider health consequences. *Planning:* Enable emergency services to understand the health consequences of any evacuation so that it is not undertaken lightly.	
6	**Report/Communication:** Inform Director of Public Health. If there is a possibility of deliberate release, attend the Strategic Coordinating Group and communicate upwards within more specialised health protection departments. Consider communication regarding risk perception, for instance possible or putative exposure to blood of victims or contaminants of explosion sites, such as asbestos.	
7	**Disease Trends, Clusters, and Significant Situations:** Will depend on situation and exposure. The public is not commonly exposed to explosions in the UK, although they occur in occupational settings. Blast injuries from pressure changes can affect air-filled organs (ears, lungs and gastrointestinal tract) and organs surrounded by fluid-filled cavities (e.g. brain and spinal cord). Exposure to chemicals in smoke can give acute and delayed health effects (upto 36 hours from corrosive chemicals; bronchiolitis two to three weeks from nitrous oxides) if the exposure is concentrated (e.g. in a confined space). However, the risk of developing long-term physical effects from a single acute exposure is very small relative to the other risks experienced in normal life. There may be short-lived psychological reactions to the incident. Some workers or public exposed to explosion and death and injury may suffer some complicated psychological effects (e.g. Post Traumatic Stress Disorder) and require suitable mental health interventions. Inhalation of acetylene may resuls in a drunken-like state (euphoria, excitement, slurred speech) with gastrointestinal disturbance and headache. However, exposure is unlikely outside the workplace.	

Further reading

Public Health England (PHE). 2005. *Health effects of explosions and fires*. https://www.gov.uk/government/publications/health-effects-of-explosions-and-fires

Public Health England (PHE). 2014. *Acetylene: properties, incident management and toxicology*. https://www.gov.uk/government/publications/acetylene-properties-incident-management-and-toxicology (accessed 31 December 2015).

A2.8 **Fire with smoke SIMCARD**

		Yes/No
1	**Situation:** Report of fire with smoke plume (contents known as 'products of combustion').	
2	**Incubation Period (Lead Time):** Immediate effects noticed by vulnerable people (with respiratory conditions). Some effects delayed 1–2 days, dependant on chemical.	
3	**Mode of Transmission (Exposure):** Inhalation. Smoke contains cocktail of gases, droplets and particles; changes with temperature and interaction with other chemicals.	
4	**Confirmation (Criteria):** Confirm details of incident (start time, site of fire, wind direction, strength, whether plume is airborne or touching ground ('grounding'), likely duration of incident, population under plume), and current response.	
5	**Action** *Immediate:* Public information should be released immediately by emergency services through all available media. Initial advice, even before details of incident are known: 'Go in, stay in, tune in' to reduce exposure, and give access to media and internet community health messages. Consider more active involvement if the fire is from worrisome sites such as old tyre depositories, scrap metal yards, old buildings with asbestos containing roofing materials. Note: Smoke is always harmful; the level of harm depends on exposure. Toxins can be asphyxiants (displace oxygen), irritants (to airways), or unusual organic compounds. *Public Health:* Check information, including health advice, already released; then make public health risk assessment based on all available information: review local map, taking wind direction into account. Countering incorrect messages should be done carefully. Obtain specialist toxicological advice for smoke and any chemicals in fire. Consider whether multi-agency major incident should be declared. Health protection teams can declare if public health response would be enhanced, even if other agencies do not see a major incident for themselves. Ask emergency services to release the public health advice through agreed multi-agency response, or directly through public health communication teams. Smoke plumes which do not ground do not pose a risk to health; be alert to fallout of particles from plumes causing anxiety and issue health advice with public information. *Planning:* Incorporate into thinking behind multi-agency plans and emergency responses that all smoke is harmful. Build in appropriate actions and alerts. Ensure clear communication channels between front-line health protection teams and regional or national toxicological support. Spend regular time together to understand each other's approaches and needs.	
6	**Report/Communication:** Inform Director of Public Health, appropriate health protection colleagues. Any reports should be shared within the wider public health team.	
7	**Disease Trends, Clusters, and Significant Situations:** Depends on pollutants inhaled, dose and length of exposure. Smoke inhalation mortality is between 45–80% for those within burning buildings, mainly immediate due to carbon monoxide (see Carbon monoxide SIMCARD) or cyanide poisoning.	

Further reading

Health Protection Agency. 2002. *Products of combustion*. www.who.int/hac/techguidance/tools/PRODUCTS%20OF%20COMBUSTION%20-%20HPA.pdf (accessed 21 April 2016).

A2.9 **Flooding SIMCARD**

		Yes/No
1	**Situation:** Excess water from fluvial (river), pluvial (rain) and coastal sources in the wrong place at the wrong time, disrupting daily life, travel and provision of services. Groundwater flooding occurs when the water table rises, days or weeks after heavy rainfall, possibly elsewhere. Any flood may persist for weeks. See chapter 15 for further details.	
2	**Incubation Period (Lead Time):** Immediate effects (e.g. drowning); delayed effects after flood has receded, during clean up and later (e.g. mental health issues); may be few days warnings from Met Office, but the resulting flood may differ from that expected.	
3	**Mode of Transmission (Exposure):** Immersion in water, isolation due to flood waters cutting access, hypothermia, carbon monoxide exposure.	
4	**Confirmation (Criteria):** Visual, reports from members of the public or emergency services, news reports.	
5	**Action** *Immediate:* Check any emergency plans (including dam and riverbank failures). Provide immediate relief to the population (by emergency services). Save lives (emergency services plus military plus voluntary agencies), protect essential services, property and livestock. *Public Health:* Support evacuation (see Evacuation SIMCARD) if necessary. Run Scientific and Technical Advice Cell for Strategic Coordination Group. Support local environmental health officers with public health advice to aid first line responders and for dissemination to local community (see also Carbon Monoxide SIMCARD). Consider own business continuity issues. Hold debrief and identify lessons learned; apply these in preparation for further floods. Surveillance and evaluation of health impacts (acute; medium to long term; academic research to improve knowledge of interventions and flooding). *Planning:* Support multiagency and community resilience plans with flood warning systems: Met Office Flood Forecasting Centre: Flood Guidance Statement; Environment Agency flood alerts. Ensure agencies and partners understand their own and others' roles and responsibilities (Local Resilience Fora; emergency services; Environment Agency; local authorities; health services; community).	
6	**Report/Communication:** Support public communications through Strategic Coordination Group: written (leaflets/booklets/posters on community notice boards/bus shelters); traditional media (press releases/interviews); social media; public meetings). Report to own senior management. Disseminate lessons learned and encourage other areas to apply appropriately.	
7	**Disease Trends, Clusters, and Significant Situations:** Health issues not well characterized. Hypothermia, loss of essential provisions, unlikely but possible exposure to microorganisms or chemicals in the waters. Carbon monoxide poisoning a danger from indoor use of generators or barbecues for heat. Drowning due to results of entrance into flood waters on foot or in vehicles. Early and late onset distress may persist beyond the incident with some people presenting with post-traumatic stress disorder.	

Further reading

Public Health England (PHE). 2014. *Flooding: health guidance and advice.* https://www.gov.uk/government/collections/flooding-health-guidance-and-advice (accessed 31 December 2015).

Public Health England (PHE). 2014. *Flooding: planning, managing and recovering from a flood.* https://www.gov.uk/government/publications/flooding-planning-managing-and-recovering-from-a-flood (accessed 31 December 2015).

PHE in Partnership with Environment Agency. 2015. *Flooding: Advice for the Public.* https://www.gov.uk/government/uploads/system/uploads/attachment_data/file/401980/flood_leaflet_2015_final.pdf. PHE publications gateway number: 2014622 (accessed 21 April 2016).

A2.10 **Fuel spills SIMCARD**

Fuel: leak or spill from fixed site of heating oil (kerosene, paraffin), diesel; also petrol station leaks (also note Spills of Unknown Type SIMCARD A2.1)

		Yes/No
1	**Situation:** Possible fuel spill near residential properties, or petrol-like taste or smell from drinking water. Domestic oil tanks usually leak from tank, the fittings, pipe into property, or during refilling. Leaks can be gradual or sudden, localized or cross property boundaries. Leaks from fuel/petrol stations may be found when digging at distance. Flooding may cause fuel contamination of an area.	
2	**Incubation Period (Lead Time):** Respiratory symptoms progress over 24–48 hours. Pulmonary oedema is delayed for 24–72 hours.	
3	**Mode of Transmission (Exposure):** Inhalation of vapours; ingestion of contaminated water, vegetables or vomit; skin contact or eye splashes from pooled fuel. Heating oil vapours less toxic than petrol, but unpleasant. Tolerance differs; some report headaches, nausea, dizziness, irritation of eyes, nose, throat, after inhaling vapour. Skin contact causes mild irritation. Symptoms are short-lived and disappear as odour recedes.	
4	**Confirmation (Criteria):** Confirm spillage (observation, fuel stains, check pipes, utility company test of water) and likely type of fuel: petrol lightest and most volatile, then diesel, then paraffin. Odour good indicator of spill. Consider air sampling, particularly if odours persist, to determine health risk.	
5	**Action** *Immediate:* Remove people from exposure. Ventilate enclosed spaces where vapours collect; ensure all flames extinguished. Environmental health visit site: can be helpful to accompany them. Supplier may be able to remove remaining fuel urgently. If swallowed, obtain medical advice immediately to reduce the risk of lung damage (chemical pneumonitis) if droplets are inhaled (e.g. vomiting after ingestion). *Public Health:* Discuss with environmental health department how to estimate quantity, extent in space, time. Consider if evacuation (see Evacuation SIMCARD) of any domestic or other nearby property is necessary while leak is found and remediated. Get toxicological assessment of any air sampling results. Encourage householders to check oil tank and lines periodically.	
6	**Report/Communication:** Inform local public health team, toxicological colleagues, local authority.	
7	**Disease Trends, Clusters, and Significant Situations:** At low doses, fuel oil vapour irritates. Higher concentrations may produce staggered gait, slurred speech, confusion. Prolonged skin exposure to liquid petrol or inhalation of vapour associated with renal dysfunction. Prolonged skin exposure to diesel may cause variety of skin conditions, generally from inadequate or inappropriate use of personal protective equipment. Although petrol is classed as a possible human carcinogen (diesel only to animals), it is unlikely that short-term, low-level occasional exposures pose any risk of cancer.	

References

Public Health England (PHE). 2014. *Petrol: properties, incident management and toxicology.* https://www.gov.uk/government/publications/petrol-properties-incident-management-and-toxicology

Public Health England (PHE). 2014. *Diesel: properties, incident management and toxicology.* https://www.gov.uk/government/publications/diesel-properties-incident-management-and-toxicology (accessed 31 December 2015).

Public Health England (PHE). 2012. *Kerosene: health effects, incident management and toxicology.* https://www.gov.uk/government/publications/kerosene-properties-incident-management-and-toxicology (accessed 21 April 2016).

A2.11 **Mobile incidents (leak—tanker) SIMCARD**

To be used when responding to Mobile Incident (e.g. leaking road tanker)—(note also Spills of Unknown Type SIMCARD A2.1)

		Yes/No
1	**Situation:** Where there has been a leak from a moving vehicle, perhaps over several miles?	
2	**Incubation Period (Lead Time):** Depends on the chemical released but likely to be short (minutes to hours)	
3	**Mode of Transmission (Exposure):** Inhalation; may be skin exposure to or ingestion of splashed liquid.	
4	**Confirmation (Criteria):** A commercial tanker will have chemical codes: numbers and letters on a prominent orange-brown sign. Fire services carry the codes and can inform public health what the chemical is.	
5	**Action** *Immediate:* Isolate the vehicle. Cover spill patches if possible. Identify exposed people, including possibly, but not certainly, the driver of the tanker. Consider if similar vehicles have a fault. *Public Health:* Have the chemical identified if possible; the Fire Service Hazmat team will confirm the meaning of the HazChem sign (coded orange-brown sign on tanker). Confirm that ambulance is able to assess those exposed to identify those needing A&E evaluation. Register the exposed people if feasible for follow up. Consider if public warnings need to be put out on all media; alert A&Es and walk-in centres in relevant areas of possible self-presenters. Alert neighbouring health protection teams if the spill trail crosses administrative boundaries. *Planning:* Ensure multi-agency plans are available, either as stand-alone, or as part of overarching plans, so that a fully integrated response can be made. The spill may cross administrative boundaries: plans should take this into account.	
6	**Report/Communication:** Director of Public Health; relevant environment agency; communication team. A press statement may need to be prepared.	
7	**Disease Trends, Clusters, and Significant Situations:** Will depend on chemical and exposure. There are more tanker spills than health protection teams are aware of since most are small and do not constitute a large hazard to public health.	

A2.12 **Non-top-tier COMAH (lower tier) sites incident SIMCARD**

For incidents at a lightly regulated (non-top-tier COMAH) or non-regulated site

		Yes/No
1	**Situation:** A fire, leak, explosion, or other incident at 'lower-tier' COMAH site. These sites are covered by Containment of Major Accident Hazards regulations but such lower-tier COMAH sites do not need to have off-site plans to use in incident. Response may be less formal, or multi-agency interaction less well organized. The hazards at unregulated sites may remain unknown for some time during the incident, but there may also be a risk of explosion (see Explosion SIMCARD).	
2	**Incubation Period (Lead Time):** Public health alert can be immediate. However, delays of several hours in the notification to health protection are known, sometimes due to the low-level categorisation of incident site within emergency services.	
3	**Mode of Transmission (Exposure):** Inhalation of smoke or gas; skin or eye contact or ingestion of splashes. Decontamination on site by ambulance or fire service may be needed.	
4	**Confirmation (Criteria):** The alert may come through the emergency services or another route (e.g. general public health colleague asking health protection for support or advice). Consider what other information you need (place, time, what has happened, who has responded, what has been done) and obtain from emergency services through your usual channels.	
5	**Action** *Immediate:* Emergency services will respond and assess situation, establishing local (bronze) command under control of fire service. Alerts for multi-agency response (if needed) should go through the normal, agreed channels. *Public Health:* Consider the size of the incident: is it a major incident for public health? If yes, then call a multi-agency response: activate your own major incident plan. If not, then respond from your base, obtain specialist regional or national toxicological and environmental advice and support emergency services and local authority. Questions about decontamination (see Decontamination SIMCARD) and evacuation (see Evacuation SIMCARD) may arise. Consider on their merits. Support local authority recovery group with health advice as necessary. *Planning:* Ensure the local multi-agency incident plan is kept up to date and exercised regularly. Learn from incident debriefs. Review business continuity plan similarly.	
6	**Report/Communication:** Inform health protection colleagues (including communication staff) and Director of Public Health.	
7	**Disease Trends, Clusters, and Significant Situations:** Disease outcomes depend on chemical, exposure and dose. There are usually more incidents at non-COMAH sites than at lower-tier sites, which may be more common than upper-tier sites.	

Further reading

Your own major incident plan.

Your own business continuity plan.

Public Health England (PHE). 2016. *Recovery, remediation and environmental decontamination.* https://www.gov.uk/government/collections/recovery-remediation-and-environmental-decontamination (accessed 21 April 2016).

A2.13 **Ionizing radiation incident SIMCARD**

For radiation leak during use or transport

		Yes/No
1	**Signs & Symptoms:** Radioactive materials are used in industry, medicine and research with many transport movements each year. They are also found in large industrial sites (REPPIR) as part of the nuclear industry. Large sites have emergency plans with alert systems through the emergency services to health protection. Other situations may be alerted through a wide variety of routes.	
2	**Incubation Period (Lead Time):** Earlier (deterministic) effects arise soon after exposure to radiation, but only if this dose exceeds relevant threshold values. Their severity, but not probability of occurrence, depends on dose level: damage to body tissues e.g. marrow, gastrointestinal tract, central nervous system, lung, skin; death within a short period at very high doses. Deterministic effects that are generally non-fatal include nausea, vomiting and impaired lung function. For a given total dose, severity of effect tends to be less if the exposure period is longer than if it is received in a short time. Delayed (stochastic) effects are long delayed and are important in clinical surveillance and population epidemiology. Their overall probability depends on dose to exposed groups/populations. There is no lower safe limit. The main types, which may arise many years after exposure, are induction of cancer in those exposed, and gene-related disease in subsequent generations.	
3	**Mode of Transmission (Exposure):** Radiation (shine) direct to organs; skin and clothes. Contamination by radioactive particles; inhalation or ingestion of radioactive particles.	
4	**Confirmation (Criteria):** Typical severe clinical findings presenting within 24 hours of exposure to high doses: Smaller doses give gastrointestinal effects (nausea, vomiting) and symptoms related to falling blood counts (infection, bleeding). Relatively larger doses can produce neurological effects and rapid death. Linking individual cancers to prior radiation exposure is difficult.	
	Confirmation (Laboratory Investigation): An absolute lymphocyte count can estimate radiation exposure dose roughly. Time from exposure to vomiting can also estimate exposure dose levels.	
5	**Action** *Public Health:* Confirm details of incident. Contact radiation specialists in Public Health England for expert radiation advice, and implement appropriate radiation plan (there are several, each for a different situation) and coordinate public health response. If an isolated case or small incident, support emergency responders and local authority with specialist advice coupled with local knowledge. If a major incident, attend multi-agency incident control (Strategic Coordinating Group) along with radiation expert; support Scientific and Technical Advice Cell. Initiate appropriate radiation response plan (if no other agency has done). Provide multi-agency group with public health advice for general public. Initiate register of exposed persons for long-term health follow-up. Consider the scale of the incident and initiate your local business continuity plan if necessary.	
6	**Report/Communication:** Local health protection and public health colleagues, including Director of Public Health, and emergency service colleagues. Regional and national health protection colleagues. Prepare media statements and interviews in conjunction with Strategic Coordinating Group. Be prepared in large incidents for Central Government interest (COBR (Cabinet Office Briefing Room) will sit).	
7	**Disease Trends, Clusters, and Significant Situations:** Clusters of disease related to large incidents (e.g. atomic bombs in Japan, nuclear power accident at Chernobyl) have been recorded and followed up for decades.	

Further reading

Public Health England (PHE). 2013. *Radiation incidents: public health preparedness and response.* https://www.gov.uk/government/collections/radiation-incidents-public-health-preparedness-and-response (accessed 30 December 2015).

Public Health England (PHE). 2013. *National arrangements for incidents involving radioactivity (NAIR).* https://www.gov.uk/guidance/national-arrangements-for-incidents-involving-radioactivity-nair (accessed 21 April 2016).

Health Protection Agency. n.d. *Understanding radiation.* http://webarchive.nationalarchives.gov.uk/20140714084352/http://www.hpa.org.uk/Topics/Radiation/UnderstandingRadiation/ (accessed 21 April 2016).

A2.14 **Swimming pools chlorine incidents SIMCARD**

To be used when responding to incidents where cleaning chemicals releasing chlorine have been wrongly mixed

		Yes/No
1	**Situation:** Chlorine containing compounds for water purification in swimming pools are constituted by mixing different precursors. Sometimes this goes wrong and chlorine gas is released.	
2	**Incubation Period (Lead Time):** Immediate; may be late (up to 36 hours)	
3	**Mode of Transmission (Exposure):** Inhalation and eye exposure. Chlorine gas is irritant to eyes, respiratory tract and skin. Skin irritation or burning usually only occurs from exposure to concentrated chlorine gas or in the immediate vicinity of a release of pressurized liquid (unlikely at a swimming pool). Optic neuropathy has been reported following acute inhalation (probably unlikely at swimming pool concentrations).	
4	**Confirmation (Criteria):** Confirm details of situation. Chlorine is a greenish gas, but lack of colour does not mean that it is absent.	
5	**Action** *Immediate:* Evacuation of site (whole or partial, depending on local situation). Turn off/stop any source of chemicals. Decontamination by copious amounts of water for anyone who has had skin or eye exposure. Do not use swimming pool showers unless advised to by emergency services. Ask site operator to make list of users/staff and their contact numbers before they leave for any further information advice. *Public Health:* Obtain specialist toxicological advice from regional or national health protection colleagues. Ensure ventilation of building. Advise anyone suffering symptoms to seek medical attention. Consider possible concentrations of exposure since pulmonary oedema (with increasing breathlessness, wheeze, hypoxia, cyanosis) may take up to 36h to develop following exposure to high levels (>40 ppm). *Planning:* Support local authority in ensuring swimming pool has an action plan for future situations like this one.	
6	**Report/Communication:** Director of Public Health, local environmental health department. Consider a joint press release.	
7	**Disease Trends, Clusters, and Significant Situations:** Mass disease is unlikely in this scenario; long-term effects at these concentrations are unlikely.	

References

Public Health England (PHE). 2014. *Chlorine: properties, incident management and toxicology.* https://www.gov.uk/government/publications/chlorine-properties-incdent-management-and-toxicology (accessed 30 December 2015).

A2.15 **Top-tier COMAH (Containment Of Major Accident Hazards) sites incident SIMCARD**

To be used when responding to an incident at a Top-tier COMAH site

		Yes/No
1	**Situation:** COMAH (Containment Of Major Accident Hazards) sites are regulated under the COMAH regulations because they store and use named chemicals above a volume/hazard threshold. Significant off-site release of chemicals will initiate the plan. Upper-tier sites are regulated by the Health and Safety Executive (lower tier sites (see Non-top-tier COMAH site incident SIMCARD) by the local authority).	
2	**Incubation Period (Lead Time):** Health effects of an incident may be immediate or delayed, depending on the chemical released.	
3	**Mode of Transmission (Exposure):** Inhalation is the main mode of exposure for the public; ingestion and skin and eye contact are more likely in those exposed on site.	
4	**Confirmation (Criteria):** The activation of the off-site emergency plan should inform emergency services of the problem, time of starting and immediate response.	
5	**Action** *Immediate:* Emergency services will attend the site and initiate the Strategic Coordinating Group (SCG). The health protection team should be alerted through agreed local procedures. Examine the health protection team's copy of the off-site plan (know how to access the plan). *Public Health:* Note details and consider business continuity implications for health protection team resources. Contact regional environmental and toxicological colleagues for advice and support. Alert relevant Director of Public Health. Attend the SCG, and contribute to STAC (Scientific and Technical Advice Cell) to support the SCG with health advice and public information. Support local authority during recovery phase with health advice and media statements. The Air Quality Cell can be mobilised to measure/estimate off site chemical and exposure levels. *Planning:* The site must exercise its emergency plans every three years. Support the local authority with the plan review and join exercising of the site off-site plans.	
6	**Report/Communication:** Attend hot debrief and report any relevant lessons to health protection emergency planning manager for incorporation into the plan. Similarly, attend later multi-agency debrief and report lessons. During incident, communicate with Director of Public Health and upwards in health protection as necessary. Prepare health media statements for SCG and, during recovery stage, local authority as necessary.	
7	**Disease Trends, Clusters, and Significant Situations:** Outcomes are related to the type of incident, the chemical released and the dose of exposure. COMAH sites are often found together; in some cases, an incident at one site may put a neighbouring site at risk (domino site); plans should take this into account.	

Further reading

Health and Safety Executive. n.d. *Control of major accident hazards (COMAH).* http://www.hse.gov.uk/comah/ (accessed 30 December 2015).

Health and Safety Executive. 2011. *Buncefield: Why did it happen? The underlying causes of the explosion and fire at the Buncefield oil storage depot, Hemel Hempstead, Hertfordshire on 11 December 2005.* http://www.hse.gov.uk/comah/buncefield/buncefield-report.pdf (accessed 31 December 2015).

Public Health England (PHE). 2016. *Recovery, remediation and environmental decontamination.* https://www.gov.uk/government/collections/recovery-remediation-and-environmental-decontamination (accessed 21 April 2016).

A2.16 **Waste transfer site fires SIMCARD**

		Yes/No
1	**Situation:** Waste transfer (storage) sites are common because of increased community recycling. Many thousands tons of mixed plastics and paper stored in bales on site, regulated by relevant environment agency; permit conditions may be breached: bales stored in fire breaks, into roof spaces, presenting fire risk. Fires may burn for weeks, especially if inert plastic coating is induced at waste surface by cooling, possibly from fire service water. Waste under this layer may smoulder, releasing smoke; very difficult to extinguish. Dilemma: slow burn, with ongoing smoke; or attempt to extinguish, with possible contamination off-site from copious amounts of polluted fire-water. See chapter 14 for more details.	
2	**Incubation Period (Lead Time):** Unknown: spontaneous combustion possible when ambient temperatures are high, but negligence or arson also possible. While burning, unlikely that cause will be established; thereafter, may become crime scene.	
3	**Mode of Transmission (Exposure):** Inhalation of smoke.	
4	**Confirmation (Criteria):** Report from emergency services or local authority.	
5	**Action** *Immediate:* Emergency services respond to fire. Issue 'Go in, stay in, tune in' message on local radio and other media to reduce community exposure to smoke. Discourage sightseers. *Public Health:* Liaise with emergency services, local authority and environment agency. Consider calling major incident, establishing multi-agency Strategic Coordination Group; when not done early, can lead to ongoing communication and decision-making difficulties. Obtain specialist environmental and toxicological advice from regional or national colleagues. Support Strategic Coordination Group's dissemination of health advice to community. Advice needs repeating and tailoring (daily) by weather as fire continues. Be realistic: sheltering cannot be continued for weeks. Undertake site visit. Respond sensitively to community concerns with timely information and sensible advice: use local knowledge. Be honest about risks identified. Public may worry about dioxins (unlikely to be released in quantity; toxicity is largely by ingestion of contaminated dietary components; reassurance monitoring might be worthwhile) or vermin moving off-site. *Planning:* Consider pre-emptive multi-agency meeting to agree response to any site that may become a risk due to weather or other considerations.	
6	**Report/Communication:** Director of Public Health, national health protection colleagues. The community (often, using short, practical, realistic, simply stated communications by all means possible).	
7	**Disease Trends, Clusters, and Significant Situations:** Disease outbreak unlikely. People with pre-existing respiratory disease should avoid smoke plumes, which may exacerbate their condition. Vermin around waste sites are a nuisance for local authority attention rather than established cause of disease.	

Further reading

Health Protection Agency. n.d. *Products of combustion.* http://www.who.int/hac/techguidance/tools/ PRODUCTS%20OF%20COMBUSTION%20-%20HPA.pdf (accessed 30 December 2015).

Appendix 3

SIMCARDs for dealing with environmental hazards and situations

A3.1 **Air pollution SIMCARD**

		Yes/No
1	**Situation:** Raised air concentrations of regulated pollutants (mainly nitrous oxides and particles; also benzene, 1,3-butadiene, carbon monoxide, lead, ozone, sulphur dioxide). Indoor air pollution from particles from solid fuel a leading global risk factor for disease burden: largely open fires in developing countries; solid fuel burners becoming more common in the UK. See chapter 16 for further details.	
2	**Incubation Period (Lead Time):** Immediate (days) or delayed (months-years)	
3	**Mode of Transmission (Exposure):** Outdoor air, particularly traffic related, power generation, industry, waste recycling, heath, moorland, natural sources (volcanoes, deserts). Indoor air, particularly particles, cigarette smoke, also volatile organics from new carpets, paint.	
4	**Confirmation (Criteria):** Air Quality Standards: scientifically acceptable concentrations recorded over given time period; benchmarks pollution changes (details in Table 16.1 and 16.2). Exceedence: defined time period where concentration higher than Standard. Objective: target date when exceedences of Standard must not exceed specified number. Indoor air pollution has no limit values. Static outdoor monitoring sites run by local authority and national consultants. Data modelled at national, occasionally local, level. Particles classed by diameter (microns): PM_{10} includes $PM_{2.5}$; PM_{10} without $PM_{2.5}$: coarse particles; $PM_{2.5}$ fines; PM0.1 ultrafines.	
5	**Action** *Immediate:* With public health, health protection, environmental health professionals, clinicians, consider priority areas for air quality: transport, waste recycling, industry, power generation. *Public Health:* Support and strengthen local authority air quality strategy: transport, traffic, highways, planning. Support local environmental health officers with public health advice. Consider regular meetings with local air quality officers to review on-going situations, develop strategy. Encourage Local Authorities to prioritize air pollution. Public health action on air pollution (including increasing exercise, active transport, using public transport) benefits diabetes, cardiovascular disease, obesity. Support air quality objective introduction into local authority's strategy. Support systematic health impact assessments for appropriate planning applications. Identify, encourage and support appropriate local, regional, national actions.	
6	**Report/Communication:** Within local public health team, local authority, specialist health protection teams. Consider using local authority website and other public-facing links for real-time, local air quality data, interpretation.	
7	**Disease Trends, Clusters, and Significant Situations:** Depends on pollutant, local pollution patterns, demography, health status: effects higher nearer main roads, in deprived communities. Diseases include respiratory, cardiovascular, cerebrovascular, liver, metabolic disorders, diabetes, premature births, impaired foetal development, lung cancer.	

(continued on the next page)

Further reading

Lim SS, T Vos, AD Flaxman, et al. 2012. A comparative risk assessment of burden of disease and injury attributable to 67 risk factors and risk factor clusters in 21 regions, 1990–2010: a systematic analysis for the Global Burden of Disease Study 2010. *Lancet*, **380**: 2224–60.

Straif K, A Cohen, J Samet (eds). *Air Pollution and Cancer*. IARC Scientific Publications, 161. Lyon: International Agency for Research on Cancer. http://www.iarc.fr/en/publications/books/sp161/

WHO. n.d. *Air pollution*. http://www.who.int/topics/air_pollution/en/ (accessed 31 December 2015).

WHO. 2012. *Burden of disease from household air pollution for 2012*. http://www.who.int/phe/health_topics/outdoorair/databases/FINAL_HAP_AAP_BoD_24March2014.pdf (accessed 30 December 2015).

WHO. 2012. *Burden of disease from ambient air pollution for 2012*. http://www.who.int/phe/health_topics/outdoorair/databases/AAP_BoD_results_March2014.pdf (accessed 30 December 2015).

WHO. 2013. *Review of Evidence on Health Aspects of Air Pollution—REVIHAAP: Final Technical Report*. http://www.euro.who.int/en/health-topics/environment-and-health/air-quality/publications/2013/review-of-evidence-on-health-aspects-of-air-pollution-revihaap-project-final-technical-report (accessed 31 December 2015).

A3.2 **Arsenic SIMCARD**

		Yes/No
1	**Situation:** Raised concentrations of arsenic in contaminated land (UK) or water (including USA, SE Asia) and as an antifungal wood preservative (tanalized wood). Has been used (historically) as medicine. Inorganic compounds in fish and shellfish. Found in tobacco smoke and smelters.	
2	**Incubation Period (Lead Time):** Acute toxicity: hours. Chronic ingestion: long (>10 years as carcinogen)	
3	**Mode of Transmission (Exposure):** Ingestion; inhalation uncommon. Skin contact does not give rise to the skin lesions characteristic of arsenic poisoning, they arise from ingestion. Ingestion of small quantities of organic arsenic from seafood does not pose a health risk.	
4	**Confirmation (Criteria):** Acute: garlic smell to breath and tissue fluids; vomiting, abdominal pain and diarrhoea, followed by numbness and tingling of the extremities, muscle cramping and death, in extreme cases. Chronic: pigmentation changes with hard patches on soles and palms; characteristic skin hyperkeratosis ('dew drops on a dusty road'); peripheral neuropathy: painful, glove-stocking symmetrical paraesthesia; hepatic and renal damage; diabetes, cardiovascular disease ('blackfoot disease' Taiwan). Trans-placental toxin: spontaneous abortion, stillbirth, preterm birth; lung cancer and bronchiectasis later in life.	
	Environmental Investigation: Concentration measured in water (WHO health based standard >10 ug/l), soil (national standards), food, occasionally air.	
5	**Action** *Immediate:* Remove source, if possible. Soil: Cover soil to reduce dust hazard. Plan long-term remediation strategy in conjunction with other professionals and agencies. Water: Consider alternative supplies of water, including rain water. *Public Health:* Land: averaged concentrations in defined area (e.g. garden) above health criterion value (defined nationally in many countries) need further consideration and may need further investigation by environmental health department in association with health protection professionals Water: averaged concentrations over time and space above WHO standard need further investigation by environmental health department in association with health protection professionals and environmental specialists: difficult problem to resolve. Install arsenic removal systems (central or domestic): ensure appropriate disposal of removed arsenic. May need central government action.	
6	**Report/Communication:** Local community, clinicians, local authority, public health community, central government.	
7	**Disease Trends, Clusters, and Significant Situations:** Disease directly attributable to arsenic contaminated land or water has not been demonstrated in the UK; in Southeast Asia, arsenic poisoning is common due to the high intake from contaminated water and crops.	

Further reading

Public Health England (PHE). 2014. *Arsenic: properties, incident management and toxicology.* https://www.gov.uk/government/publications/arsenic-properties-incident-management-and-toxicology (accessed 31 December 2015).

WHO 2010. *Exposure to arsenic: a major public health concern.* http://www.who.int/ipcs/features/arsenic.pdf (accessed 30 December 2015).

A3.3 **Asbestos SIMCARD**

Fires, waste, clean-up exposures

		Yes/No
1	**Situation:** Asbestos: several naturally-occurring silicate minerals with long, fine, parallel fibres; previously used for fire resistant properties: found in roofing cement, insulation, ceiling and floor tiles, textured paint. Contaminates land. Two main types: serpentine—soft, malleable, can be woven (chrysotile: white asbestos: most common); amphiboles—brittle (several sub-types: crocidolite: blue asbestos, amosite: brown asbestos; anthophyllite: no commercial value; tremolite: contaminant of other asbestos: no commercial value; actinolite: contaminates chrysotile and talc deposits).	
2	**Incubation Period (Lead Time):** Long (often >20 years for cancer)	
3	**Mode of Transmission (Exposure):** Inhalation: most asbestos products pose little risk if intact; when damaged may release fibres into air. Fibres also naturally occurring: likely daily exposure to low levels by everyone. Very unlikely that the general population is exposed to concentrations high enough, over sufficient period of time, to cause adverse health effects. Short-term high level exposure may cause cancer. Secondary exposure (to someone in direct contact with asbestos containing materials), particularly short-term, unlikely to pose an elevated public health risk. Occupational exposure remains important. Ingestion not a risk.	
4	**Confirmation (Criteria):** Soft tissue asbestosis considered a feature of high occupational exposure. Pleural disorders, mesothelioma and lung cancers more commonly associated with long-term, but low level, exposure.	
	Laboratory Investigation: No human laboratory confirmation of asbestos exposure. Characterize environmental asbestos type to facilitate risk assessment.	
5	**Action** *Immediate:* Consider source removal or isolation: collect obvious lumps of free asbestos containing material to reduce risk of later weathering or breakages. *Public Health:* Discuss with environmental health department and specialist toxicological colleagues. Form action plan (surveillance, remediation, removal, isolation) at appropriate level to risk.	
6	**Report/Communication:** Local community, clinicians, local authority, public health community.	
7	**Disease Trends, Clusters, and Significant Situations:** Size and shape of fibres appear to play major role in toxicity:	

Asbestos-induced effect	Length of fibre (μm)	Width of fibre (μm)
Asbestosis	> 2 μm	> 0.15 μm
Mesothelioma	> 5 μm	< 0.1 μm
Lung cancer	> 10 μm	< 0.15 μm

Lung cancer may develop up to 40 years after exposure; however, in the UK there is an unexplained increase in incidence in younger women without obvious occupational or other exposure. Household cases of asbestos-induced cancer are thought to be due to household exposure to contaminated work clothing. Mesothelioma may have other causes than asbestos exposure. Smoking increases the risk of cancer from asbestos.	

References

Public Health England (PHE). 2014. *Asbestos: properties, incident management and toxicology*. https://www.gov.uk/government/publications/asbestos-properties-incident-management-and-toxicology (accessed 31 December 2015).

Further reading

Lemen RA, JM Dement, JK Wagoner. 1980. Epidemiology of asbestos-related diseases. *Environmental Health Perspectives*, **34**: 1–11.

A3.4 **Disease Cluster SIMCARD**

Investigating putative clusters of chronic disease, including cancer

		Yes/No
1	**Situation:** Reported increase in disease prevalence or incidence by clinician, member of public or other professional. Even if the report seems unlikely to be true, a systematic approach to investigating the circumstances will help ascertain the known facts and alleviate any anxiety. See chapter 17 for further details.	
2	**Incubation Period (Lead Time):** Depends on the disease reported. Search for other cases (initially by asking the reporter; consider using surveillance or GP data) and confirm diagnoses. Consider the spread of onset/diagnosis dates for all cases.	
3	**Mode of Transmission (Exposure):** Worry about other local environmental or social conditions may cause the concern about the cluster to spread in the local community. There may be other drivers such as personal interest.	
4	**Confirmation (Criteria):** Confirm diagnoses are all the same and create a case definition (person, time, place). Search widely for other confirmable cases. Take a stepped approach with clear criteria allowing the investigation to be stopped when no further information adds to the understanding. Step 1: define the case/disease or situation. Step 2: accepting there is a need for further investigation, proceed to determine if the observed/expected ratio is greater than one and significant. Step 3: assuming further investigation is warranted, check for a plausible explanation and consider hypotheses to investigate. Step 4: if continuing, check for possible exposures. Step 5: any further investigation should examine concentrations of any possible exposure. Information for different steps may be acquired at the same time.	
5	**Action:** Take the complaint seriously but do not let anxiety cause over-investigation. Be prepared to stop but be able to justify and explain your reasons. If the cluster is not confirmed, communicate clearly with the complainant. If the cluster is confirmed, consider what multi-agency actions (by public health, environmental and other local authority staff, clinicians and others) are needed to investigate and possibly manage the situation further.	
6	**Report/Communication:** Report in writing or verbally to the complainant; consider a report to the Director of Public Health. There may be a need for media messages.	
7	**Disease Trends, Clusters, and Significant Situations:** Calls for cluster investigations are frequent, usually with small numbers of cases. Investigating can be time consuming. In terms of scientific, clinical of epidemiological discovery, they usually offer little, but in terms of community or professional anxiety, they are very supportive of good relationships and for alleviating anxiety and concern.	

Further reading

Abrams B, H Anderson, C Blackmore, et al. 2013. Investigating suspected cancer clusters and responding to community concerns: guidelines from CDC and the Council of State and Territorial Epidemiologists. Recommendations and reports. *Morbidity and Mortality Weekly Report*, **62**(RR08):1–14.

Coory MD, S Jordan. 2012. Assessment of chance should be removed from protocols for investigating cancer clusters. *International Journal of Epidemiology*, **42**(2): 440–47.

Goodman M, JS Naiman, D Goodman, et al. 2012. Cancer clusters in the USA: what do the last twenty years of state and federal investigations tell us? *Critical Reviews in Toxicology*, **42**(6): 474–90.

A3.5 **Composting sites SIMCARD**

		Yes/No
1	**Situation:** Composting sites (large licenced commercial site; open, on-farm wind-rows; small community sites; home garden): all but the latter need to be registered with the relevant environment agency. Composting relies on micro-organisms; high concentrations of bacteria and fungi are present in composts. When composting materials are moved (e.g. during turning), micro-organisms can become airborne as bioaerosol; complaints of odours and ill-health can arise due to worries about bioaerosol exposure. The major components of bioaerosols are bacteria, endotoxin (bacterial cell wall toxins), peptidoglycan (murein) (an amino acid-sugar mix), fungi, moulds, volatile organic compounds (e.g. terpenes).	
2	**Incubation Period (Lead Time):** Immediate: allergic reactions; later: infections (rare). Air concentrations of bioaerosols usually decrease to background levels over 200–250m distance from composting, although occasional reports indicate that, in unfavourable meteorological conditions, concentrations may remain slightly raised beyond that.	
3	**Mode of Transmission (Exposure):** Inhalation. Most inhaled particles cause allergic reactions: bacterial spores may cause allergic lung disease (not = asthma), endotoxins may cause both acute illness (flu-like symptoms, fever, myalgia and malaise, e.g. organic dust toxic syndrome) and chronic illness (bronchitis, chronic obstructive airways disease, decreased lung function). *Aspergillus fumigatus* is particularly linked to composting, but is ubiquitous in air, exposing everyone: the immune-suppressed at most at risk. Invasive aspergillosis is the commonest mould infection worldwide. Legionaires disease has also been linked to composting sites.	
4	**Confirmation (Criteria):** Bioaerosol levels from different processes are difficult to compare as there is no standard way to measure exposure: concentrations are probably highly variable.	
5	**Action:** Review situation with environmental health officers and environment agency staff. Consider distance from site of those possibly affected. Obtain permission and medical history from GP and discuss immunosuppression and possible allergic disease. Discuss with micro-biological colleagues as necessary. Consider bioaerosols, as well as chemicals and other hazards, when requests to assess planning and permitting applications are presented for health protection review. Odours may need consideration (see Odours SIMCARD). Multiple cases may need a multi-agency review meeting.	
6	**Report/Communication:** Communicate with the complainant, local environmental health and environment agency in single cases. If multiple cases, report to Director of Public Health.	
7	**Disease Trends, Clusters, and Significant Situations:** Respiratory problems (eye, upper airway irritation, decreased lung function) occur far more commonly in site workers (exposed to concentrations 10–1,000 times ambient air) than in the general public. There is no evidence of ill health in nearby residents when bioaerosols are above background concentrations at greater than 250 m distance from the composting site.	

References

Latge JP. 1999. Aspergillus fumigatus and Aspergillosis. *Clinical Microbiology Review*, **12**(2): 310–50.

Swan JRM, A Kelsey, B Crook, et al. 2003. *Occupational and Environmental Exposure to Bioaerosols from Composts and Potential Health Effects—A Critical Review of Published Data*. Health & Safety Executive Research Report 130. Norwich: Her Majesty's Stationery Office.

A3.6 **Contaminated land SIMCARD**

		Yes/No
1	**Situation:** Contaminated land advice is usually sought by the local authority which, under the Environmental Protection Act (1990) Part IIA, undertakes a risk-based approach to prioritize and assess potentially or actually contaminated sites. A risk-based approach is also required as part of planning process for new developments. Government has target of 60% new-build on previously used land ('brownfield sites'), possibly contaminated from previous industrial use.	
2	**Incubation Period (Lead Time):** Much of the contaminated land in the UK is a legacy of earlier industry. Planning regulations have changed many times since, so land identified in the risk assessment could already be used for housing or another function. Toxicity from contaminated land is difficult to demonstrate in the UK but probably has a long incubation period (years). Management is important as one way of reducing exposure to toxins, contributing to wider public health measures. Acute toxicity is possible, particularly in heavily contaminated land to which small children have access.	
3	**Mode of Transmission (Exposure):** Consider three pathways: Ingestion: direct ingestion of soil contaminating hands after working on land (garden, allotment etc.). Young children may ingest 100–200g soil per day. Children with pica are at greater risk. Inhalation: Dust generated by weather (dry, windy), land use or recreational use may be of respirable size and deposited in airways; particulate toxins can be absorbed. Skin contact: Some toxins can be absorbed directly through the skin or conjunctiva. Risk assessments protect the 0–6-year-old girl (longest potential lifetime exposure; carries eggs that will become her children, thus potentially exposing herself, her children and perhaps grandchildren).	
4	**Confirmation (Criteria):** Environmental health departments undertake a phased assessment: initial review of borough history identifies potentially contaminated land. Specific sites are selected for review. Phase 1: Desk Study qualitatively identifies potentially sensitive receptors (human users of the land; buildings; water). A conceptual model identifies any significant pollutant links between setting (source) and receptors. Phase 2: Intrusive Investigation investigates in detail each aspect highlighted in Phase 1 with a quantitative analysis.	
5	**Action** *Local Authority:* Leading and planning investigation, tendering for environmental consultant to undertake phased studies; application for national funding for urgent remediation of seriously contaminated land (cover, removal); remediation design, execution and verification. *Public Health:* Support local authority through health risk assessment of inhabitants of contaminated land through comparison of relevant routine health data at the lowest possible geography (e.g. ward, Lower Super Output Area) with other similar geographies. Direct health studies are unlikely to have power to detect health issues. Devise health messages for local authority communications with residents, users of land, general public, local health services, elected members.	
6	**Report/Communication:** Local community, clinicians, local authority, public health community.	
7	**Disease Trends, Clusters, and Significant Situations:** Contaminated land is common wherever industry operates/has operated without efficient controls. Some of the worst contaminated land is in developing countries.	

Further reading

Pure Earth/Blacksmith Institute has produced an annual report on the worst contaminated sites globally since 2007. http://www.worstpolluted.org/ (accessed 31 December 2015).

A3.7 **Delusional environmental toxicity SIMCARD**

For investigating possible fixed delusional complaints presenting as environmental issues

		Yes/No
1	**Situation:** Delusional environmental toxicity has only recently been recognized. It is parallel to delusional infestation (formerly delusional parasitosis). Patients present with common environmentally related complaints expressed in strange ways, or with unusual complaints that are just about environmentally plausible. Likely to be two forms: primary, an isolated, mono-symptomatic delusional disorder: patients are otherwise mentally healthy and argue rationally when discussing other issues; secondary to another defined neurological or psychiatric disorder or intoxication.	
2	**Incubation Period (Lead Time):** May develop quickly (days-weeks) from a genuine environmental experience. Duration: minutes (secondary to toxic psychosis or delirium), months, years (chronic).	
3	**Mode of Transmission (Exposure):** Shared beliefs within a family occur, with other family members growing into the delusional belief; Munchausen-by-Proxy Syndrome (the fabrication or exaggeration of symptoms in another) may possibly develop in family members (occurs sometimes in delusional infestation).	
4	**Confirmation (Criteria):** Easier to suspect than prove. There is a fixed belief out of keeping with the patient's cultural background. Delusions are (a) an 'extraordinary conviction' and an 'incomparable, subjective certainty', (b) which cannot be influenced by experience or logical conclusions, although (c) 'their content is impossible' (Jaspers, quoted by Freudenmann and Lepping 2009). Clinical and environmental evaluations must go hand in hand with. There are few clinicians who are experienced in this diagnosis at this point.	
	***Environmental Investigation*:** Appropriate environmental investigations should be undertaken, in conjunction with the clinical review. The patient may become a nuisance caller to environmental health and other agencies and will need careful support.	
5	**Action** *Immediate:* Take the complainant seriously; evaluate complaint fully and appropriately, remembering that there may be a genuine environmental problem even if there is a delusional disorder. *Public Health:* Do not suggest psychiatric investigation early, but as a result of failure of all other explanations. Consider 'stress' as the diagnosis for this discussion. Obtain permission and liaise early with the patient's General Practitioner. Treatment with anti-psychotics is likely to help some, particularly secondary cases.	
6	**Report/Communication:** Environmental health officers, General Practitioner, Mental Health services.	
7	**Disease Trends, Clusters, and Significant Situations:** The incidence is unknown: delusional infestation may be about 6/1M people, with a higher prevalence (83/1M) (Freudenmann and Lepping 2009).	

References

Freudenmann RW, P Lepping. 2009. Delusional infestation. *Clinical Microbiology Reviews*, **22**(4): 690–732.

A3.8 **Electromagnetic fields SIMCARD**

To be used when investigating complaints concerning electromagnetic fields

		Yes/No
1	**Situation:** Enquiries from members of the public, clinicians or environmental health officers about possible adverse health effects from visible or buried power lines, usually high voltage, may be general or ask specifically about cancer, including leukaemia.	
2	**Incubation Period (Lead Time):** Overall evidence for adverse effects on health at levels of exposure normally experienced by the general public is weak. The least weak evidence is around the exposure of children to power frequency magnetic fields and childhood leukaemia. The lead (incubation) time remains unknown.	
3	**Mode of Transmission (Exposure):** Electric and magnetic fields created by power supplies (at 50 or 60 Hertz) cause electrical currents inside the body. Faint flickering visual sensations can occur at field strengths many thousands of times higher than those encountered in buildings.	
4	**Confirmation (Criteria):** Some studies show an association between exposure to magnetic fields in the home (and/or living close to high voltage power lines) and a small excess of childhood leukaemia; however, magnetic fields do not have sufficient energy to damage cells and thereby cause cancer. The overall balance of evidence is towards no effect for other conditions such as Alzheimer's disease; the evidence is even weaker than that for childhood leukaemia.	
5	**Action:** Take the enquiry seriously and discuss the above findings with the enquirer to reassure. Refer to the HPA archive web page (see references). If the enquirer raises strange questions (e.g. the neighbour's rewiring is affecting their health) or discusses the issue in an unusual or fixated manner, consider the possibility of delusionals (see Delusional environmental toxicity SIMCARD).	
6	**Report/Communication:** Single enquiries are unlikely to need wider communication but may need a confirmatory email or letter.	
7	**Disease Trends, Clusters, and Significant Situations:** While it is estimated that 2–5 cases of childhood leukaemia each year, from a total of ~500 cases (UK), could be attributable to magnetic fields, the evidences is not strong. At present there is no clear biological explanation for the possible increase in childhood leukaemia from exposure to magnetic fields. The evidence that exposure to magnetic fields causes any other type of illness in children or adults is far weaker.	

References

HPA archives, 2014. *Health effects of electric and magnetic fields.* http://webarchive.nationalarchives.gov.uk/20140714084352/http://www.hpa.org.uk/Topics/Radiation/UnderstandingRadiation/UnderstandingRadiationTopics/ElectromagneticFields/ElectricAndMagneticFields/HealthEffectsOfElectricAndMagneticFields/ (accessed 31 December 2015).

A3.9 **Landfill sites SIMCARD**

		Yes/No
1	**Situation:** Enquiries about health effects sites, dust, water run-off or leachate (water or other liquid passing through landfill extracts solutes, suspended solids or other components) may come to any public health or environmental health professional. UK waste traditionally went to landfill; suitable sites are becoming scarcer. Old sites: used quarries, gravel or sand pits, marsh land; may become 'land-raise' when waste overtops surrounding land level.	
2	**Incubation Period (Lead Time):** May be decades between waste disposal and questions about health. Older landfill sites do not have impermeable lining: possible pollutant movement into or through surrounding land. Dust generation is possible at working sites.	
3	**Mode of Transmission (Exposure):** Movement of pollutants into air (mainly landfill gas (~65% methane, ~35% carbon dioxide), land or water, with pathways to population of inhalation, ingestion and skin contact. Traffic-related emissions and waste blow from transport and site. Vermin problems on poorly managed site.	
4	**Confirmation (Criteria):** Confirm facts with other professionals and agencies: landfill site, age, content (if known), possible source of fill, current land use; nearby population, industry, infrastructure, geology, hydrogeology, pollutant movement; draw model of movement of pollutant and pathways to potentially affected population. Modern landfills are subject to regulatory controls, requiring site design and operation such that there is no significant impact on human health.	
5	**Action:** Meet and discuss with environmental health colleagues. Agree a plan of investigation to answer environmental and health questions (may involve environmental measurements) that remain unanswered from the confirmation criteria above: may include convening a multi-agency health advisory group (environmental and public health professionals, specialist health protection professionals, environmental or toxicological scientists, Environment Agency, relevant others). Health studies of nearby population are unlikely to have enough power for significance. Agree terms of reference and an end-point, guide resulting investigations, interpret findings, and support communications from the Director of Public Health to residents, media and local health professionals.	
6	**Report/Communication:** Director of Public Health, local community, local health professionals.	
7	**Disease Trends, Clusters, and Significant Situations:** Odours (see Odour SIMCARD) may affect nearby residents; may be more physiological than pathological. Bioaerosols unlikely to travel >250m. Living close to a well-managed landfill poses little if any risk to health. Old landfill sites may release harmful pollutants: some studies have suggested raised incidence of cancer or congenital abnormalities near landfills but methodological problems exist, questioning findings which have not been confirmed.	

Further reading

Public Health England (PHE). 2011. *RCE– 18: impact on health of emissions from landfill sites.* https://www.gov.uk/government/publications/landfill-sites-impact-on-health-from-emissions (accessed 25 April 2016).

A3.10 **Mould SIMCARD**

Complaints concerning mould

		Yes/No
1	**Situation:** Complaints of damp in houses may be referred by the local environmental health department for advice on the health effects. Mould is a particular problem after flooding but is also found in composting piles, cut grass and wooded areas: anywhere warm and moist. Most complaints related to mould are associated with respiratory symptoms.	
2	**Incubation Period (Lead Time):** Unknown but relatively short (days, weeks).	
3	**Mode of Transmission (Exposure):** Inhalation of mould spores and toxins from mould cell walls.	
4	**Confirmation (Criteria):** Examination of the building can confirm damp, with visible mould on walls, ceilings and furnishings.	
5	**Action:** Support improvement of local housing conditions: control humidity, fix leaky sites, clean and dry after flooding, ventilate shower, laundry, and cooking areas. Advise susceptible people to avoid areas likely to support mould growth. Current evidence does not support measuring specific indoor microbiologic factors to guide health-protective actions.	
6	**Report/Communication:** Involve local community and media in raising awareness and encouraging action.	
7	**Disease Trends, Clusters, and Significant Situations:** Dampness and mould are associated with increases of 30–50% in a variety of health outcomes (upper respiratory infections and allergies, cough, wheeze, respiratory infections) in a variety of populations (young children and the elderly); those with existing skin problems (e.g. eczema), respiratory problems (e.g. allergies, asthma, chronic disease), immunosuppression.	

Further reading

Fisk WJ, Q Lei-Gomez, MJ Mendell. 2007. Meta-analyses of the associations of respiratory health effects with dampness and mould in homes. *Indoor Air*, **17**: 284–96.

Mendell MM, AG Mirer, K Cheung, et al. 2011. Respiratory and allergic health effects of dampness, mold, and dampness-related agents: a review of the epidemiologic evidence. *Environmental Health Perspectives*, **119**: 748–56.

Public Health England (PHE). 2013. *Cold Weather Plan for England 2013: Making the Case: Why Long-term Strategic Planning for Cold Weather Is Essential to Health and Wellbeing.* https://www.gov.uk/government/uploads/system/uploads/attachment_data/file/252854/Cold_Weather_Plan_2013_Making_the_Case_final_v2.pdf (accessed 31 December 2015).

WHO Europe. 2009. *Damp and Mould: Health Risks, Prevention and Remedial Actions.* Copenhagen: WHO. http://www.euro.who.int/__data/assets/pdf_file/0003/78636/Damp_Mould_Brochure.pdf (accessed 30 December 2015).

WHO Europe. 2009. *WHO Guidelines for Indoor Air Quality: Dampness and Mould.* Copenhagen: WHO. http://www.euro.who.int/en/health-topics/environment-and-health/air-quality/publications/2009/who-guidelines-for-indoor-air-quality-dampness-and-mould (accessed 30 December 2015).

A3.11 **Noise SIMCARD**

Complaints concerning noise

		Yes/No
1	**Situation:** Complaints about noise are usually made to environmental health departments, who may ask health protection staff for support and advice. The noise may be industrial or commercial or, occasionally, domestic. Planning and permitting applications may have noise sections about which health protection advice is sought.	
2	**Incubation Period (Lead Time):** Immediate (e.g. nuisance, social disruption); long-term (e.g. cardiovascular).	
3	**Mode of Transmission (Exposure):** The health effects of noise are divisible into auditory (impairment of hearing: occurs almost exclusively in industrial settings) and non-auditory (commonly, annoyance; also sleep disturbance, interruption of speech and social interaction, disturbance of concentration (hence of learning and long-term memory), hormonal and cardiovascular effects (chronic exposure)). It is not clear to what extent these effects are actually harmful. Some evidence suggests that noise-sensitive people are more prone to mental illness and that the effects of noise may be more pronounced in mentally ill people.	
4	**Confirmation (Criteria):** Ambient noise can easily be measured. There are known effects at known levels.	
5	**Action:** Support the local authority who will organize measurements if appropriate; most noise complaints can be dealt with under nuisance rather than public health legislation.	
6	**Report/Communication:** Local Director of Public Health, environmental health department.	
7	**Disease Trends, Clusters, and Significant Situations:** Long-term effects are not as well understood as they could be. Complaints about low frequency noise come from a small number of people but the degree of distress can be quite high. There is no firm evidence that this type of sound causes damage to health, in the physical sense, but some people are certainly very sensitive to it. In some situations, but by no means all, a source can be identified and controlled.	

Further reading

Chartered Institute of Environmental Health. 2015. *Noise and health.* http://www.cieh.org/policy/noise_health.html (accessed 31 December 2015).

Health Protection Agency. 2014. *Environmental Noise and Health in the UK. A report by the Ad Hoc Expert Group on Noise and Health.* http://webarchive.nationalarchives.gov.uk/20140714084352/http://www.hpa.org.uk/ProductsServices/ChemicalsPoisons/Environment/Noise/ (accessed 31 December 2015).

A3.12 **Odour SIMCARD**

		Yes/No
1	**Situation:** Complaints usually made to environmental health departments; health protection asked for support. Complaints: around waste disposal (landfill, composting sites), water treatment, industry, chemical incidents, food processing, agriculture, homes. Planning and permitting applications may discuss odour.	
2	**Incubation Period (Lead Time):** Odours smelled immediately; effects may take time, depending on combination of type, duration, strength of smell (pungent odours less well tolerated than pleasant, which can become nuisance if strong).	
3	**Mode of Transmission (Exposure):** Unpleasant odours affect quality of life. Responses range from ignoring, annoyance, nuisance, to health effects. Odiferous activities regulated by local authorities, or Environment Agency, to ensure insignificant amounts of odours released.	
4	**Confirmation (Criteria):** Human nose very sensitive to odours, detecting many substances below harmful concentrations. Odours can cause annoyance, sometimes leading to stress and anxiety. Some people experience symptoms (nausea, headaches, dizziness) as reaction to odours from non-harmful substances. Odour threshold concentrations known for some chemicals. A very few guideline values exist showing levels below which toxic effects do not occur.	
5	**Action:** Confirm the situation. Consider other issues, particularly if complaint relates to commercial premises. Discuss with the environmental health department, or Environment Agency. Consider if acute risk other than the odour exists: gas leak or chemical spill? (HPA 2014) checklist can help assessment http://webarchive.nationalarchives.gov. uk/20140629102627/http://www.hpa.org.uk/ProductsServices/ChemicalsPoisons/ ChemicalRiskAssessment/ChemicalIncidentManagement/OdourIncidents/Guidelines/. Undertake site visit if possible; consider meeting the public to ascertain wider issues. Discuss with local public health team, specialist health protection staff, and toxicological colleagues. Agree approach, with appropriate investigations, remediation and exit strategies. Try to distinguish between physiological (minor but irritating symptoms, e.g. nausea, headaches, dizziness) and toxicological effects (adverse effects resulting in damage to health). Community health investigations unlikely to be helpful (resist requests with reasons: problem of small numbers, case definition issues); personal diaries of when the odours are noted (with effects), and timeline of complaints to health services (before or after the publicizing of the situation?) may help.	
6	**Report/Communication:** Inform local public health and environmental health departments, specialist environmental and toxicological colleagues; consider a holding media statement. Responding can be difficult; may end with little satisfaction for anyone.	
7	**Disease Trends, Clusters, and Significant Situations:** There can be a full range of outcomes, from indifference to actual ill health. Pathological/ toxicological outcomes need a multi-agency health response supporting the relevant regulatory authority; physiological responses best dealt with by local authority through nuisance legislation.	

Further reading

Health Protection Agency. 2014. *HPA archive. Guidance for odour complaints.* http://webarchive. nationalarchives.gov.uk/20140629102627/http://www.hpa.org.uk/ProductsServices/ChemicalsPoisons/ ChemicalRiskAssessment/ChemicalIncidentManagement/OdourIncidents/Guidelines/ (accessed 31 December 2015).

Kreis IA, A Busby, G Leonardi, et al. 2012. *Essentials of Environmental Epidemiology for Health Protection: A Handbook for Field Professionals.* Oxford: Oxford University Press.

WHO. 2000. *Air Quality Guidelines for Europe.* 2nd edition. Copenhagen: WHO European series, 91.

A3.13 **Planning or permitting applications SIMCARD**

		Yes/No
1	**Situation:** New developments need planning approval, by local authority, or central government (national infrastructure issues). Permission covers new building or extension and change of use; determines if development is an acceptable use of land. They may also need environmental permit (from Environment Agency) which determines if an operation can be managed so as to minimize pollution. Any part of public health may be approached for advice for either application: local public health team, specialist health protection team, and/or specialist environmental and toxicological staff within national public health organizations.	
2	**Incubation Period (Lead Time):** Both planning and environmental permits have tight timetables, outlined in consultation document.	
3	**Mode of Transmission (Exposure):** The documents may come physically or through electronic link. Health may be affected by ingestion, inhalation or skin contact with contaminants related to the development. Health may be affected by aspects other than pollution (see below).	
4	**Confirmation (Criteria):** Liaise with the other local and national teams to coordinate response. Local health protection teams are ideally placed to support interactions between national specialists and local public health professionals. Liaison with the local environmental health department and local planners is of great benefit.	
5	**Action:** Establish and maintain good relationships with national and local colleagues, including specialist environmental support, local public health and environmental health departments. Ensure specialist review of technical aspects of application is undertaken, including any potential for pollution (air, land, water) with possible or actual pathways to local population. Ensure relevant authority is given summary of local demography and epidemiology, taken from routine data at the lowest relevant and available geography; do not undertake fresh studies. Highlight important issues in the light of the application, local knowledge and technical review. Other issues beyond any direct effects of pollution should be considered with the wider public health team, including traffic-related pollution (see Air pollution, Noise, Odour SIMCARDs), and accidents; pressure groups' and elected member's interest; employment opportunities; and house price worries.	
6	**Report/Communication:** Ensure relevant authority has a written report covering relevant issues. Remember: this report will go into the public domain.	
7	**Disease Trends, Clusters, and Significant Situations:** Applications for environmental permits and planning permission are refused or granted (often with conditions) by other agencies. They will take into account timely and appropriate information from public health bodies, but are not bound by that information.	

Further reading

Environment Agency. 2012. *Guidance for developments requiring planning permission and environmental permits.* https://www.gov.uk/government/publications/developments-requiring-planning-permission-and-environmental-permits (accessed 31 December 2015).

A3.14 **Radon SIMCARD**

Possible radon exposure

		Yes/No
1	**Situation:** Enquiry about possible radon gas entry into a building. Radon is a colourless, odourless radioactive gas formed by the radioactive decay of the small amounts of naturally occurring uranium in all rocks, particularly granite, and soils. The distribution in the UK is uneven but well mapped. A risk map of the UK is available at 1 km grid square resolution for initial risk assessment (http://www.ukradon.org/information/ukmaps).	
2	**Incubation Period (Lead Time):** Lead time from exposure to lung cancer (only health risk) is unknown (many years).	
3	**Mode of Transmission (Exposure):** Radon gas enters houses from the ground through cracks in concrete floors and walls and around drains, pipes, and small pores of hollow-block walls. Levels are usually higher in basements, cellars and ground floors. Radon particles are inhaled and are retained in lung tissue where they decay, releasing alpha particles (two protons plus two neutrons) which damage the lung.	
4	**Confirmation (Criteria):** Radon gas concentrations in buildings can be measured over a three month period (http://www.ukradon.org/information/measuringradon); the results are adjusted for seasonal variations. Currently, there is no known way to recognize a radon-induced cancer, although advances in genomics may change this.	
5	**Action:** The UK action level for radon is 200 Bq/m^3. Actions to be instigated at or above this level should include remedial work by the building owner, usually through increasing air-flow through improved under-floor ventilation or creating a sump (http://www.ukradon.org/information/reducelevels).	
6	**Report/Communication:** For single properties, there is no need for further communication beyond pointing the enquirer to the UK Radon website (http://www.ukradon.org/). For public buildings and radon reduction programmes, communications with local public health and environmental health teams is essential. Media statements with partners (local authority; general public health) should be prepared.	
7	**Disease Trends, Clusters, and Significant Situations:** Radon increases lung cancer risk, in proportion to exposure, through radioactive decay (alpha particles) within the lungs. Radon is estimated to cause >1,100 deaths from lung cancer each year in the UK, half occur among smokers since smoking and radon exposure are synergistic. There is evidence that the risk of lung cancer exists equally for all groups (men, women, young, old, non-smokers, smokers) below the UK action level (200 Bq/m^3) and even below 100 Bq/m^3. Like other sources of radiation, it is probable that there is no safe dose, although the risk decreases with decreasing concentration since the dose-response relationship appears linear.	

References

Public Health England (PHE). n.d. *UKRadon.* http:// www.ukradon.org/ (accessed 31 December 2015).

Further reading

Public Health England (PHE). 2009. RCE– 11: *Radon and Health: report of the independent Advisory Group on Ionising Radiation.* https://www.gov.uk/government/publications/radon-and-public-health (accessed 26 April 2016).

A3.15 **Ultra-violet light SIMCARD**

		Yes/No
1	**Situation:** Exposure to UV light (UV radiation) is generally outdoors to sunshine or indoors to tanning machines. UV light is not seen by the human eye. Solar UV reaching the earth's surface is divided into two types, ultraviolet B (UVB) and the less energetic ultraviolet A (UVA). UV light is strongly linked to the induction of skin cancers, probably to eye disorders, in particular cataract, and suppression of the body's immune system. Any UV exposure is associated with an increased individual risk of health effects. A completely safe level of UV exposure cannot be demonstrated.	
2	**Incubation Period (Lead Time):** Sunburn can arise during, or within a few hours after, sun exposure; skin cancers can take many years to develop.	
3	**Mode of Transmission (Exposure):** Sunbeds emit UV and can cause tanning and sunburn; their uncontrolled use is a risk for skin cancers. The risk of melanoma (main cause of death from skin cancer) is related, among other things, to the number of intense exposures to UV. Such exposures may be particularly damaging in children, although skin cancers usually develop in adult life. Since there is no evidence to suggest that any type of sunbed is less harmful than natural sun exposure, there are restrictions on sunbed use in the UK by those aged under 18 years.	
4	**Confirmation (Criteria):** Discuss sunbed parlours with the local environmental health department as they should be licensed by the local authority. Daily UV indices for different areas of the UK to help guide public health advice re skin protection whilst outdoors can be seen at http://uk-air.defra.gov.uk/data/uv-index-graphs.	
5	**Action:** Protection from UV light by clothing, sunscreens and shadow, particularly when the sun is likely to be at its strongest, between 11am and 3pm. The use of sunbeds for cosmetic tanning should be discouraged. Multi-agency support for UV protection campaigns in the local media.	
6	**Report/Communication:** Local Director of Public Health; local environmental health department (for licencing), media (to promote UV protection and key public health messages)	
7	**Disease Trends, Clusters, and Significant Situations:** The UK incidence of skin cancer is rising: currently ~40,000 new cases and nearly 2,000 deaths each year. However, UV light has beneficial effects: vitamin D synthesis, medical treatments for skin diseases. In the former, relatively low levels of UV are required and, in the latter, the exposures are controlled to maximize the beneficial effects of treatment.	

Further reading

Public Health England (PHE). 2008. *Ultraviolet radiation (UVR)*. https://www.gov.uk/government/collections/ultraviolet-radiation-uvr (accessed 26 April 2016).

A3.16 **Water supply—discoloured or lost supply SIMCARD**

		Yes/No
1	**Situation:** Information from utility companies indicates a problem with water supply to a defined area: may come to light due to an unexpected leak, breach of pipe, or through increased customer complaints. Water companies are legally obliged to provide safe drinking water at customer's taps, including good pressure, colour, and taste, and free from contamination. Water issues should be reported by the utility company to Health Protection.	
2	**Incubation Period (Lead Time):** Immediate.	
3	**Mode of Transmission (Exposure):** Discoloured water may taste unpleasant. Loss of supply increases risks of diarrhoeal diseases through impaired hygiene, toileting, waste disposal.	
4	**Confirmation (Criteria):** Discuss issue with water utility: What is known and how (utility workers' reports/customer complaints)? What has happened and why? Repair time expected? Any illness reports?	
5	**Action** *Immediate:* With utility company: Confirm geographical spread of problem. Confirm alternative supplies of water to residents and businesses. Agree 'boil water' or 'do not drink' notice if appropriate with water utility. *Public Health:* **Enquire** if there are any known vulnerable people, particularly those on dialysis who will need alternative safe water supplies. Utility companies should have a list. **Ensure** water testing will be carried out for micro-organisms or repeated chemical sampling once pressure is restored. **Consider** criteria for removal of any 'boil water' or 'do not drink' notice with utility company. **Respond** to enquiries from relevant drinking water inspectorate (Private Water Supplies n.d.), if required.	
6	**Report/Communication:** Utility company will report incident, causes, immediate and long-term remedial actions, and plans to prevent recurrence to the relevant drinking water inspectorate (Private Water Supplies n.d.). The inspectorate will review the reports and make recommendations for future practice. These will be copied to the local health protection team, which should review them and consider if there is any further public health action that is needed.	
7	**Disease Trends, Clusters, and Significant Situations:** Loss of water for drinking, food production and washing will not, by itself, cause disease, but may give rise to unhygienic situations which foster infectious disease. Discoloured or unpleasant tasting water will not cause disease unless the chemical concentrations are raised above standards. Even then, the contaminated water may need to be drunk in large quantities or for a long time before disease manifests, since all such standards are very protective of health and based on lifetime exposure at that level.	

References

Private Water Supplies n.d. http://www.privatewatersupplies.gov.uk/ (accessed 8 March 2016).

Further reading

Drinking water inspectorate:

England and Wales. http://dwi.defra.gov.uk/about/index.htm (accessed 8 March 2016).

Northern Ireland. http://www.doeni.gov.uk/niea/water-home/drinking_water.htm (accessed 8 March 2016).

Scotland. http://www.dwqr.org.uk/about-us (accessed 8 March 2016).

A3.17 **Water supply—private water supplies SIMCARD**

		Yes/No
1	**Situation:** Private water supply: any water supply not provided by a water company. Mainly rural. Source may be well, borehole, spring, stream, river, lake, pond, rainwater or other, and may serve one property or several. Private supplies should meet the standards and other requirements of water supply regulations.	
2	**Incubation Period (Lead Time):** Outbreaks of gastrointestinal disease have been linked to private water supplies. Incubation period depends on the organism. Concentrations of manganese, iron, lead, arsenic, nitrate and pesticides can breach standards.	
3	**Mode of Transmission (Exposure):** Mainly ingestion.	
4	**Confirmation (Criteria):** Laboratory testing (microbiological and chemical), carried out annually.	
5	**Action** *Immediate:* Approach local authority and main water utility company for support in providing alternative water supply for drinking and food preparation. A 'boil water' notice or a 'do not use' notice will be issued by the local authority, as appropriate, depending on the use and contamination. Remember to remove the notice as soon as possible and inform the users clearly. *Public Health:* Not all failures of standards by private supplies will be reported to health protection, since remediation is straight-forward. Advice may be sought for particularly high levels of a chemical or micro-organisms. The public health response is dictated by the particular failure, but should ensure a safe alternative supply is available until the private supply is either sorted or a mains supply provided. Support from specialized environmental or toxicological colleagues can assist the risk assessment and evaluate responses in chemical contamination.	
6	**Report/Communication:** The local authority will report to the relevant drinking water inspectorate. Consider informing the Director of Public Health; a media statement may be needed.	
7	**Disease Trends, Clusters, and Significant Situations:** Outbreaks of gastrointestinal disease are likely to be localized to the water supply users. Ingestion of raised levels of arsenic and lead (see Arsenic, Lead SIMCARDs) may lead to acute or chronic poisoning. Manganese and iron discolour water (see Discoloured water SIMCARD). Nitrate may lead to 'blue baby syndrome' (met-haemoglobinaemia) in infants (0–3 months) where the water is used for formula, because their normal intestinal flora contribute to the generation of met-haemoglobin; older children and adults can experience this syndrome, but at higher concentrations of nitrates. Disease risk from contamination by pesticides varies by chemical: organophosphates and carbamates cause neurotoxicity. Others may irritate the skin or eyes, be carcinogens, or affect the endocrine system.	

References

Drinking Water Inspectorate. 2014. *Private water supplies in England and Wales.* http://dwi.defra.gov.uk/private-water-supply/index.htm (accessed 8 March 2016).

Private Water Supplies. n.d. http://www.privatewatersupplies.gov.uk/ (accessed 8 March 2016).

Appendix 4

Health protection legislation (England) guidance (2010): notifiable diseases

Please note: Table A4.1 is for guidance only and each case should be considered individually. A registered medical practitioner notification form template is provided in Table A4.2.

Table A4.1 Notifiable diseases, with explanatory notes and guidance on the need for urgent notification

Notifiable diseases	Definition/comment	Likely to be urgent?
Acute encephalitis		No
Acute meningitis	Viral and bacterial.	Yes, if suspected bacterial infection.
Acute poliomyelitis		Yes
Acute infectious hepatitis	Close contacts of acute hepatitis A and hepatitis B cases need rapid prophylaxis. Urgent notification will facilitate prompt laboratory testing. Hepatitis C cases known to be acute need to be followed up rapidly as this may signify recent transmission from a source that could be controlled.	Yes
Anthrax		Yes
Botulism		Yes
Brucellosis		No—unless thought to be UK-acquired
Cholera		Yes
Diphtheria		Yes
Enteric fever (typhoid or paratyphoid fever)	Clinical diagnosis of a case before microbiological confirmation (e.g. case with fever, constipation, rose spots and travel history) would be an appropriate trigger for initial public health measures, such as exclusion of cases and contacts in high risk groups (e.g. food handlers).	Yes
Food poisoning	Any disease of infectious or toxic nature caused by, or thought to be caused by, consumption of food or water (definition of the Advisory Committee on the Microbiological Safety of Food).	Clusters and outbreaks, yes. For specific organisms see Table A1.1; 1.2; 1.3.
Haemolytic uraemic syndrome (HUS)		Yes

(continued)

Table A4.1 Continued

Notifiable diseases	Definition/comment	Likely to be urgent?
Infectious bloody diarrhoea	See also HUS in Schedule 1 and VTEC in Schedule 2.	Yes
Invasive group A streptococcal disease and scarlet fever		Yes, if IGAS. No, if scarlet fever
Legionnaires' disease		Yes
Leprosy		No
Malaria		No, unless thought to be UK-acquired
Measles		Yes
Meningococcal septicaemia		Yes
Mumps	Post-exposure immunization (MMR or HNIG) does not provide protection for contacts.	No
Plague	Yes	
Rabies	A person bitten by a suspected rabid animal should be reported and managed urgently, but if a patient is diagnosed with symptoms of rabies, they will not pose a risk to human health.	Yes
Rubella	Post-exposure immunization (MMR or HNIG) does not provide protection for contacts.	No
SARS	Yes	
Smallpox	Yes	
Tetanus		No, unless associated with injecting drug use
Tuberculosis		No, unless healthcare worker or suspected cluster or multi-drug resistance
Typhus		No
Viral haemorrhagic fever (VHF)		Yes
Whooping cough		Yes, if diagnosed during acute phase
Yellow fever		No, unless thought to be UK-acquired

Note: Registered Medical Practitioners (RMPs) are also required to notify suspected cases of other infections ('other relevant infection') or contamination ('relevant contamination') that present, or could present, significant harm to human health.

Source: Data from Department of Health. *Health Protection Legislation (England) Guidance 2010* (London: Department of Health, 2010) © 2010 Crown Copyright, http://webarchive.nationalarchives.gov.uk/20130107105354/http:/www.dh.gov.uk/prod_consum_dh/groups/dh_digitalassets/@dh/@en/@ps/documents/digitalasset/dh_114589.pdf

Table A4.2 Registered medical practitioner notification form template

Health Protection (Notification) Regulations 2010: notification to the proper officer of the local authority
Registered Medical Practitioner reporting the case

Name	
Address	
Post code	
Contact number	
Date of notification	
Notifiable disease	
Disease, infection or contamination	
Date of onset of symptoms	
Date of diagnosis	
Date of death (if patient died)	
Index case details	
First name	
Surname	
Gender (M/F)	
DOB	
Ethnicity	
NHS number	
Home address	
Post code	
Current residence if not home address	
Post code	
Contact number	
Occupation (if relevant)	
Work/education address (if relevant)	
Post code	
Contact number	
Overseas travel, if relevant (destinations & dates)	

Appendix 5

The reporting of causative agents from local laboratory to local health protection team (PHE)

As regards urgency, the key consideration will be the likelihood that an intervention is needed to protect human health and the urgency of such an intervention. The likelihood of the diagnosis of an infection being considered urgent may also increase if it is part of a known or suspected cluster, or in someone with increased risk of transmission such as enteric infection in a food handler. Table A5.1.

Table A5.1 Causative agents and guidance on the need for urgent notification

Note: This table is only for guidance and each case should be considered individually. Notifiable organisms	Definition/comment	Likely to be urgent?
Bacillus anthracis		Yes
Bacillus cereus	Only if associated with food poisoning	No, unless part of a known cluster
Bordetella pertussis		Yes if diagnosed during acute phase
Borrelia spp		No
Brucella spp		No, unless thought to be UK-acquired
Burkholderia mallei		Yes
Burkholderia pseudomallei		Yes
Campylobacter spp		No, unless part of a known cluster
Chikungunya virus		No, unless thought to be UK-acquired
Chlamydophila psittaci		Yes if diagnosed during acute phase or part of a known cluster
Clostridium botulinum		Yes
Clostridium perfringens	Only if associated with food poisoning	No, unless known to be part of a cluster
Clostridium tetani		No, unless associated with injecting drug use

(continued)

Table A5.1 Continued

Note: This table is only for guidance and each case should be considered individually. Notifiable organisms	Definition/comment	Likely to be urgent?
Corynebacterium diphtheriae	Notify without delay, before results of toxigenicity tests are known	Yes
Corynebacterium ulcerans	Notify without delay, before results of toxigenicity tests are known	Yes
Coxiella burnetii		Yes if diagnosed during acute phase or part of a known cluster
Crimean-Congo haemorrhagic fever virus		Yes
Cryptosporidium spp		No, unless part of known cluster, known food handler, or evidence of increase above expected numbers
Dengue virus		No, unless thought to be UK-acquired
Ebola virus		Yes
Entamoeba histolytica		No, unless known to be part of a cluster or known food handler
Francisella tularensis		Yes
Giardia lamblia		No, unless part of known cluster, known food handler, or evidence of increase above expected numbers
Guanarito virus		Yes
Haemophilus influenzae	Invasive, i.e. from blood, cerebrospinal fluid or other normally sterile site	Yes
Hanta virus		No, unless thought to be UK-acquired
Hepatitis A, B, C, delta, and E viruses	All acute and chronic cases.	All acute cases and any chronic cases who might represent a high risk to others, such as healthcare workers who perform exposure-prone procedures
Influenza virus		No, unless known to be a new subtype of the virus or associated with known cluster or closed communities such as care homes
Junin virus		Yes
Kyasanur Forest disease virus		Yes
Lassa virus		Yes
Legionella spp		Yes
Leptospira interrogans		No

Table A5.1 Continued

Note: This table is only for guidance and each case should be considered individually. Notifiable organisms	Definition/comment	Likely to be urgent?
Listeria monocytogenes		Yes
Machupo virus		Yes
Marburg virus		Yes
Measles virus		Yes
Mumps virus		No
Mycobacterium tuberculosis complex		No, unless healthcare worker or suspected cluster or multi-drug resistance
Neisseria meningitidis	Excluding asymptomatic cases (e.g. throat carriage)	Yes
Omsk haemorrhagic fever virus		Yes
Plasmodium falciparum, vivax, ovale, malariae, knowlesi		No, unless thought to be UK-acquired
Polio virus	Wild or vaccine types	Yes
Rabies virus	Classical rabies and rabies-related lyssaviruses	Yes
Rickettsia spp		No, unless thought to be UK-acquired
Rift Valley fever virus		Yes
Rubella virus		No
Sabia virus		Yes
Salmonella spp.	Including *S. Typhi* and *S. Paratyphi*	Yes, if *S. Typhi* or *S. Paratyphi* or suspected outbreak or food handler or closed communities such as care homes No, if sporadic case of other *Salmonella* species
SARS coronavirus		Yes
Shigella spp.		Yes, except *Sh. sonnei* unless suspected outbreak or food handler or closed communities such as care homes
Streptococcus pneumoniae	Invasive, i.e. from blood, cerebrospinal fluid or other normally sterile site	No, unless part of a known cluster
Streptococcus pyogenes	Invasive i.e. from blood, cerebrospinal fluid or other normally sterile site, or associated with necrotising soft tissue infection	Yes

(continued)

Table A5.1 Continued

Note: This table is only for guidance and each case should be considered individually. Notifiable organisms	Definition/comment	Likely to be urgent?
Varicella zoster virus		No
Variola virus		Yes
Verocytotoxigenic *Escherichia coli*	Including *E. coli* O157	Yes
Vibrio cholerae		Yes
West Nile Virus		No, unless thought to be UK-acquired
Yellow fever virus		No, unless thought to be UK-acquired
Yersinia pestis		Yes

Source: Data from Department of Health. *Health Protection Legislation (England) Guidance 2010* (London: Department of Health, 2010) © 2010 Crown Copyright, http://webarchive.nationalarchives.gov.uk/20130107105354/http:/www.dh.gov.uk/prod_consum_dh/groups/dh_digitalassets/@dh/@en/@ps/documents/digitalasset/dh_114589.pdf

Glossary

Absolute risk The probability of disease/outcome in a group.

Active immunity Immunity acquired following infection or stimulation of an individual's immune system (e.g. by vaccination).

Active TB Disease caused by a member of the Mycobacterium TB complex family, determined by positive smear or culture from any part of the body or when there is sufficient radiographic, clinical, or laboratory evidence to support a diagnosis for which treatment is indicated. (See Chapter 12)

Acute respiratory illness Clinical diagnosis of acute-onset symptoms usually including at least one of the following signs or symptoms: cough, sore throat, shortness of breath, nasal discharge.

Air quality cell (AQC) Multi-agency group convening experts to assess air pollution for major chemical incidents such as fires, explosions and major chemical releases. (See Chapter 14)

Air Quality Management Area (AQMA) Geographically and legally defined areas where local authorities estimate air pollution levels above regulatory standards. Part IV Environment Act 1995 requires UK local authorities to conduct Local Air Quality Reviews with Action Plans for each AQMA. (See Chapter 16)

Alcohol acid fast bacilli (AAFB/AFB) Mycobacteria, which resist decolourization using acid or alcohol following staining.

Ambient air Average outdoor air conditions (over a time period, e.g. 15 minutes, month, year) typically measured away from air pollution. (See Chapter 16)

Antigenic drift The accumulation of mutations in genes that code for antibody binding sites on viruses leading to new progeny viruses that are less likely to be recognised by the same antibodies, i.e., antigenically different. (See Chapter 8)

Antigenic shift A sudden, major change in the influenza virus Haemagglutinin and/ or Neuraminidase surface proteins, resulting in a new influenza virus subtype. When shift happens, most people in the community lack immunity to the new subtype causing an epidemic or pandemic. (See Chapter 8)

Antibody Antibodies (synonym immunoglobulins) are produced as part of the immune response to antigens or immunogens. IgM antibodies are produced early in an infection (may indicate acute infection), IgG are produced later after IgM and persist for longer (may indicate chronic infection).

Antigen (Ag) An antigen is any substance that causes the production of antibodies as part of an adaptive immune response - it is an ANTIbody GENerator.

Anti-tuberculosis treatment (ATT) The treatment for active TB is usually given in two phases, an initial four-drug course (isoniazid, rifampicin, pyrazinamide, and ethambutol) for two months, then isoniazid and rifampicin alone for a further four months or longer. (See Chapter 12)

Association A relationship between two factors under study in which one varies statistically with another. An association may arise without a causal relationship between the factors.

Attributable risk The incidence of disease/outcome within a group with a specific risk factor that can be directly attributed to that risk factor.

Atypical mycobacteria Mycobacteria that do not belong to the MTB-complex family. Also referred to as 'environmental' mycobacteria. They may cause disease that clinically resembles TB, but that is not usually transmissible from person-to-person. (See Chapter 12)

Bacteraemia The presence of bacteria in the blood, detected by a positive blood culture. (See Chapter 7)

Bacille Calmette-Guèrin (BCG) Live vaccine against TB, containing a strain of Mycobacteria bovis. (See Chapter 12)

Bias A systematic error in a study, which can lead to an incorrect estimation of the outcome. Studies which reduce the risk of bias more effectively are less likely to yield distorted results.

Cancer registry Inventory of all malignant tumours in residents of an area. (See Chapter 17)

Carrier A carrier is a person who is carrying an infectious organism but is well (asymptomatic). Carriers have the potential to infect others. In relation to gastrointestinal illness, a carrier is someone who has excreted pathogenic organisms in faeces (also occasionally urine in salmonellosis) (continuously/intermittently) for more than 12 months. (See Chapter 6)

Causation A relationship between events in which one is the result of the other.

Chemoprophylaxis The prevention of a disease using drugs. Commonly it is used to describe the use of anti-tuberculosis treatment to treat latent TB, or to prevent TB in children who have been exposed to TB, or antibiotics given to close contacts to prevent further spread of meningococcal disease. (See Chapter 11 and Chapter 12)

Chest X-ray (CXR) A routine investigation, frequently used in the diagnosis of active pulmonary TB. Features of TB include: lymphadenopathy, parenchymal changes, pleural effusion (primary TB); fibrosis and cavitation (active post-primary TB); multiple small shadows (miliary TB). The presence of cavities on CXR is associated with increased infectivity. Patients with HIV-TB co-infection can have a normal CXR in spite of sputum-smear-positive TB.

Cluster Refers to two or more probable or confirmed cases with an epidemiological link (place, person, and time) which warrants further investigation.

Colonization Isolation of bacteria from a non-sterile site (skin, nose, rectum etc.). (See Chapter 7)

Confounding A factor associated with both an exposure and an outcome but not an intermediate causal step between them. For example, in a study assessing the impact of air pollution on lung disease, smoking may be a confounding factor as smoking can contribute to air pollution and can lead to lung cancer.

Contact A person with significant risk of direct or indirect exposure to a case of a disease. The definition of a contact will vary depending on the condition. Many conditions consider household contacts as those most at risk of contracting the condition. The definition of a contact depends on the infectivity of the condition (e.g. for measles a contact is anyone who has had face-to-face contact with a case or been in the same room for 15 minutes). In contrast, a contact for TB requires cumulative contact of over eight hours with the case. (See Chapter 5; Chapter 11)

Controlled burn A restricted or controlled use of water/foam on fires to reduce potential environmental impacts of chemical or contaminated fire water run-off. (See Chapter 14)

Chronic Obstructive Pulmonary Disease (COPD) A collection of lung diseases including chronic bronchitis, emphysema, and chronic obstructive airways disease. People with COPD have difficulties breathing, primarily due to airflow obstruction.

Community-acquired infection An infection that results from an exposure to a pathogen that is not related to a healthcare intervention in a hospital.

Culture Growing micro-organisms in the laboratory from patient specimens. It can provide information on identification and drug sensitivities of bacteria. (See Chapter 4)

Descriptive epidemiology Summary of disease/situation by person, place, and time.

Directly observed therapy (DOT) The patient is observed taking each and every dose of their TB treatment. Usually applied in the UK only to patients who have previously been non-adherent to treatment, and those with multi-drug resistant (MDR) TB. (See Chapter 12)

Directly observed therapy, short-course (DOTS) The World Health Organization (WHO) control strategy for TB, which includes microscopy-based diagnosis, standardized treatment administered by DOT, a secure supply of quality drugs and equipment, monitoring and supervision, and political commitment.

DNA viruses Viruses whose genetic information is coded in deoxyribonucleic acid.

Droplet precautions The use of personal protective equipment (PPE) to prevent transmission of droplet infections. This includes a face mask, gloves, and apron for contact with the patient or their environment. Eye protection should also be worn for aerosol-generating procedures. (See Chapter 11 and Chapter 18)

Environment Agency (EA) An executive non-departmental public body, which works to create better places for people and wildlife, and support sustainable development.

Epidemic The widespread occurrence of an infectious disease in a community at a particular time.

Epidemic curve A histogram that describes the distribution of cases in a defined population, location, and time period. Usually, the date of onset is presented on the X-axis and the number of cases on the Y-axis. An epidemic curve can help to determine the peak of disease occurrence (mode), possible incubation period, and the type of disease propagation. (See Chapter 22)

Epidemiologically-linked case An individual with disease who has had a significant exposure to a confirmed case of a disease.

Excreter Asymptomatic individual excreting pathogenic organisms in their faeces or urine for less than 12 months.

Exclusion period The period of time that cases would be required to not attend school or work environments to prevent onward transmission of a disease. In the case of diarrhoea, the exclusion period is generally 48 hours after the last normal stool, although this may be longer for certain conditions that require proof of microbiological clearance for high-risk contacts. (See Chapter 5)

Exposure Contact with a risk factor for developing a condition. (See Chapter 17)

Exposure Prone Procedures (EPPs) Exposure prone procedures (EPPs) are those where there is a risk that injury to the worker may result in exposure of the patient's open tissues to the blood of the worker. These procedures include those where the worker's gloved hands may be in contact with sharp instruments, needle tips or sharp tissues (spicules of bone or teeth) inside a patient's open body cavity, wound, or confined anatomical space where the hands or fingertips may not be completely visible at all times.

Extended-spectrum beta-lactamases (ESBLs) A type of resistant organism that produces enzymes that inactivate penicillin and cephalosporin antibiotics. They are often linked to other resistant genes such as resistance to quinolone antibiotics. ESBLs occur in bacteria such as *E.coli* and *Klebsiella species*.

Extensively drug resistant TB (XDR TB) TB that is resistant to isoniazid and rifampicin (MDR) and any fluoroquinolone and at least one of three injectable second-line drugs (kanamycin, capreomycin, or amikacin).

Extra-pulmonary TB TB in any part of the body outside of the lungs (e.g. meningeal or renal TB).

Flood guidance statement (FGS) Issued by the Flood Forecasting Centre (FFC) and provides a daily flood risk assessment up to five days in advance by county for responders in England and Wales. (See Chapter 15)

Flood warnings Issued by the Environment Agency and available to the public. These outline three levels of risk: flood alert (flooding possible, be prepared); flood warning (flooding expected, immediate action required); severe flood warning (severe flooding, danger to life). (See Chapter 15)

Fomite An object or substance (e.g. furniture, clothing or door handle) that can carry infectious organisms and is implicated in transmitting infection from one individual to another.

Foodborne disease Any disease of microbiological origin caused by, or thought to be caused by, the consumption of food or water.

Geographic Information System (GIS) Visualization tools that allow users to create interactive queries, analyse spatial information, edit data in maps, and visually present relationships, patterns and trends. (See Chapter 14)

Gram-negative bacteria (Gr-ve) Bacteria that do not retain crystal violet dye in the Gram-staining process such as *E.coli, Klebsiella pneumoniae* and *Pseudomonas aeruginosa*. (See Chapter 4; Chapter 7)

Gram-negative diplococci(us) A round bacterium that typically presents in the form of two joined cells (e.g. *Neisseria meningitidis*). (See Chapter 4; Chapter 11)

Hazard Something that can threaten health.

Healthcare-associated infection An infection that occurs following or during a healthcare intervention undertaken either in the community (including the patient's home) or in a healthcare setting.

Health and safety prohibition notice A legal notice, using health and safety legislation, to prohibit any activity which poses a risk of serious injury. (See Chapter 5)

Health criterion- values Benchmark concentrations of chemicals that are unlikely to lead to ill health and be protective of human health. (See Chapter 17)

Health register A rapid way to collate basic details of individuals affected by an incident in the immediate aftermath of an event. (See Chapter 15)

Herd protection Occurs when a high percentage of the population is immune to a virus or bacteria, which makes it difficult for a disease to spread as there are very few unprotected people. This provides a degree of protection to individuals without individual immunity. (See Chapter 10)

High-risk contact (for gastrointestinal infections) A person at increased risk of transmitting gastrointestinal infection to contacts: people with doubtful personal hygiene who cannot practise good personal hygiene (group A); children aged 5 years old or under who attend school, preschool, nursery or other similar childcare or minding groups (group B); people whose work involves preparing or serving unwrapped foods not subjected to further heating (group C); clinical, social care, or nursery staff with direct contact with highly susceptible patients or persons for whom a gastrointestinal infection could have serious effects (group D)

Holding press statement Prepared press statement that can be released upon request.

Hospital-acquired infection An infection that results from an exposure to a pathogen following or during a healthcare intervention in a hospital.

Hospital Episode Statistics A data warehouse containing details of all admissions, outpatient appointments, and A&E attendances at NHS hospitals in England.

Host Person or animal that affords subsistence or lodgement to an infectious agent under natural conditions.

Human immunodeficiency virus (HIV) HIV causes HIV infection and AIDS by diminishing host immunity. Decreased immunity results in increased susceptibility to infection including TB.

Iatrogenic Disease resulting from the actions of a healthcare professional (e.g. disease caused following use of a medical device, using prescribed medications, or surgical interventions).

Incident In communicable disease control, an incident refers to one case of a serious disease (e.g. Ebola/plague/anthrax).

Incubation period The time between exposure to the organism and date of onset of the first signs and/or symptoms.

Index case The first case to come to the attention of the investigator; not always the primary case. (See Chapter 5; Chapter 10; Chapter 20)

Infection The presence of micro-organisms in the body causing adverse signs or symptoms.

Infectious period The time period during which someone can transmit an infection.

Smear positive TB (infectious TB) Usually refers to patients with pulmonary TB that are sputum-smear-positive with evidence of acid-fast bacilli on microscopy. TB of other parts of the respiratory tract or oral cavity is also considered infectious and in some cases (e.g. laryngeal TB) can be very infectious. The presence of a productive cough and lung cavitation on chest X-ray increases the risk of the person being infectious.

Influenza illness An acute viral respiratory illness due to infection with the influenza virus. (See Chapter 8)

Influenza-like illness (ILI) Sudden onset of fever (>38 °C) with cough or sore throat. This is a clinical diagnosis made on the presenting symptoms. There are many viruses which can cause ILI. (See Chapter 8)

Inoculation injury Inoculation injury is an injury that exposes an individual to the blood or body fluids of another individual via a break in the skin such as a needlestick, bite or scratch. The term includes mucocutaneous exposure, i.e. splashes to the eyes, mucosa, or non-intact skin. (See Chapter 6)

Interferon gamma release assay (IGRA) A blood test measuring immune reaction to *M. tuberculosis*. It is used to diagnose latent TB infection. The antigens used in IGRA tests are absent from the BCG vaccine-strain hence unlike tuberculin skin testing, IGRA testing is not made positive by previous BCG vaccination. (See Chapter 12)

Isoniazid The main mycobacterial killing drug, used for anti-tuberculosis treatment.

Latent TB infection (LTBI) Evidence of infection with mycobacterium TB complex but with no symptoms or signs of TB disease. Individuals with LTBI are at risk of progressing to active disease and may be offered chemoprophylaxis with anti-TB drugs. (See Chapter 12)

Legionellosis The collective term for syndromes caused by infection with Legionella. (See Chapter 9)

Microbiological clearance The reduction of the number of pathogenic organisms in a specimen below that detectable by conventional means. (See Chapter 5)

Multi-drug resistant organisms (MDRO) Any organism that is resistant to multiple drugs (e.g. extended-spectrum beta lactamases; carbapenemase-producing *Enterobacteriaciae*, multi-drug resistant TB).

Morbidity Illness or disease.

Multi-Agency Flood Plan (MAFP) A plan developed by the Local Resilience Forum (LRF) in England to support the complex and sustained response required for floods. (See Chapter 15)

Multi-drug resistant TB (MDR TB) TB resistant to isoniazid and rifampicin, with or without other drug resistance. (See Chapter 12)

Mycobacterium tuberculosis (MTB) complex Organisms causing latent TB infection and TB disease. The important members of the complex are *Mycobacterium tuberculosis, M. bovis*, and *M. africanum*. (See Chapter 12)

Neonate (neonatal) An infant less than four weeks old. (See Chapter 7)

Neutropenia Low neutrophil count (white blood cells that fight infections caused by bacteria and fungi). The lower the neutrophil count, the greater the risk of infection.

National Health Service England (NHSE) A non-governmental public body which supports the commissioning of NHS services in England.

Nosocomial Infection Is synonymous with hospital-acquired infection. An infection that is acquired in a hospital or other healthcare setting.

Notifiable diseases A list of diseases that a registered medical practitioner (RMP) in England must legally notify to Local Authority Proper Officers (Consultants in Communicable Disease Control (CCDC)), on suspicion, in order that action can be taken to protect public health from a risk of significant harm from infection. See Appendix 4 for a list of notifiable diseases. Similar arrangements exist in Norhtern Ireland, Scotland, and Wales.

Outbreak An observed number of cases greater than that expected for a defined place and time period, or two or more cases with a common exposure.

Outbreak Control Team (OCT) A multi-agency group of professionals convened when an outbreak is declared, whose functions include risk assessment of the situation, development of a management strategy, and allocation of responsibilities.

Pandemic An epidemic occurring worldwide, or over a very wide area, crossing international boundaries and usually affecting a large number of people. (See Chapter 8)

Particulate matter (PM) Small respirable particles that may penetrate into lungs to alveolar levels. The diameter of the particle is described in the name and is measured in microns: PM_{10} = <10 microns; $PM_{2.5}$ = <2.5 microns; $PM_{0.1}$ = <0.1 microns. (See Chapter 16)

Passive immunity Immunity produced by the transfer or administration of antibodies. It is divided into natural (transfer of antibodies across the placenta during pregnancy) and acquired (administration of antibodies into a susceptible individual).

Passive surveillance system A surveillance system that relies on the routine reporting of event or disease data by those individuals or organizations involved in the diagnosis or detection (e.g., notifiable diseases surveillance). This system relies on cooperation; provides basic information about an event or diseases; is less expensive; and may suffer from underreporting. (See Chapter 13; Chapter 21)

Phage typing Subtyping of bacteria based on their susceptibility to lysis by a panel of bacterial viruses known as bacteriophages. This can be helpful in identifying and investigating outbreaks.

Public Health England (PHE) An executive agency, sponsored by the Department of Health in England. It protects and improves the nation's health and wellbeing, and reduces health inequalities.

Pontiac fever Mild non-pneumonic, self-limiting influenza-like illness caused by Legionella infection. (See Chapter 9)

Post-exposure prophylaxis (PEP) Drugs/vaccines/immunoglobulins offered to provide protection from infection or illness after exposure. (See Chapter 6; Chapter 8; Chapter 10)

Postherpetic neuralgia (PHN) PHN is a nerve pain due to damage caused by the *Varicella zoster* virus. Typically, the neuralgia is confined to a dermatomic area of the skin and follows an eruption/invasion of *Herpes zoster* (commonly known as of shingles) in that same dermatomic area.

Primary case The case that introduced the disease into the group or population. (See Chapter 10; Chapter 20)

Prodrome The period during which a particular infectious disease has become symptomatic but the typical clinical features have not yet appeared.

Prophylaxis Protection from infection before exposure. (See Chapter 6; Chapter 11)

Public Health Risk Assessment Assesses the risk of a situation incorporating the relevant contexts (e.g. site or community history, legislation), interests, and perceptions of community and relevant bodies and technical/scientific risk assessments (e.g. incidence). (See Chapter 3)

Pulmonary TB TB disease that affects the lungs, usually producing a cough that lasts longer than two weeks. (See Chapter 12)

Pyrexia/Fever Elevated body temperature above normal (around 37°C). Between 37 and 38 °C is classed as a mildly elevated but above 38°C is deemed a high temperature.

Ro (Basic reproductive number) The average number of new cases generated by one infectious case (secondary cases) over the course of its infectious period, in an entirely susceptible population. (See Chapter 10)

Receptors People potentially affected by an incident. (See Chapter 14)

Recovery coordinating group (RCG) Multi-agency group which manages the return to normality after incident. (See Chapter 14)

Relative risk The ratio between incidence of disease within an exposed group and a non-exposed group.

Reservoir Animal/plant/place where an infectious agent normally lives and multiplies, and from which it is transmitted to a susceptible host.

Responders Category 1 responders assess risks to communities and plan to deal with emergencies (e.g. emergency services, local authorities, public health); Category 2 (e.g. utilities) responders support Category 1 (Civil Contingencies Act 2004). (See Chapter 3; Chapter 14; Chapter 15; Chapter 20)

Rifampicin A drug used to treat tuberculosis.

Rising tide incidents Emergency increasing from an initial steady state over a period of time. (See Chapter 13)

Risk Probability that a substance/hazard will cause harm under specific conditions. (See Chapter 17)

RNA viruses Viruses whose genetic information is coded in ribonucleic acid.

Science and Technical Advice Cell (STAC) Multi-agency group that brings together experts to provide a single point of scientific and technical advice to the Strategic Coordinating Group, during a major incident. (See Chapter 14; Chapter 15; Chapter 20)

Secondary case The case that contracted the infection from the primary case.

Secondary stressor An event/policy indirectly related to the primary event that results in psychosocial stress (e.g. loss of possessions, resources, infrastructure failure, interruption of daily life). (See Chapter 15)

Septicaemia (blood poisoning) The presence of numerous actively dividing bacteria in the blood overwhelming the immune system causing serious life-threatening illness. It is unlike bacteraemia, which refers to presence of bacteria in the blood usually with no systemic effects.

Standardized incident ratio (SIR) The ratio between the observed number of new cases in a study population and the number of new cases expected, taking age and sex into consideration, over a specific time period.

Standardized mortality ratio (SMR) The ratio between the observed number of deaths in a study population and the number of deaths expected, taking age and sex into consideration, over a specific time period.

Sputum Phlegm that is coughed up from inside the lungs. To diagnose TB, sputum samples are examined microscopically for mycobacteria using a smear and are cultured which, if positive, will confirm the species of mycobacteria.

Strain typing Laboratory method useful in identifying linked cases in an outbreak.

Strategic Coordinating Group (SCG) Multi-agency group composed of all relevant agencies to agree high-level objectives and guide response during a major incident; led by Strategic Coordinator (usually police, but may change as incident progresses). (See Chapter 14; Chapter 15; Chapter 20)

Sub-clinical infection Infection with no symptoms or signs, i.e. infected person does not know they have it.

Syndromic surveillance The collection, analysis, and interpretation of health data about clinical pictures (sign and symptoms) to provide early warning for action of public health threats. (See Chapter 13; Chapter 14; Chapter 21)

Tactical Coordinating Group (TCG) Multi-agency group providing tactical support during a major incident.

Toxicity Biological effect of a substance. (See Chapter 17)

Tuberculin skin test (TST) A skin test for determining if a person is infected with mycobacteria. The test, also called Mantoux test, is performed by injecting tuberculin into the inner surface of the forearm and is read between 48 and 72 hours after administration. Reading the test means measuring the diameter across the forearm of the raised, hardened and inflamed area.

Typing Molecular methods such as variable number tandem repeats (VNTR) to determine relatedness between organisms of the same species.

Urinary antigen test Testing urine for legionella surface antigen, specific to *L. pneumophila*. (See Chapter 9)

Vehicle An inanimate object that becomes contaminated (e.g. food/toys) allowing transfer of an infectious agent to a host.

Vero cytotoxin (shiga-like toxins) A toxin that damages red blood cells associated with Shigella spp and some diarrhoea producing E.coli. The toxin can cause the haemolytic uraemic syndrome (HUS) with renal failure. (See Chapter 5)

Viraemia The presence of viral particles and viruses in the bloodstream.

Vulnerable individual A non-immune individual in whom infection is likely to be more severe and subject to a higher complication rate (e.g. pregnant women, infants, and the immunocompromised).

Worried well Concerned individuals who are not exposed and not at risk of contracting infection/disease.

Index

Page numbers in bold signify main coverage

WITHDRAWN
FROM LIBRARY

WITHDRAWN
FROM LIBRARY

BMA LIBRARY
BRITISH MEDICAL ASSOCIATION